PRAISE
THE PURPOSEFU

"Marty Gallagher has produced an absolute classic! I couldn't put it down... packed with real no b.s info from real ironmen. I am proud to be included with the outstanding athletes and their stories... A breath of fresh air!"
—Dorian Yates, 6-time IFBB Mr. Olympia

"I would venture to say that I have read every book pertaining to weightlifting over the last three decades, and I have probably read the majority of the articles in this area. There are two things I can say unequivocally about what I have read. One, Marty Gallagher is the best writer in the world of physical fitness and strength, bar none, and two, Gallagher's newest book ***The Purposeful Primitive*** is the best manuscript ever produced in this field.

Teeming with esoteric information on training, biomechanics, nutrition, and sport psychology, ***The Purposeful Primitive*** is a wealth of information that every serious lifter needs to read. You are going to like this book. NO! You are going to LOVE it. I promise you that. It's Gallagher's best work, and that means it is strictly world class."
—Dr. Judd Biasiotto, author of 46 fitness and health-related books, world powerlifting champion

"I really only have two things to say about Marty Gallagher that bear on his new book, ***The Purposeful Primitive***. The first is that there are two classes of writers in powerlifting: 1) Marty Gallagher and 2) all others. The second is that one day, ten years ago, Marty called to say he knew a Russian guy who he thought might be a good writer for ***MILO***, so we invited the guy to submit an article: It was called ***Vodka, Pickle Juice, Kettlebell Lifting and other Russian Pastimes***, the author was Pavel Tsatsouline, and rest, as they say, is history."
—Randall J. Strossen, Ph.D, Publisher and Editor-in-chief, *Milo* Magazine

"For those who buy or judge reading material by size, number of pages, volume, or distance able to be thrown and cause damage, Marty has your back on this one. For the intellectual athlete who actually thirsts for knowledge and sees content as King, you will get 30 years of genius and experience in the Iron Game mixed with the passion and ability of Hemmingway all wrapped up in one book and the result is ***The Purposeful Primitive***. From me to you—Go buy the book and enjoy!!"
—Rickey Dale Crain, IPF/WPC/AAU World Champion, 2000 Powerlifting Hall of Fame Inductee

"As a student, athlete, teacher, researcher, professional coach, and businessman I have spent over 60 years in health, fitness and sport, devoted to 'how to become the best you can be'. ***The Purposeful Primitive*** has been a very interesting journey for me... back-to-the-future...

Marty does a wonderful job bringing out the art and science of training, extracting many of the critical universal and specific principles (guiding rules to action—social, emotional, mental, physical and spiritual) that are applicable to living a productive life in general, and in training for health, fitness and sport, specifically. In addition, I like the way Marty personalizes the lives of outstanding athletes and shows how they applied these fundamental, can't-miss principles in their training to help them become the best they could be in their sport. My recommendation: if you want to achieve something 'great in your life', add ***The Purposeful Primitive*** to your training library... yesterday."
—Dr. Bob Ward, *Sports Science Network*, former head strength and conditioning coach, Dallas Cowboys

"Marty Gallagher has written a most interesting book that contains not only telling first hand biographies from powerlifting's heyday, but the routines and mindset of the top practitioners of the strength pursuit. His style is rich with anecdote, at the same time being right on point regarding the many divergent paths to the attainment of fitness. The basic truths underlying those paths have been distilled down to a certainty, allowing the reader to intelligently compose their own program. Good job from one who sought intensely over many years to grasp the essence of power and fitness and most importantly loves what he does."
—Hugh Cassidy, first world heavyweight powerlifting champion

"Marty Gallagher is a brilliant writer who thinks deeply about subjects he knows and loves. His manifesto/encyclopedia contains a ton of wisdom, one-of-a-kind role models, awesome color photos... a truly fascinating read."
—Clarence Bass, author of the *Ripped* series, *Lean For Life, Challenge Yourself*, and *Great Expectations*

"Gallagher takes the gems of the greatest strength athletes in history and distills the keys to success for all of us.

After reviewing profile after profile after profile of great strength trainers in history, Gallagher goes the next step: he sums up their approaches then shows that all of them are right. As a person trained in the basics of theology, I understood immediately Gallagher's great point: it's not 'either/or' when it comes to strength and body mass, it is 'both/and'. I live by the coaching point: 'Everything works...for a while,' and Gallagher breathes flesh and blood into this principle.

There is so much more to this book, of course. The mental training section blends the Western and Eastern approaches to the mind game of training. Again, we find 'both/and', but Gallagher also spends a lot of time detailing how to incorporate these tools in one's training.

But wait, there's more! There is a section on cardio training for strength athletes that really makes me more comfortable with this notion of 'doing cardio'. It's nice to see the return for the widely misunderstood teachings of Len Schwartz's Heavy Hands. Moreover, we see a commonsense approach to this whole overhyped field.

The section on diet towards the end of the book again reflects the idea of both/and'. It is simply this: refreshing. Gallagher gives clarity to the calorie conundrum. Yes, every diet approach works, but Gallagher shows us a way to link them together. Truly, this man of experience understands that success leaves footprints and every approach is worthy of discussion.

Oh, this book is a joy. I put this book next to **Tommy Kono's *Weightlifting, Olympic Style*** for sheer fun and delight and love of training. I am convinced that I will probably keep reading ***The Purposeful Primitive*** in bits and snips for years. It's just fun and funny while pounding into the reader the 'secrets' of advanced training. Many won't like the message. The secrets involve training really hard and really heavy."
—Daniel John, Head Track and Field Coach, Juan Diego Catholic High School, American Record Holder, Masters Weight Pentathlon

"What can one say with certainty about the author of this book—Marty Gallagher? Nothing other than the facts that he has 'been there and done that' as an 800-plus pound squatter! That he has written over a thousand articles about fitness and nutrition in the published print media (not to include his amazing blog). That he is not just a genius, but the best interviewer and storyteller going. And that he has not only truly trained the world's strongest athletes, but that he has distilled the most useful information from 15 of the foremost weight lifters, bodybuilders, psychologists and 'bodymaster' nutritionists of the last half century into a form that can be used by anyone from overweight, exercise-adverse beginner to world champions in their sports.

From Olympic lifting to power lifting and bodybuilding, whether muscle gain or fat loss, from cooking to supplements, from changing exercise and eating habits to molding the psychology of a champion (whether one is even remotely interested in competition or not), Marty has covered it all. I only wish I had had a book like this when I was growing up and trying my best to get bigger and stronger. Marty has demonstrated, without question, that he is the current and undeniably best 'trainer of champions' and 'ultimate guide to physical—and mental—transformation.' This book not only provides the simplest instructions and cheapest financial and lifestyle requirements, it is absolutely the single best book ever written on being the best you can be physically and otherwise."
—James E. Wright, Ph.D, former Director of Sports Science, U.S. Army Physical Fitness School; former Health and Science Editor, *Flex* Magazine

"Absolutely magnificent. What a breathtaking book on a life with iron. Marty Gallagher delivers an outstanding, comprehensive book with a writing style worthy of Hemingway himself. This book takes you on a journey through the iron-history of the great ones and in the most sophisticated way Marty presents probably the best ever written material on life, iron and mental fortitude.

This book is impossible to put down once you start reading it. It should be the first read of any who aspire to lift weights and be healthy. There are not enough words in the English language

(or Danish for that matter) to describe how excellent this book is. It is an absolute must to any Strength & Health enthusiast. I give it my highest recommendation!!"
—Kenneth "*the Dane of Pain*" Jay, MSc, Sr. RKC

"*The Purposeful Primitive* both inspired me, and also challenged some of my long-held notions about strength and athleticism. In the foreword, Pavel calls Marty Gallagher his mentor, and once you read this book, you'll understand why. The Purposeful Primitive is the most significant strength-training book I've read in 10 years."
—Charles Staley, Staley Training Systems

"Marty's literary style intrigued me and I could not put the book down!! I was drawn into being educated by a powerlifter that made points that would make me a better high school teacher/coach as well as an excellent Olympic weightlifting coach.

I was hooked by page 263, with Marty's 'physical and psychological weak points'. "What's the toughest lesson to learn in all of fitnessdom? I would nominate prioritizing weaknesses and not continually playing to our strength.' There it is! That did it! If nothing else, this chapter needs to be read by all coaches and by all athletes and all trainers in the fitness world...

I highly recommend *The Purposeful Primitive* as a must read."
—Mike Burgener, Senior International Weightlifting Coach, Coach for the Junior World Women's Weightlifting Team

"Marty Gallagher has convincingly presented the concept that successful people in all domains 'stand upon the shoulders of those who have gone before them.' He has accurately indicated that most of the fitness gurus and elite athletes of today are chasing after the *golden fleece* instead of following the tried, true and scientifically and empirically proven and validated principles of physical training, cardiovascular training, nutrition and psychology.

Marty characterizes this by stating; 'Old school methodology is the modern solution for achieving true physical transformation.' Readers will sink their teeth into the substance and procedures of the masters found between the covers of *The Purposeful Primitive*.

The Purposeful Primitive is an enlightening read, filled with great insights into the masters of the last century in Olympic Lifting, Powerlifting, Bodybuilding, Cardiovascular Training, Nutrition and Psychology.

Great job Marty Gallagher, master of: writing, powerlifting, physical training, cardiovascular training, nutrition and psychology."
—Dr. Paul Ward, PED, QPT Publications

"WOW! My old friend Marty knocked this one out of the park.
I was so fascinated I could not put the book down. These are exactly the routines most of us experienced in those days. It brought back a lot of memories.

For all you young powerlifters out there who want to build real power like we did it in the old days this is the book to get. Thank you so much Marty."
—Dan Wohleber, former national powerlifting champion, multiple world record holder, 1st man to deadlift 900 pounds

"When Marty called and asked if I could pose for a few photos for his new book, I knew I didn't have to worry about associating myself with anything he was writing. I knew it would be a quality book focused on proven, basic training principles and based on Marty's vast store of real, first-hand knowledge. What I didn't know until receiving my copy and really giving it a close look, was that I was stumbling across a small role in one of the most comprehensive, well-written, and above all else, entertaining, books on weight training that's ever been written.

I have a pretty extensive strength training library, and Marty's book belongs on the top shelf with Dreschler's Weightlifting Encyclopedia, Starr's The Strongest Shall Survive, McCallum's Keys to Progress, and McRobert's Brawn. I realize now how lucky I am to have been in the right place at the right time to be a small part of Marty's crowning achievement and lasting contribution to the Iron Game. Thanks so much Marty for not letting these great stories and this wealth of information fade away with the old masters!"
—Chuck Miller, attorney, journalist, C.S.C.S., AAU world and national powerlifting champion

"I enjoyed Marty Gallagher's new book and particularly liked his 'resurrection' of the methods of the Iron Masters. So much of that Old School training wisdom has been forgotten or discarded in our modern era. The training philosophies of men like Bill Pearl and Ed Coan are timeless and grounded in principles that have stood the test of time. These philosophies are based in the idea that first and foremost, hard and sustained physical effort must be implemented for a protracted period. This requires using lots of Old School discipline.

I agree with Marty's premise that to modify the human body, to improve it, to make it more muscular and leaner, requires real work. Too many individuals in this day and age want to believe that some miracle method exists that can magically bypass the requisite pain and struggle. By spotlighting men from a simpler era, Marty shows that real gains can be gotten from methods that need not be unduly complicated. I would hope that modern readers could absorb some of the iconic lessons he relates in his own unique way."
—John Parrillo, CEO Parrillo Performance Products

"I have been studying the industry for 20 years. Marty is in a class of his own. Combine his fitness knowledge with a unique talent for writing and one has an unbeatable combination."
—Larry Christ, multi-time national master powerlifting champion

"Once again, Marty Gallagher has proven that he is powerlifting's most articulate and informative writer. ***The Purposeful Primitive*** is an outstanding read, with credible and essential information for beginners and elite lifters alike. I will be honored to promote the book at my gym and the many contests we host each year."
—Dr. Spero S. Tshontikidis, R.A.W. United, Inc.

"Wow! Marty Gallagher did a tremendous job! Not only was it a very interesting and entertaining read, but can be used as a reference manual. A must read for anyone interested in fitness and or strength."
—Bob Gaynor, WPC World Record holder

"***The Purposeful Primitive*** is Marty Gallagher's *magnum opus*. It's the most entertaining book about physical culture I've read in a long time. The hilarious over-the-top reminiscences of Old School powerlifting and powerlifters is combined with the basic, bare-bones, best-practice information needed to dramatically change your physical appearance and become radically bigger and stronger as long as you are willing to sacrifice your blood, sweat, and tears to the *loa* of ***the Purposeful Primitive.***"
—Steve Shafley, Powerlifter and Highland Games thrower

"Marty Gallagher has laid out simple tried and true old school principles that yield results. I believe that is what this book is all about; results. In a world full of bells and whistles, this book is a great reminder of what training should look like. I think this is an outstanding resource for physical transformation. I would recommend this book to anyone who is serious about building a real-world body."
—Tim Anderson, RKC Level II, CPT

The Purposeful Primitive

From Fat and Flaccid to Lean and Powerful

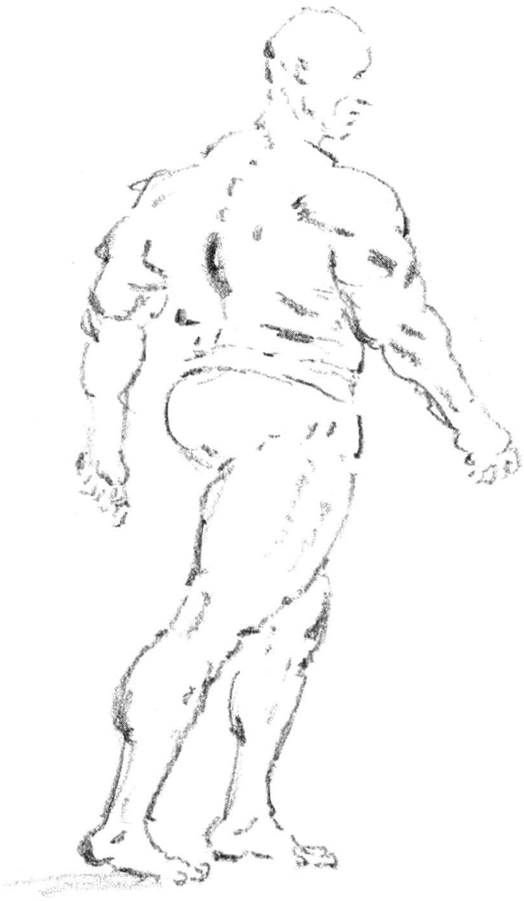

Using the Primordial Laws of Fitness to Trigger Inevitable, Lasting and Dramatic Physical Change

Marty Gallagher

THE PURPOSEFUL PRIMITIVE

MARTY GALLAGHER

Published in the United States by:
Dragon Door Publications, Inc
P.O. Box 4381, St. Paul, MN 55104
Tel: (651) 487-2180 • Fax: (651) 487-3954
Credit card orders: 1-800-899-5111
Email: dragondoor@aol.com • Website: www.dragondoor.com

ISBN: 13 digit: 978-0-938045-71-7 10 digit: 0-938045-71-7

This edition first published in June 2008

Printed in the United States of America

Book design, Illustrations and cover by Derek Brigham
Website http//www.dbrigham.com
Tel/Fax: (763) 208-3069 • Email: dbrigham@visi.com

DISCLAIMER
The author and publisher of this material are not responsible in any manner whatsoever for any injury that may occur through following the instructions contained in this material. The activities, physical and otherwise, described herein for informational purposes only, may be too strenuous or dangerous for some people and the reader(s) should consult a physician before engaging in them.

TABLE OF CONTENTS

Foreword by Pavel "Thinking Simply and Seeing Clearly" IX

I Prometheus 3
The Purposeful Primitives 4
There Is No School Like Old School 6
Standing On the Shoulders of Giants 7

IRON MASTERS 9
Paul Anderson—Primitive Patriarch 11
Typical Paul Anderson Workout 15

Bill Pearl—Anti-Aging Role Model 17
Bill Pearl's Classical Bodybuilding Training Regimen 20
The Anti-Aging Role Model 23

Bob Bednarski—Iron Icarus 25
Clash of the Titans: Barski goes to work for "The Man" 26
Training 27
Bob Bednarski Training Template 28
Aftermath: The Iron Icarus melts his wings 30

Hugh Cassidy—Iron Master Renaissance Man 31
Eat Your Way Through Sticking Points! 32
All Aboard the Pain Train! 33
Hugh Cassidy Training Split 34
Lift Big, Eat Big, Rest Big, Grow Big! 35

Mark Chaillet—Powerlifting Ultra Minimalist 37
How Little can you do and still get Super Strong? 38
Mark Chaillet's Super Simplistic System 39
Competition Training Cycle 39
8 Week Periodization Cycle 40
Stopping Machine Gun Sales at Chaillet's "House of Pain" 41

Doug Furnas—The Athlete's Athlete 45
Near Death Experience Leads to Iron Introduction 47
Dennis Wright: "Simplistic Genius" 50
Coaching Coan, Furnas and Chaillet Simultaneously 52
How did Doug train? 53

Ed Coan—The Greatest Powerlifter Of All Time... 55
How the Greatest Powerlifter in History Trained 61
Coan Trains 62

Ken Fantano—Power Theoretician 65
Powerlifting Architecture 68
"The Weight Don't Care; It Has Only One Friend: Gravity!" 70
Power Enduro 72
Fantano Phase II Competition Training Template 73

Dorian Yates—The Iron Monk 75
The Quantum Leap Forward 76
Blood & Guts: Film Noir Extraordinaire 78
My Day with Dorian 80
Bodybuilding, Blood & Guts Style 82

Kirk Karwoski—Prototypical Purposeful Primitive 85
Karwoski's Four Day/Week Power Training Program 89
Karwoski 4 Day Training Split 90
Karwoski Reemerges 91

IRON METHODS 95
The Purposefully Primitive Resistance Training Amalgamation 97

Recapitulation of Modes and Methods 100

What the Iron Masters Have in Common 104
How to Build Muscle 105
Getting Started 106

Primary Exercises 108
Squat 108
Bench Press 110
Deadlift 112

Secondary Exercises 114
Overhead Press 114
Biceps Curl 115
Triceps Extension 116

Tertiary Exercises 117
Romanian Deadlift 117
Calf Raise 118
Decline Sit-up 118

Auxiliary Exercises 118
Legs 119
Chest 121
Back 123

Two Day A Week Training 125
Two Day Split: Simplistic, Time Efficient, Deadly Effective! 126
Three Day A Week Training 126
Three Day Split: Work the Whole Body Thrice Weekly 127
Four Day A Week Training 127
Four Day Split: Ground Zero Split Routine 128
Five Day A Week Training 129
Five Day Split: Iron Immersion 129
Six Day A Week Training 130
Six Day Split: Volume Over Intensity! 131
The Purposefully Primitive Training Week 131

Periodization and Preplanning 133
4 Week Peaking Cycle 134
Periodization and Creeping Incrementalism 135
8 Week Beginner Periodization Cycle 136
Logging Entries 137

IRON ESSAYS

IRON ESSAYS 141
Primitive Roots 143

Build a Retro Home Gym 151
Stone-Age Tools for Accessing the Third Dimension of Tension 153

You've Got About An Hour 156
Capacity is a Shifting Target 159

Progress Multiplier: The Training Partner 161

How Simple can the Physical Renovation Process be made Without Losing Effectiveness? 164

Ebb and Flow 168
Thesis, Antithesis, Synthesis Embrace Change, Legislate Contrast 170
No One System, Mode or Method Trumps All Others 171
Better To Use a Lousy System with Great Intensity Than A Sophisticated System Halfheartedly 172
Don't Turn a Once Effective System into a Religion 172
Legislating Contrast 173
Contrast Is King 174

Direct Muscle Soreness and Deep Muscle Fatigue 176

Progressive Pulls 179
Six Week Progressive Pull Periodization Cycle 181

Base Strength 186

The Seductive Siren Song of Machine Exercise 188

Spawning Season 192

Back in the Day 197

What Not To Do How Not To Train 205

Remembrances of Days Past 209

MIND MASTERS 217

Mental Mentors 219
  The Functions of the Human Brain 223

Jiddu Krishnamurti—Intuitive Primitive 225

Aladar Kogler—Iron Curtain Brain Train Grand Maestro 229

MIND METHODS 233

The Tao of Fitness 235
  Shikantaza Checklist 237
  Auto-Visualization Ideo-Motor Checklist 239
  Suggested Reading 241

A 10 Step Program Based on the Kogler Brain Train Approach 242

MIND ESSAYS 247

Purposefully Primitive Psychology

Reprogram the Central Processing Unit of the Soft Machine 255

Making the Mind/Muscle Connection 258

Physical and Psychological Weak Points 263

Brain Train 266

The Psychology of a Champion Athlete 269

Purposeful Layoffs 273

Brain Train Feats and Tactics 277

Want to Change Your Physique? Start by Changing the Way You Think 280

CARDIO MASTERS 283

Purposefully Primitive Cardiovascular Exercise 285
- Mr. Analogous Strikes Again 285
- Many Roads Lead to Cardio Rome 286
- Getting Our Cardio Facts Straight 287

Leonard Schwartz, M.D.—Aerobic Avatar 291
- Birth And Death Of An Exercise Craze 293
- Len Sets Me Straight 294

CARDIO METHODS 297

The Three Types of Cardio 299
- The 1st Way: Steady-State 299
- The 2nd Way: Burst or Interval 302
- The 3rd Way: Burst or Interval 305
- Muscle Fiber Nuts and Bolts 307
- Muscle Fiber Reference Guide 308
- The 1st, 2nd and 3rd Way Cardio Modes 309

Every Self-Respecting Purposeful Primitive Needs this High-Tech Gadget 310
- The Three Benchmarks of Aerobic Activity 311
- Six Week 1st Way Periodization Cycle 312
- Nine Week 1st Way Periodization Cycle 313
- The Heart Rate Monitor Allows Aerobic Mode Cross Comparisons 314

CARDIO ESSAYS 317

Aerobic Exercise Is Irreplaceable 319
- Step Outside the Cardio Box 320

Walking for Exercise is Different Than Normal Walking 328

Zen and the Art of Walking 333

The 1,000 Calorie Cardio Burn 337

The Carefree Psychotic Peeks Inside Ali's "Near Room" 341

Hammer Time! 347

Martial Artists and 3rd Way Hybrid Cardio 349

In Praise of Steve Justa Sustained-Strength Grand Maestro 353

Nutrition Masters 357

No Need to Square the Nutritional Circle 359

John Parrillo 363
- Bigger and Leaner 366
- Build the Metabolism 367
- A Day In The Life Of A Parrillo-Style Dieter 369
- Parrillo On Manipulating The Insulin/Glucagon Axis 370

Ori Hofmekler 373
- The Warrior Diet Template 379
- "Avoid Extreme Low Calorie Diets." 379
- "Detoxify the Body" 380

Nutrition Methods 383

The Nutritional Amalgamation 385
- The Right Tool for the Right Job at the Right Time 386
- Which Way to Jump? 387
- Jumping into the Deep End of the Pool 388
- A Hypothetical 12 Month Rotational Nutritional Macro Cycle 389
- The Psychology of Taste 389
- Where and How to Start 391
- Purposefully Primitive Performance Eating 391
- Thermodynamic Reality Check 392
- Periodized Nutritional Rotation 393

Parillo Nutritional System Synopsis 394

Warrior Diet System Synopsis 395

NUTRITION ESSAYS 398

The Anabolic Effect of Food 399

Post-Workout Smart Bomb 403
Ori's Take on the Window of Opportunity 405

Getting in Touch with Hunger 407

My Meal with Mongo 411

The Diesel Leads the Way 416
  Dorian Yates Daily Meal Schedule Pre-Competition Phase 419

Holiday Hedonism Setting Up the Anabolic Burst 421

What's the Biggest Myth in ALL of Fitness? Spot Reduction! 425
  Where Body Fat Is Drawn Down From Is Beyond Your Control 426
  Want a Ripped Waist? Reset the Metabolic Thermostat 427
  Ab Exercise Heretic 428
  The Caloric Cost of Exercise is Vastly Overrated 428
  The Procedural Consensus of the Iron Elite 429

Food Tricks 430

Magnificent Mini-Me! 437

EPILOGUE 441

The Purposefully Primitive Manifesto Doing Fewer Things Better 443
An Inch Wide and a Mile Deep 445
Rationalization, Visualization, Actualization 446
Fitness from Big Pink 451

RESOURCE GUIDE 459

INDEX 465

ABOUT THE AUTHOR 473

"Thinking Simply and Seeing Clearly"

Foreword by Pavel

Ten years ago a gruff voice left a message on my answering machine inviting me to write for a muscle magazine. The caller signed off as Marty Gallagher. He would become the big brother I never had and my mentor.

Since their overwhelmingly warm reception of Paul Anderson half a century ago, Russians have always been respectful of American strength and I am no exception. Anywhere Marty and I met, be it in a powerlifting meet where he was my "corner man", on a meditative walk through the mountains, over a glass of wine at the Ritz in Washington or a fine Mennonite-raised steak at Marty's country compound, I prodded and cajoled my friend for more knowledge. What I have learned has blown me away by its beauty and simplicity. I invite you to be equally blown away from your reading of *The Purposeful Primitive*.

The author of the book you are about to enjoy is the best writer in the iron game, period. He is so far ahead of the competition, both in his inner and outer knowledge of his subject and in his masterful delivery, that he is in a league of his own and the second best is not even in sight. It only took him forty years to reach his overnight success.

Marty was twelve when his father, an Irishman of few words, bought him his first barbell set. Like many, the boy learned how to weightlift from photos in *Strength & Health*. Like few, the self-coached weightlifter went on to win a national teen title and set a record in one of the lifts—even though he had not seen a live snatch or clean-and-jerk until his first meet! Then he found powerlifting and never looked back. Like mixed martial arts today, powerlifting in the sixties was an aggressive, anti-establishment sport. It was populated by rough characters like Don Blue who had to get a permission to leave prison for a day to compete in the World's—with a barely healed knife wound. Marty the juvenile delinquent was inevitably drawn in.

The young street tough apprenticed under another Irishman, Hugh Cassidy, a world champion and a legend of the strength sport. Weighing less than 300 pounds, Hugh benched 570 raw with a two-second pause! How many men could do it today? Far from a stereotypical musclehead, Cassidy was, among other things, fluent in German and an accomplished sculptor. It was this Renaissance man who would encourage the young gun to write his first powerlifting article. It was Cassidy's training methodology that would become the foundation of Gallagher's "purposefully primitive" method.

Training and competing alongside the iron elite, men like Mark Chaillet and Doug Furnas, Marty Gallagher kept learning, adding what was useful and discarding what was useless. His analytical mind, raw talent, and grim determination rapidly propelled him to the top.

Marty got strong. Very strong. He squatted 840 and had a clear shot at breaking the 871-pound world record. Then, like a tragic twist in the plot of one of Gallagher's beloved dark Russian novels, came the accident. Aided and abetted by a well meaning but unskilled gym member, a fully loaded barbell shattered the contender's leg...

His victorious comeback as a master lifter decades ahead of him, Marty Gallagher stayed in the game as a coach. And what a coach he was! His stable of athletes reads like "Who's Who" of the sport. Ed Coan. Introverted and enigmatic, he has brought down over a hundred world records and is undisputedly recognized as the greatest powerlifter in history. Kirk Karwoski. Explosive and bigger than life, this über-champion is admired by the hard to impress Russians. Making his Jedi master Cassidy proud, Gallagher has carried on the Old School legacy and continued an impeccable iron lineage.

This coach extraordinaire kept "polishing the chrome" of the Method until it met French aviator and writer Antoine de Saint Exupéry's criterion for perfection. "In anything at all, perfection is finally attained not when there is no longer anything to add, but when there is no longer anything to take away, when a body has been stripped down to its nakedness." Enter *The Purposeful Primitive.*

Gallagher has two passions, lifting and literature. He is as good as anyone in either. Bring the two pursuits together, and he has no equals and no runners-up.

In this one of a kind volume he brings you the hard won strength discoveries from the golden age of powerlifting, the seventies and the eighties. Filtered, systematized, and refined by one of the best coaching minds anywhere. It is a method second to none, even today. Consider this. As this book is going to print, the deadlift world records in four weight classes stand unbroken since they were set between 1982 and 1992. These records were set by American athletes who followed the Method revealed in *The Purposeful Primitive.*

The Method is at least as good as anything new out there. Its edge is its beautiful simplicity, something that contemporary methodologies, American and Russian, are lacking. For instance, the Russian national powerlifting team bench presses up to eight times a week. "Purposefully primitive" lifters do it only once or twice a week. The new generation of American athletes practices a great variety of esoteric exercises. The old school lives on a monastic diet of the basics. "If two methods deliver similar results," reasons Gallagher, "I will pick the more efficient one".

I would be kidding myself if I believed that more than a handful of readers have dreams of listening to the "Star Spangled Banner" standing atop the champions' podium at a powerlifting world championship. Most simply want to transform their physiques, build muscle and lose fat. Again, *The Purposeful Primitive* delivers.

When it comes to building muscle—prime meat, strong as it looks—powerlifters are the ultimate experts. Although endless pumping allows bodybuilders to develop huge fake muscles, it easy to tell these pretenders by their inflated, rather than dense, look. Real muscle, on the other hand, is rock hard and the person carrying it walks with an unmistakable presence of power. He draws attention because everyone is subconsciously recognizing him as the leader of the pack, not because he looks like a freak. Ironically, even in competitive bodybuilding the top dogs are rarely pumpers. Arnold Schwarzenegger and Franco Columbo are former powerlifting champions. Dorian Yates and Ronnie Coleman are powerlifting strong.

Building muscle the powerlifting way has many advantages over the popular pump artist routines. First, you get strong. If you see no benefit in that, may I suggest that you put this book away and join a Pilates class? Second, strong muscles don't shrink in a couple of days away from the gym. "Some years ago a certain Mr. America came to New York to give an exhibition," reminisces professional strong man Sig Klein in his old age. "I always admired his photos and asked him to show me his arm. He refused, saying that he had just made the long flight from California and this could have shrunken his arms. I was flabbergasted. If a few hours trip or a few days layoff from training makes that much difference in his muscles, then those muscles were useless and I didn't care to see them."

Third, the "purposefully primitive" method demands very little of your time and even less of your money. Most hobbyists buy the highest quality professional grade equipment if they have the means. No self-respecting chef would pick Walmart knives over Williams & Sonoma's. Yet amazingly, when it comes to fitness, people shun the tools and the techniques of the professionals and opt for mass market choices, the equivalent of cheap plastic. It is especially bizarre, since, unlike in any other endeavor, a strength professional tool kit is a lot less expensive than the amateur alternatives! Compare the price tags on a barbell and on some fancy exercise machine. Ditto for the membership at a no frills gym like YMCA as opposed to a ritzy health spa. When you are listening to Gallagher, you are getting Williams & Sonoma quality at Walmart prices.

You might argue that while powerlifters may be masters of piling on thick slabs of muscle, what do they know about getting lean? A good point. Fortunately, Gallagher is no ordinary powerlifter, he is a Renaissance man of all around fitness. Not content with just being muscular and strong, he is also lean and athletic. Recently on a bet this baby boomer smoked a local high school football star in a sprint! Marty's sensei, Hugh Cassidy had shown his apprentice the way when he cut down from 300 pounds to ripped 190. The Method stands on a balanced tripod of Iron, Cardio, and Nutrition. The author has spent decades researching the most effective and reliable methods of getting lean and this book features cutting edge recommendations from experts like nutrition visionary Ori Hofmekler and master of lean Bill Pearl.

You might suspect that, akin to those academic elite who remain completely out of touch with the People, world class coach Gallagher has nothing to offer to a regular Joe or Jane such as yourself. Wrong again. A true training system can be scaled up or down. If it can't be, it is not a system but a collection of tips. One Russian powerlifter has said this about the system of Marty's Russian counterpart, the national team coach Boris Sheyko: "the methodology was... attractive... primarily because it was a system built from the bottom up on the same principles. Which is why beginners, masters, and the elite 'train Sheyko' basically the same way. The only difference is in the load and volume." The author of *The Purposeful Primitive* has had remarkable success with extremely obese regular folks. I have had the privilege of watching him train some of them. I have heard women cry, grateful about the many pounds they had shed, thanks to his tough love.

Last but not least of the arrows in Gallagher's quiver is the "brain train" section of the book. Don't expect beaten to death clichés about "positive thinking". The author's "purposefully primitive psychology" is as far removed from the psychobabble which has thoroughly discredited mind power techniques in this country, as a world record squat attempt from a half-hearted set of leg extensions. And it does not matter whether your goal is to add pounds to your deadlift or subtract them from your spare tire, these techniques will dramatically shorten your journey to wherever you desire to be.

In addition to learning some of the most effective techniques of body and mind transformation, you are about to treat yourself to some of the best writing the English language has to offer. Gallagher is a samurai, equally adept in the manly and the literary arts. Since his teens Marty has been inhaling Hemingway, London, Chekhov, and Turgenev. After four decades of voracious reading and hard living, the brooding Irishman has become their equal. He retreated to the country where he, in the words of Jack London, could be "living close to the earth, thinking simply and seeing clearly", and wrote the Great American Novel of Strength.

Ladies and gentlemen, I am honored to present Marty Gallagher's *The Purposeful Primitive.*

A writer's job is to tell the truth. His standard of fidelity should be so high that his invention, out of his own experience, should produce a truer account than anything factual can. For facts can be observed badly; but when a good writer is creating something, he has time and scope to make of it an absolute truth.

—Ernest Hemingway

I am bringing fictional techniques to reportage.

—Truman Capote

I Prometheus

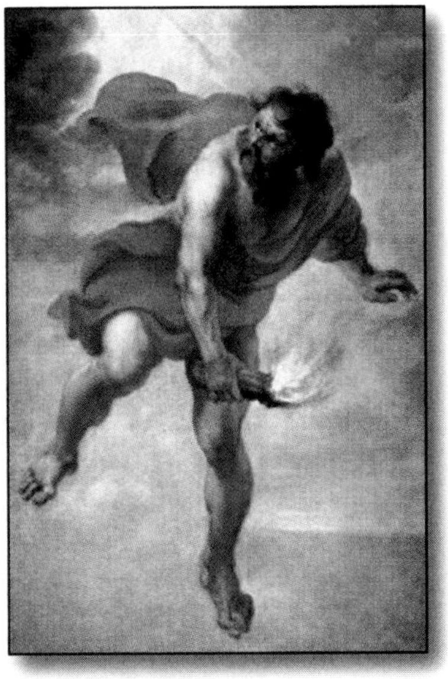

Like Prometheus I stole fire from the Gods. In my case, I stole from the athletic Gods, in order to help normal people in their quest to physically transform themselves.

My role is that of fact gatherer and interpreter. I assemble data, I codify and identify ideas; I explain theories and philosophies. I sort through and restate profound methods, making them user-friendly. As a Purposeful Primitive my prime directive is to reveal the irreducible training and nutrition methods used by elite athletes to build muscle and reduce body fat. Implement these methods and you will create a stronger, leaner body. Stronger and leaner makes any athlete better at what they do, regardless of the discipline or sport.

I am an athlete, a lesser athlete, just as Prometheus was a lesser God. I have stood on the 1st place pedestal in a foreign country at a World Championship and heard the National Anthem played. Still, my athletic achievements are Lilliputian compared to the Gods I write about. My achievements were sufficient enough to allow me access to the realm of the elite. Still, I was always an athletic overachiever, in that my accomplishments vastly exceeded my limited genetic gifts. In one sense this was a blessing: as art critic David Gelertner once observed, *"Some great artists (say Raphael, Degas, Rodin or Picasso) are born with great technique. Others like Cezanne are born with more will and insight than technical means. If you are an artist in the second category, your work gains in depth, integrity and power from your dogged technical struggles. Lack of fluency concentrates the mind."* I engaged in dogged technical struggles and my lack of athletic fluency concentrated my mind.

I was a physiological overachiever whose lack of genetic gifts caused me to overcompensate in ways that eventually resulted in a certain uniqueness that set me apart from my athletic contemporaries.

My limitations meant I had to train smarter, research deeper, learn and figure harder, riddle longer and ponder more on how to improve and further my own athletic quest. I continually searched to find ever-better methods and mentors. This book is the summation of the modes and methods I gleaned from the Masters with whom I came into contact. This book is my very own version of G.I. Gurdjieff's *Meetings with Remarkable Men.* This book is an accumulation of ideas, a treatise on the commonalities and particularities that draw together and differentiate the true Masters.

The rationale, the *raison d'etre* for this book is profound: how best to stimulate, trigger, ignite or instigate tangible, irrefutable, undeniable physical progress? How do we transform the human body? The athletic elite *know* how to reconfigure the body. The average fitness acolyte who seeks physical renovation needs to access and incorporate these elite tactics.

Being an athlete interested in improving my own game, being in a position to quiz and grill top athletes about the training and eating protocols that got them there, I made the most of the opportunity. I talked long, often, and in great depth to hundreds of top athletes. My job was to write articles about the tactics they used to excel. My fate was to be a good, not great, competitor. As a journalist I knew enough to ask the right questions and then shut up and listen (in awe) as the great ones took the time to talk and share the training, nutrition or mental tactics that made them great.

I knew their language and I knew how to interpret often arcane abstractions into readable prose regular folks could understand and utilize. Too many interviewers make the mistake of trying to impress the interviewee instead of letting them tell their tale. As one curmudgeon said, "I never learned a damn thing listening to myself talk." Like Prometheus, I stole fire from the Gods. I now pass along their accumulated wisdom for use in your own transformational quest. Be smart enough to use and apply their methods. Their ways are the proven ways and their ways will allow you to morph from what you *are* into what you *want to be*. And that, my friend, is truly incredible.

The Purposeful Primitives Masters, Modes & Methods

Transformational Techniques & Tactics

Physical transformation is made way too complicated. When people talk about "fitness" or "diet" they are really talking about physical transformation. They are dissatisfied with how they look and feel and they want to do something about it. In actuality what people seek, though they may not think of it in this way, is *transformation*. They want to morph their physique, change it, modify it, and improve upon its current state.

What constitutes a better body? The irreducible core definition of what people seek from fitness could be boiled down to two things: decreased body fat and more muscle. There are lots of other benefits they might seek from a diet or exercise plan, but at the root core, the reason all those diet books are sold and all those abdominal devices are purchased is that people want to lose body fat. The reason people belong to gyms and purchase exercise equipment is they want to build muscle.

Unfortunately in this day and age, the Information Age, we are awash in a sea of health and fitness confusion and contradiction. *This* approach contradicts *that* approach, this diet plan claims incredible results, yet is precisely the opposite of another diet plan, both of which present powerfully persuasive arguments and (pseudo) science to back up their claims. One school of exercise will champion one approach for sculpting the physique that stands in stark contrast to another school of exercise; both schools have compelling arguments and trot out radically transformed adherents that tell you how this particular system transformed their physiques in no time flat with a minimum amount of time, effort and expense. Everything related to fitness nowadays comes with a price tag. In order to lure you into purchasing one mode or method over another, be it diet-related or exercise-related, the manufacturer will claim that radical physical transformation can be yours and can be made both *quick* and *easy*—assuming you buy their magical product.

If radical physical transformation were truly quick and easy any outfit that produced such a product, system or method, one that *truly* delivered quick and easy results would rule the world. There is no such thing as quick and easy physical transformation. We'll call this the 1st truism of the Purposefully Primitive Philosophy.

Human nature wants desperately to believe that a mode or method, a pill or potion exists that will magically shortcut the sweat, toil, tears, blood, time and teeth-grinding effort it takes to trigger tangible transformation. Human nature wants desperately to believe that a magical system exists—but you just haven't found it yet. So you keep looking and you keep buying, you keep hoping and wishing, you keep purchasing books, DVDs, gym memberships, dietary food plans, exercise equipment, fat burning pills, nutritional supplements of every type and kind; anything that promises you what you want to hear. All in the hope of finding that magical method, mode or substance that will enable you to undergo a significant physical makeover with a minimum investment of time, money and especially effort. You want nothing less than to undergo a phantasmagoric metamorphosis, from ugly earth-bound caterpillar into a gorgeous celestial butterfly. So you buy and buy and you try and try—yet still you stay the same. Understand that true transformation is difficult, arduous, prolonged and intense. You need discipline, grit, tenacity, perseverance and patience. That's the bad news. The good news is that certain systems, methods and modes can and will transform the human body. Certain disciplines, done diligently, radically reduce body fat and create new muscle tissue. My task is to share with you the battle-tested modes and methods of the true Masters.

There Is No School Like Old School

The human body is subject to biological imperatives, cause and effect, i.e. do *this* and *that* will happen. Biological cause and effect is not about *new, better, improved, revolutionary or double your money back if not satisfied within 14 days of purchase!* True biological imperatives are about science.

Scientifically speaking, if a muscle, any muscle, is subjected to a specific resistance protocol of sufficient intensity, the target muscle *must* grow larger and stronger if that muscle is then fed and rested. That is science.

Another biological imperative informs us that if the human body operates in *negative energy balance* (NEB) for a protracted period, a resultant loss in bodyweight *must* occur. This is basic caloric thermodynamics. Furthermore, if the body operates in NEB for a protracted period, and if other specified procedures and protocols are enacted, the human body preferentially calls up its body fat reserves (stored energy) and uses body fat to fuel activity. Enact specific training and eating procedures and the human body *must* grow new muscle and *must* oxidize stored body fat.

Cause and effect is objective: enact certain procedures and certain predictable results occur. The body has no choice. There are certain resistance-training protocols that have been used for decades and have been proven to deliver real results. These training procedures were invented and refined by Master resistance trainers. There are certain forms of cardiovascular exercise that have been used for decades and have been proven to deliver amazing results. There are certain nutritional modes and methods that have been used for decades and accelerate the oxidation of stored body fat while promoting recovery, healing and muscle growth. These systems work because they are rooted in science and biology. They have proven track records and have been used by elite athletes for decades. All are battle-tested with irrefutable, empirical, earned-in-the-trenches pedigrees. These systems produce results: the human body is transformed when these methods and modes are methodically applied.

In this book I introduce you to the absolute Masters of four interrelated modes of transformation: resistance training, cardiovascular training, nutrition and psychology. This is the age of fitness confusion. What actually works? What is patently bogus? How is the average civilian to differentiate between the truly profound and the slick commercial product draped in sly, sultry seductive garb? What better way to introduce you to truly effective modes and methods than to introduce you to the absolute Masters of the four realms.

Every intelligent fitness regimen needs a progressive resistance element, a cardiovascular element and a nutritional element. I add a psychological element because mental recalibration is the most neglected aspect of the transformational process. If you want to get your facts straight about resistance training, learn from a resistance Master. If you want to get your facts straight about cardiovascular training, quiz a cardio genius. If you want to get your facts straight about nutrition, listen to those who have decades of experience in that arena. If you want to get your facts straight about recalibrating your brain to better aid the transformational effort, expose yourself to hardnosed psyche Masters.

I have selected fifteen Giants, men who've made indelible marks in their respective fields of expertise. You can see a hell of a lot further standing on the shoulders of Giants: the vista is not obscured by the fitness dwarfs and pygmies that clutter the view at ground level.

In this day and age everyone frantically seeks the next breakthrough, innovation or angle. I say unequivocally: Old School methodology is the modern solution for achieving true physical transformation. Be done with the jive seduction. Be done with the illusion that somewhere there exists an effortless way. Sink your teeth into something substantive. The transformational procedures of the true Masters lie between the two covers of this book.

Standing On the Shoulders of Giants

In 1927 G.I. Gurdjieff wrote *Meetings with Remarkable Men*. In it he spoke of his encounters with various mystics: the Armenian Sarkis Pogossian, the Russian Prince Yuri Lubovedsky, Ekim Bey, Professors Karpenko and Skridlov, plus an odd assortment of seers and occultists. In describing these characters Gurdjieff wove their stories into his own story. He tells of his interactions with spiritual masters in Central Asia and calls this group "The Seekers of Truth."

Since 1962 I too have been on my own journey. I too am a seeker of truth. I too have experienced my own version of Meetings with Remarkable Men. Instead of mystics and seers, I was introduced to a succession of remarkable men; Masters of resistance training, nutrition, cardiovascular training and performance-related psychology. My idea was to introduce readers of this book to the Masters, modes and methods that I have been exposed to over the past four and a half decades. My idea was to spotlight these men and their purposefully primitive systems. The modes, techniques and tactics taught and used by the various Masters are incredibly beneficial when used by regular individuals who are on their own quest for physical transformation. In addition to offering up brief resumes on these remarkable men, I also present their philosophies and offer my own interpretation on how best to utilize, incorporate and apply the methods of these Masters. I act as an interpreter and guide. I also present related essays, ideas and methods.

Each man I write about is, in their own way, a *Purposeful Primitive*. There is a discernable connection between all these men, a subtle link that binds them. Their individual methods share a commonality; a commonality that oddly links Krishnamurti to Bednarski, Pearl to Parrillo, Fantano to Schwartz—each man's approach, within their particular area of expertise, is rooted in science and biology. Each man stresses diligent application and each offers a method to induce progress. By challenging the status quo, by offering radical alternatives to the existing orthodox protocols, each man contributed something completely unique to their specific arena.

In order to create something of true significance, the first allegiance must be to factual results. Within every discipline there exists a bedrock foundation. Each man selected is a foundational Master who has amplified and imbued the ultra-basics with his own tactical idiosyncrasies. As I became familiar with their distinct approaches, be it body or mind, I was struck by the fact that on an elemental level, each approach was deceptively simple. All used simplistic yet innovative methods powered by gut-busting physical or mental effort.

Tenacity, discipline and ferocity are politically incorrect concepts in an age where dazzling complexity and continual innovation are the name of the game. My contention is that just because a mode or method is new doesn't mean it automatically trumps what came before it. To the contrary, Old School methods, doing fewer things better, consistently exceeds results delivered by modern fragmented fitness systems.

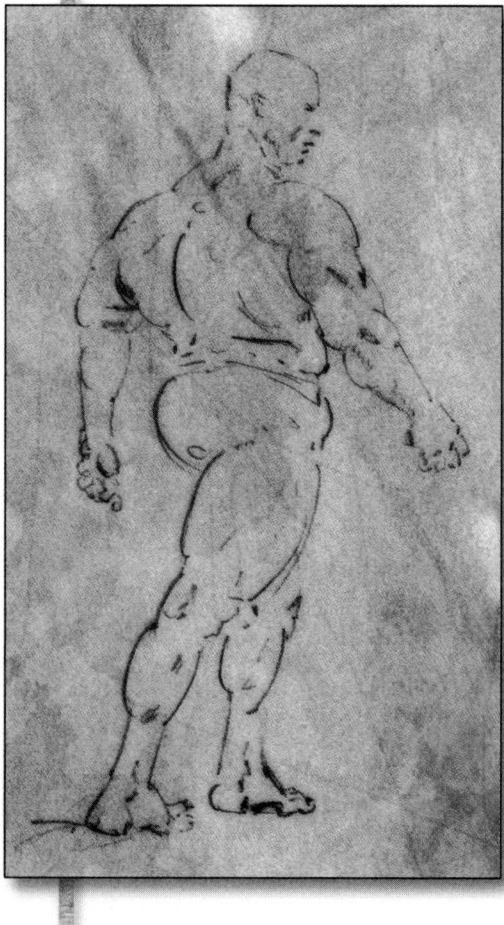

The human body is a remarkable machine and I am fascinated with the idea of improving it and making it better. William Burroughs labeled the human body "The Soft Machine" and I think that is the most amazing and appropriate description of the incredible human apparatus. In this book I relate the resistance training systems of ten legendary resistance Masters representing three separate and distinct iron disciplines. I spotlight two nutritional geniuses and two mind Masters. I introduce to the reader a cardiovascular *grand maestro* without peer. I intersperse the modes and methods of these giants with tales of my own. I relate the profundities of the Masters, designed to aid you in your own unique situation. I offer up Purposefully Primitive Masters, modes, methods, techniques and tactics that you can and should expropriate for use in your own transformational quest.

Iron Masters

The human body will not favorably reconfigure itself in response to ease and sameness. Systematic struggle and stress are required to trip the hypertrophy trigger.

Hypertrophy is not a gradual or gentle event—rather the cellular equivalent of a nuclear explosion.

PAUL ANDERSON

Primitive Patriarch

Paul Anderson roared out of the Tennessee hill country at the same moment another deep-fried, backwoods southern country boy was roaring out of Tupelo, Mississippi. Both men would forever change their respective worlds. At the same time Paul Anderson was demolishing all strength and power preconceptions, another young man the same age, Elvis Aaron Presley, was doing likewise in his field of expertise: music. Both men emerged from total and complete rural isolation. They mysteriously developed great insight within their respective crafts. Paul and Elvis destroyed every convention, demolished everything "held most sacred," shattered every orthodox belief, desecrated every ritual and decimated every cherished notion. Nothing would ever be the same after the appearance of these two hillbilly savants.

> ***Barbarians at the gate: into the breach surged battalions of converts,***
> ***Emerging from swamps and backwoods,***
> ***To blow up everything held most sacred,***
> ***They sweated, roared and swaggered to the limit,***
> ***They tore down the temple and razed it to the ground.***
>
> **—Nik Cohen**

Nothing would ever be the same after Paul and Elvis. They were cut of the same cloth: backwoods boys, uncouth, unsophisticated hicks, off-spring of honest-to-God hillbillies. Viewed first with repugnance and yawning disdain, later with pure fear and terror, these two evoked vitriolic reactions on the part of entrenched defenders of the status quo. Unconscious revolutionaries operating in different venues, they moved mountains and changed entire worlds.

Anderson shifted the gravitational pull of his world as surely as Elvis Presley changed the musical world...irrevocably, forthwith and forever. Anderson's world did not have the high societal profile that Elvis' did—but that was strictly fate and circumstance, the luck of the cosmic draw. Paul had as profound an impact on all things strength-related as The King had on all things music-related. The fact that American society placed a financial premium on pop music and assigned negligible value to strength pursuits was predictable and irrelevant. That was life's lottery.

Both men died early. I saw Anderson lift in 1966 at the Silver Spring Boy's Club. He put on a mind-blowing exhibition that changed the direction of my life. Paul began with the power clean and overhead press. He worked up to an effortless 420 pounds. The world record at the time was 418 by Russia's Yuri Vlasov. The ease and speed of his lifting blew my young mind. His pulling techniques were awkward, yet powerful. Once he shouldered a weight, he simply lay back a tad before blasting the barbell overhead. He used none of the knee jerk trickery that eventually got the overhead press banned from Olympic lifting. Another Purposeful Primitive, Clarence Bass, recalls seeing Anderson lift in his prime:

> ***"I saw him {Anderson} lift in 1958 at the Russian-American match held in Madison Square Garden. Anderson had turned professional by then and appeared as a special attraction. At the conclusion of the contest, the Russian champion Medvedev had pressed about 350. Anderson created a sensation by cleaning and pressing 425 for two reps and just failing with a third."***

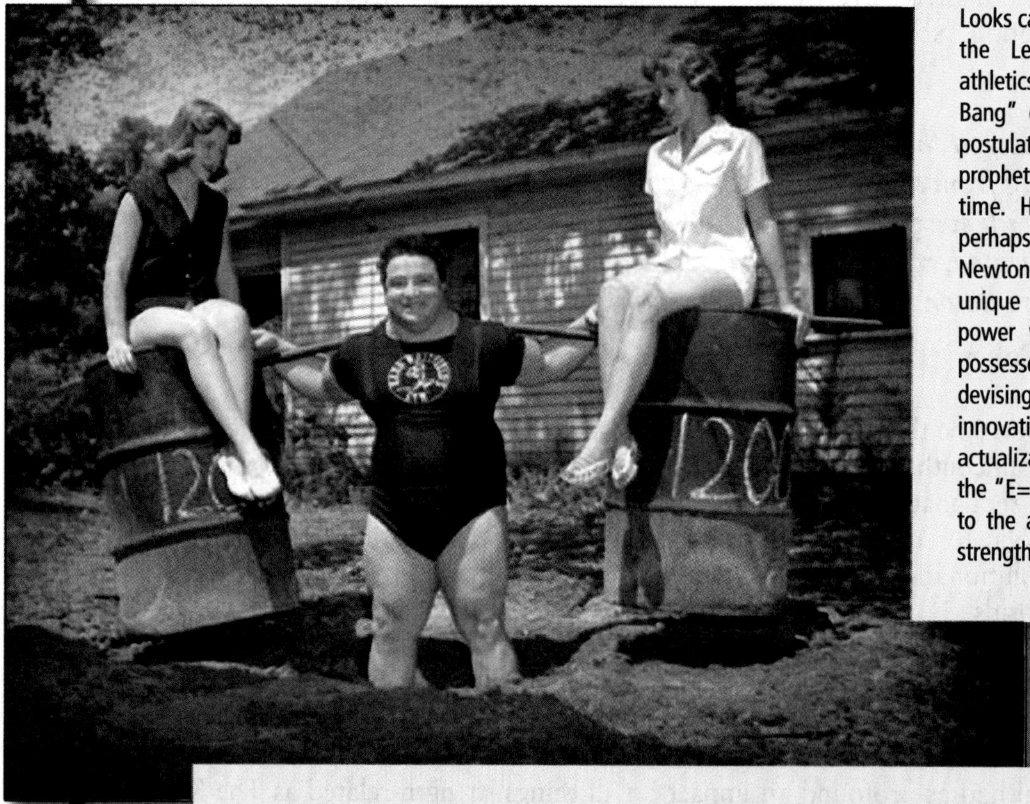

Looks can be deceiving: Does this look like the Leonardo Di Vinci of strength athletics? Paul Anderson was "The Big Bang" of modern strength training. His postulations and theorems were profound, prophetic and light years ahead of his time. He was the Albert Einstein, or perhaps more accurately, the Sir Isaac Newton of modern strength training. His unique approach towards building raw power was born in rural isolation. He possessed an idiot savant-like ability for devising systems and methods. His fertile, innovative mind produced realizations and actualizations that formed the foundation, the "E=MC squared" of all things related to the acquisition of power, muscle and strength.

Revolutionary, counterintuitive and unorthodox, Paul was a strength theoretician who experimented on himself with incredible results. This camp, jive photo actually portrays something quite profound: the invention of the power rack and partial rep training. Taken in 1954, out back of his family home, this photo depicts a groundbreaking innovation, figuratively and literally. It was but one small sliver of the Andersonian genius. Squatting in a hole reduced the range-of-motion. Over time he put all the dirt back into the hole and ended up doing deep squats with 1200 pounds. His creative mind effortlessly generated heretofore unheard of strength building modes and methods that are still in use today.

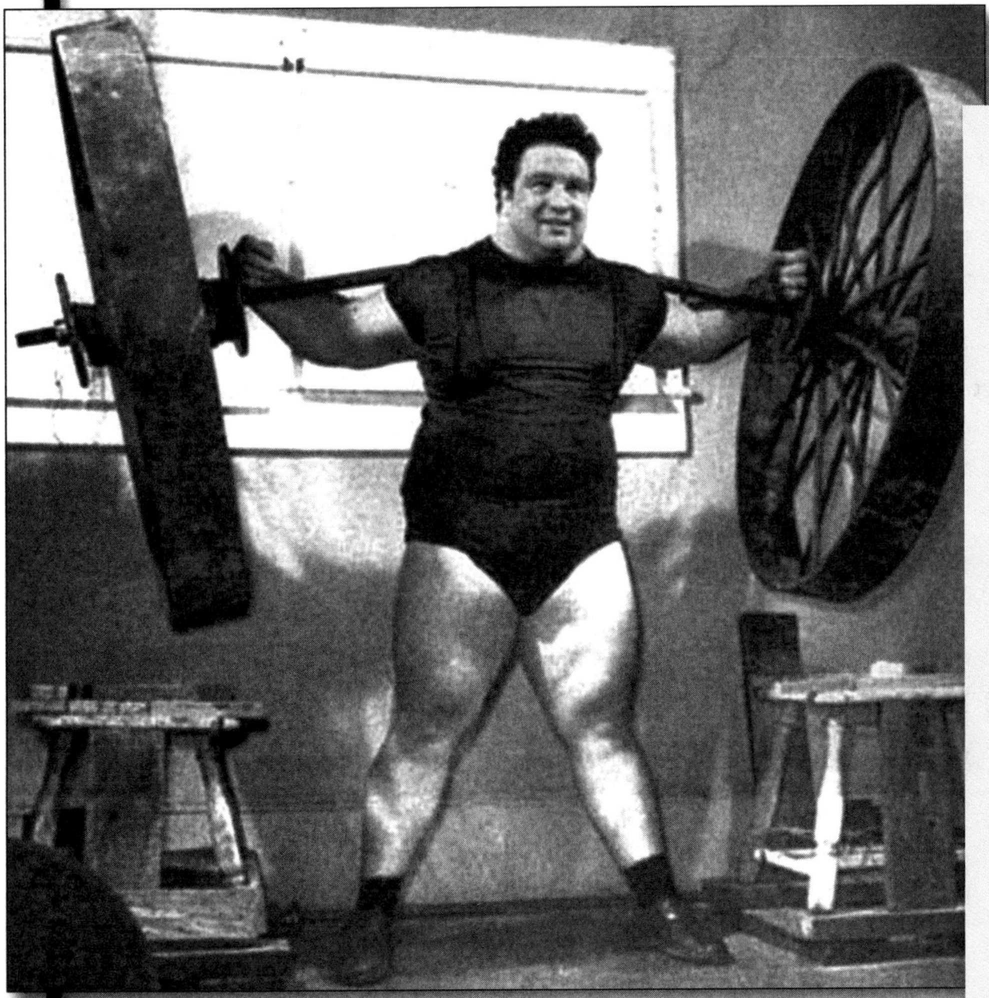

Big Paul reportedly liked to golf and had two holes set up on his farm. He would take his driver, crack the ball 300 yards, chip up, putt in and walk to an outdoor weightlifting platform set up adjacent to the green. There, a 400 pound barbell sat in a rack apparatus. Big Paul would dip under the barbell, step back and press the 400 pound barbell overhead 3-5 times before replacing it. He would tee-up, drive back, chip up to the first green, putt in and walk to a second weight lifting platform set adjacent to that putting green. A barbell loaded to 800 pounds sat in a squat rack. Paul would squat the weight for 3-5 reps and replace the bar. Back and forth he'd go, drive, chip, putt, lift...this could go on all afternoon. Paul liked the walking interspersed with the lifts. Afterwards he would have a cool drink on the farmhouse porch.

At the Silver Spring exhibition Paul wore his combat boots while pressing. Paul shed the boots and performed squats wearing black socks and a bathing suit. He used his special squat bar and wore a tee-shirt. No lifting belt for either lifts. He squatted 900 pounds for 5 reps. I thought it was the most incredible event of my life. His performance was shattering, jarring, disconcerting, unbelievable and done with eerie ease. The speed, the nonchalance with which he handled 900 was science fiction stuff. I never saw a big man squat with that velocity until Shane Hamman appeared on the power scene thirty years later.

Afterwards Paul talked about the Lord to the crowd then headed off to another whistle stop somewhere down the line. I heard he was doing four shows a week and what we witnessed required no real exertion on his part; he had many weekly shows to perform and could not afford to extend himself at any particular exhibition.

Late in his life I had the pleasure to talk with him on numerous occasions at his home in Georgia. He was stricken hard by Bright's disease and wheelchair bound. I first interviewed him for a *Muscle & Fitness* feature article. He took a liking to my interview style, my knowledge of him and his career and my serious questions. I called him periodically and he liked to talk about training. He felt that he never reached his potential. During his peak physical years he traveled so much and put on so many exhibitions that he never had the opportunity to settle in and train with singular focus and purpose. He felt that had he had an inspirational goal—like lifting in the Olympic Games—he could have become much better. He applied for reinstatement prior to several Olympic Games and was always turned down flat by the steely-eyed men that ran the AAU. Had he been allowed to compete, he would have likely won the '60, '64 and '68 Olympics. Only the rise of Alexev could have ended his reign. His infractions, taking a few bucks for professional wrestling matches, are laughable by today's standards.

Paul power clean and pressing 425 for reps at Muscle Beach in 1956.

Born 1932, Anderson won the world weightlifting title in 1955 and Olympic gold medal in 1956. As a member of the first U.S. sports team to visit the Soviet Union during the Cold War, the 5'9", 360 pound Anderson lifted for 15,000 Muscovites on a 1955 State Department sponsored trip. Anderson shattered the world record in the press by an unprecedented 50 pounds, ramming 402 overhead in a drizzling rain. The Moscow newspapers called him "Chudo Prirody, The Wonder of Nature." Upon returning home, he was summoned to the White House by Vice-President Nixon.

Randy Strossen wrote that Anderson's early training was prophetic. "Paul combined short, intense workouts...throughout the day, with periods of rest. For example, he would do 10 reps in the squat with 600, rest for about 30 minutes, and then do a second set of 10. After another 30 minutes rest, he would increase the weight to 825 and do three reps, rest again and do two more reps with 845. Then he would rest again and conclude by doing half squats with 1200 for 2 or 3 reps and quarter squats with 1800. The whole routine took three hours or more. He would sip milk during the rest periods, consuming a gallon or more throughout the course of the day."

Randy writes that Paul's purposefully primitive extended training sessions were "Eerily prescient of what would become the structure of state-of-the-art weight lifting programs decades later. Most productive national teams train in a similar fashion, but in Anderson's time it was unheard of. Paul Anderson's approach was consciously developed and planned, and taken together, was quite unlike anything seen before—as were his results."

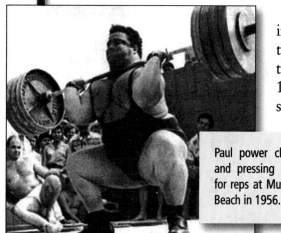

This typical Anderson workout, circa 1955, required three to four hours to complete.

Typical Paul Anderson Workout

Tuesday, Thursday, Saturday

Exercise	Poundage/Reps
Full Squat	600 x 10 (2 sets)
	825 x 2
	845 x 2
	900 x 2
Half Squat	1200 x 2
Quarter Squat	1800 x 2
Deadlift	650 x 6-8 (4 sets)

Monday, Wednesday, Friday

Exercise	Poundage/Reps
Press Off Rack	300 x 6
	400 x 2
	390 x 2
	370 x 2
Press Outs	500 x 4 (several sets from sticking point to lockout)
Press from Shoulders to Top of Head	500 x 4
Push-Press Off Rack	450 x 3
Bench Press	400-450 x 6-8 (used multiple sets)

Andy the Athlete:

- Handstand presses: He was spry enough to flip himself upside down and do repetition handstand press-ups

- Paul had a 36 inch vertical leap and could broad jump over 10 feet weighing 360. He beat a member of the US Olympic 400 meter relay team in a 20 yard dash. He then placed the man on his shoulder and ran a lap.

Paul in top shape around 1965: cut-throat politics kept him from lifting at the Olympics. He'd taken some money for pro wrestling and that was that. Free World athletes competed against state-supported Communist athletes on the most un-level of playing fields. Purity police in America purged many of our best.

Paul was the epicenter of Purposeful Primitive resistance training. His mind was inquisitive and he used overwhelming power to muscle up the press, snatch and clean and jerk; subtlety and technique be damned. He came up in a time when the training orthodoxy was uniform and aligned, i.e. to improve performance in the three lifts, the three lifts needed to be practiced exclusively. Andy, training in rural seclusion, stepped outside the box of conventional thinking (factually he was never in the box) and showed athletes the next arena of improvement. Tommy Kono wrote in Randy Strossen's book, "*The Mightiest Minister*" that Paul created quite a stir in the training hall at the 1955 Munich World Championships by doing squats "with close to 700 pounds for ten reps without any warm-up; he performed them so rapidly that it was as if free squats were being performed." Kono said Anderson would've used more weight, but that was all they could load on the bar. On Anderson's next trip to Russia, the Soviets had constructed squat racks and benches to duplicate Paul's unorthodox approach.

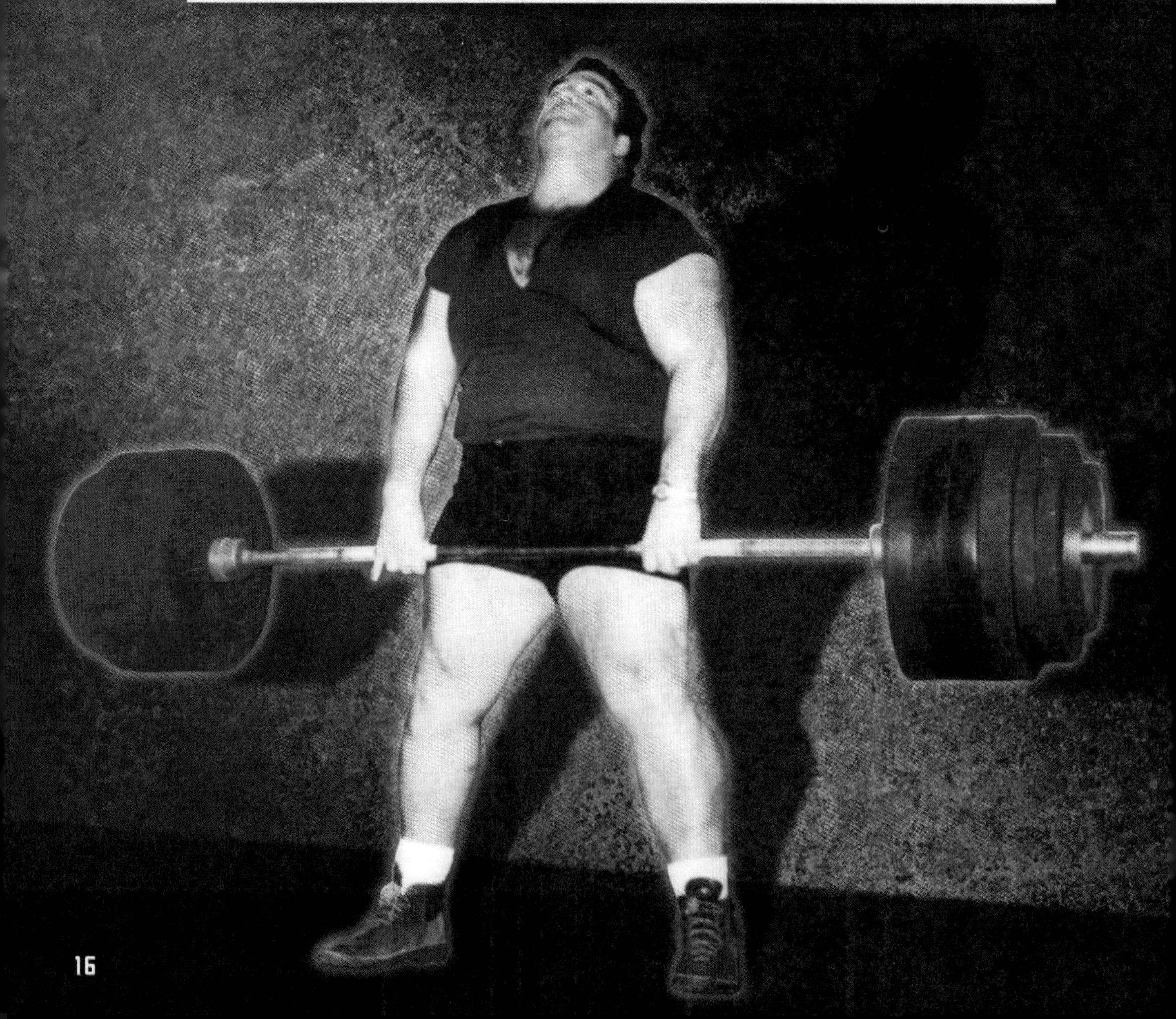

BILL PEARL

Anti-Aging Role Model

Back in the sixties, men who weight trained with any degree of seriousness practiced three separate and distinct forms of progressive resistance training: bodybuilding, powerlifting and Olympic weight-lifting.

Bodybuilding was about building muscle mass while staying lean. Powerlifting was about lifting as much as possible in the squat, bench press and deadlift. Olympic lifting was how much poundage could be hoisted overhead in the press, snatch and clean and jerk. The Amateur Athletic Union ran the Mr. America competition for forty years and controlled most local physique competitions. They awarded *athletic points* to physique competitors. If you wanted the extra points, you needed to demonstrate proficiency at some sport. Most bodybuilders picked Olympic lifting.

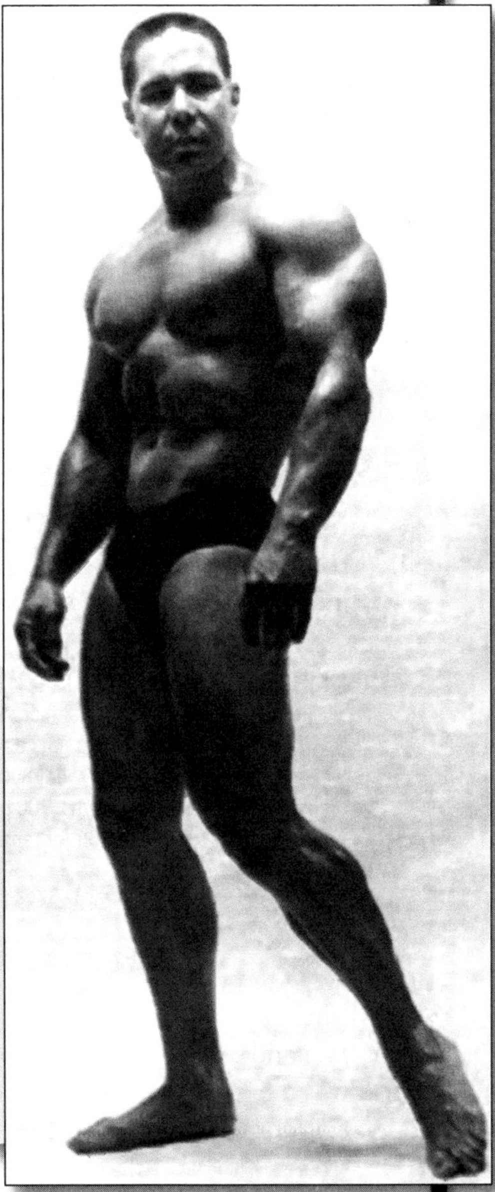

Behold the prototypical power physique. This is the body all the boys and men wanted. The Herculean look is always the preferred look amongst real men. Taken circa 1965, Bill was as strong as he looked. Weighing 240 pounds at a time when 195 was considered 'big,' Bill was the trendsetter and always the adult in the room. Pearl was principled and resolute.

I got to know him after his career was over. He was easily one of the most lucid, intelligent athletes I ever had the privilege to interview. He built his bulk using massive poundage in power movements. He later shifted to a volume regimen. Pearl was a nutritional anomaly: in a world of ravenous carnivores he was an unapologetic vegetarian.

Bodybuilders entered lifting competitions to pick up those invaluable athletic points. Powerlifters of the day often were often ex-Olympic lifters who couldn't master the subtleties of the very exacting O-lift techniques. Olympic lifters were plentiful in the sixties. Practicing the three overhead lifts produced men with thick traps, python-like erectors and rotund rhomboids. Massive backs were built by pulling on cleans and snatches; thick shoulders were built from heavy overhead pressing and jerking. Pearl came up in this cross-trained era. Genetically predisposed to thickness, he amplified his ample natural gifts.

Multiple-discipline lifting produced outstanding physiques. Men who practiced the three interrelated lifting arts, men like John Grimek, Marvin Eder and Roy Hilligen, developed incredibly rugged and functional physiques. Arnold Schwarzenegger, Sergio Oliva and Franco Columbo were later examples of Old School bodybuilders with heavy lifting backgrounds. All three were national or world level lifters before they peaked as bodybuilders.

Nowadays no one practices the three lifting arts and something has been lost. Today is the dreaded era of the resistance specialist. Physiques nowadays tend to have a predictable sameness about them. High-torque power exercises are required to develop mountainous traps, enormous erectors and overall muscle thickness. By becoming truly strong at basic compound multi-joint barbell and dumbbell exercises, muscles develop in a way unobtainable by any other mode.

Dorian Yates and Ron Coleman between them ruled the bodybuilding world for 15 consecutive years. This was largely because of their incredible leg and back development: Yates rowed with 500 for reps while Coleman deadlifted 800 for reps: there is an undeniable correlation between massive strength development and massive muscle development. Strength increases beget muscle size increases.

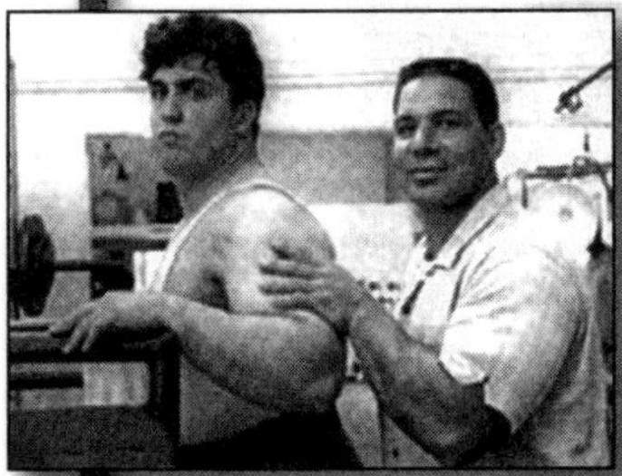

Bill stands with powerlifting immortal Pat Casey. Irish Pat was the first man to bench press 600 pounds; this in the mid-sixties. Pat pushed 622 in a t-shirt and was also the first man to squat 800 and total 2,000 in a powerlifting competition. Casey could do repetition dips with a 200 pound dumbbell strapped around his waist. Pat did seated barbell presses with 400 for reps.

Casey was the greatest West Coast powerlifter of all-time. He passed away recently.

In the 1960's two bodybuilders stood apart from the pack. Each was an immortal: England's Reg Park and America's Bill Pearl. Reg was God-like, Arnold's mentor. Bill Pearl was the American Colossus. These two men took the look that John Grimek actualized and epitomized, the power look, to the next level. Both men were big men; thick, incredibly strong yet graceful. They had functional builds and were as powerful as they looked. Both were athletic. Bill squatted 600 pounds when 400 was an excellent lift. Reg bench pressed

500 when 300 was good. While the top physique competitors of the day weighed 170 to 195 pounds, Bill weighed 240 and Reg 245. Pearl's proportions were eye-popping. Reg, slightly taller, had the shapelier physique. Reg was an Irish Wolf Hound while Pearl was a Bull Mastiff.

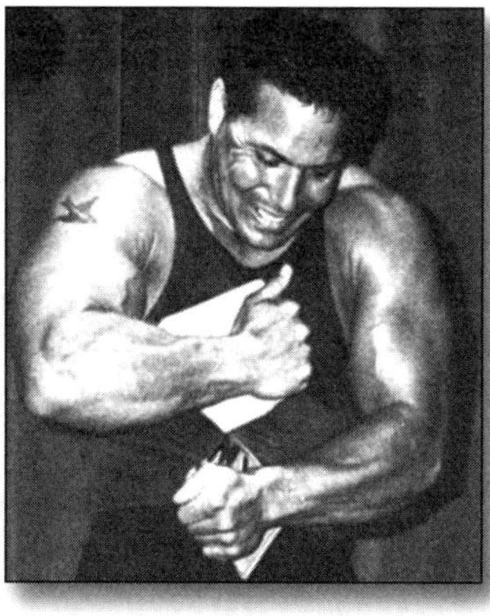

I idolized both of these men because they were manly and strong. Bill could tear license plates in half, bend spikes, lift up cars and rip phone books in half. Later in life I had the great fortune of meeting Bill and he was as friendly and open as I'd imagined him to be when I worshipped him from afar as a youngster. Pearl taught me a lot: he taught me there are no excuses. In order to fit training into his hectic life he would get up at 4am to work out. "I got into the habit of getting up early to train because if I waited until the rest of the world got up, there always seemed to be something happening that caused me to miss the day's workout. I found if I took care of myself at 4am, then I was a lot better as a person when the rest of the world woke up and I had to interact with them."

Without knowing it, he encouraged me to train early when I still worked real jobs. Eventually he unknowingly encouraged me to leave the city and move to the country. He had opted out of the lucrative rat race in order to seek the elusive, rural, "quality of life." He was a successful gym owner in Los Angeles before he moved to the bucolic bliss of rural Oregon to live on a farm. That particular city man fantasy took root in my head and eventually I did as he did. I too bailed out of the rat race and relocated to the isolation and peace of the country.

After Bill purchased his farmette, he built an amazing gym in the barn outback. He spent his time restoring antique autos, one of his many hobbies; he was a hobbyist and had innumerable collections of old things. He also had a beautiful wife, Judy, and he was totally in love with his soul mate.

Pearl seemed genuinely happy, one of the few truly happy men I've ever encountered. Eventually I followed the path of Pearl, imbued and imprinted with my own subtle variations. Pearl is 20 years older than me and since 1964 he has inspired me. He continues to inspire me. He has been my iron role model and a life role model for 44 years and counting. His training, like his life, has evolved over the years. Pearl embraces change and instead of becoming fossilized and change resistant, as people do as they age, Bill remains fluid. Early on, Bill used bar-bending poundage in basic movements to build his incomparable mass and size. Once he obtained enough beef, he switched gears and concentrated on refining, honing, chiseling and defining his incredible mountain of muscle and sinew.

Always a training innovator, in later years he added the element of *accelerated* pace to his resistance training. Pearl injects a cardiovascular element onto his weight training efforts; a Pearl version of 3rd Way cardio. Sustained strength/cardio training that builds hybrid "super muscle." Bill related to me that once he got into the swing of his two hour daily weight training regimen, his heart rate would never drop below 120 and often would spike to 170 or more. His rapid-fire workouts purposefully combine cardio training with strength training to elicit a specific effect. He no longer cared to ride the Brahma bull of huge training poundage, he had enough size. He completely changed direction. Now the name of the game was upping the intensity by moving *faster* during the workout. He positively devoured the time element of the training parameter. His current approach could be summarized as lots of exercises performed using pristine technique done at a blistering pace. He *still* burns out young training partners.

Bill Pearl's Classical Bodybuilding Training Regimen

Bill is a classical *bodybuilder*. He is credited as the one of the first bodybuilders to create and utilize the *maximum volume* training approach. Bill exemplifies one extreme of the bodybuilding training paradigm while Dorian Yates exemplifies the other extreme. Pearl's volume regimen requires the trainee perform lots of sets, reps and exercises per muscle group. Pearl typically hits a dozen or more exercises per session. He crams as many as sixty sets into each session. He hits each muscle *two* or *three* times per week. Bill never goes to failure. He talked of establishing a session rhythm; a momentum, an accelerated pace. The training partners, all following the same routine, would go one after another Bam! Bam! Bam! From commencement until conclusion, the Pearl participants are in continual rotational motion. His boys would join him at the barn at 4:30 am to commence the daily training regimen.

Bill rotated exercises religiously, periodically alternating movements to keep things fresh and vibrant. Technique is approached with reverence; making the mind-muscle connection critical. Bill stresses *feel* and muscular contraction and trains six days per week whereas Dorian would handle massive poundage in short, less frequent weekly sessions. Bill is a stickler for proper technique. A Pearl workout has a uniform evenness about it from start to finish. Bill wears a muscle down. Dorian knocks it out.

Monday and Thursday

Bodypart	Exercise	Sets/Reps
Abs	Roman chair sit-ups, db side bends, extension pull-in, twists, jackknife	300 total reps spread over the five exercises
Chest	Dumbbell inclines, nautilus pullover, pec dec, decline bench, flat bench	5 sets of 8-10 reps for each exercise
Back	Deadlift, dumbbell row	5 sets of 8-10 reps for each exercise
Forearms	Wrist curls	5 sets of 20-25 reps
Calves	Standing calf raises	9 sets of 20-25 reps
Neck	Neck raise	5 sets of 15-20 reps

Tuesday and Friday

Bodypart	Exercise	Sets/Reps
Abs	Crunch, front bend, cable in, dumbbell bend, incline knee ups	260 total reps spread over the five exercises
Legs	Leg extensions, leg curl, front squat, leg press	5 sets of 8-10 reps for each exercise
Shoulders	Seated front press, lying laterals, side laterals, front raise	5 sets of 6-10 reps for each exercise
Forearms	Seated reverse curls	5 sets of 20-25 reps
Calves	Seated calf raise	9 sets of 20-25 reps
Neck	Partner push – front, both sides, rear	One rotation

Wednesday and Saturday

Bodypart	Exercise	Sets/Reps
Abs	Incline sit-ups, twists, leg raise, scissor kicks, weighted leg raise	300 total reps spread over the five exercises
Biceps	Machine curls, incline curls, barbell curls, concentration curls	5 sets of 6-10 reps for each exercise
Triceps	Incline triceps press, pushdowns, floor press, cable extensions	5 sets of 6-10 reps for each exercise
Forearms	Wrist roll-up	From the ground up – 5 reps
Calves	Calf raise on leg press machine	9 sets of 20-25 reps
Neck	Lying neck raise	5 sets of 20-25 reps

Now that's one hell of a lot of work! It takes Bill over two hours to wade through this monster routine. This approach stakes out one end of the classical bodybuilder approach: Bill is *maximum volume/moderate intensity*. The polar opposite is Dorian Yates' *maximum intensity/moderate volume* approach. Many individuals thrive using this approach. I strongly suggest using this approach when seeking to shed the maximum amount of body fat. Going fast, using modest poundage, cramming lots of exercises into a single session jives perfectly with a lean-out phase.

"The happiest man connects the morning of his life with the evening."
—Ancient Hindu Proverb

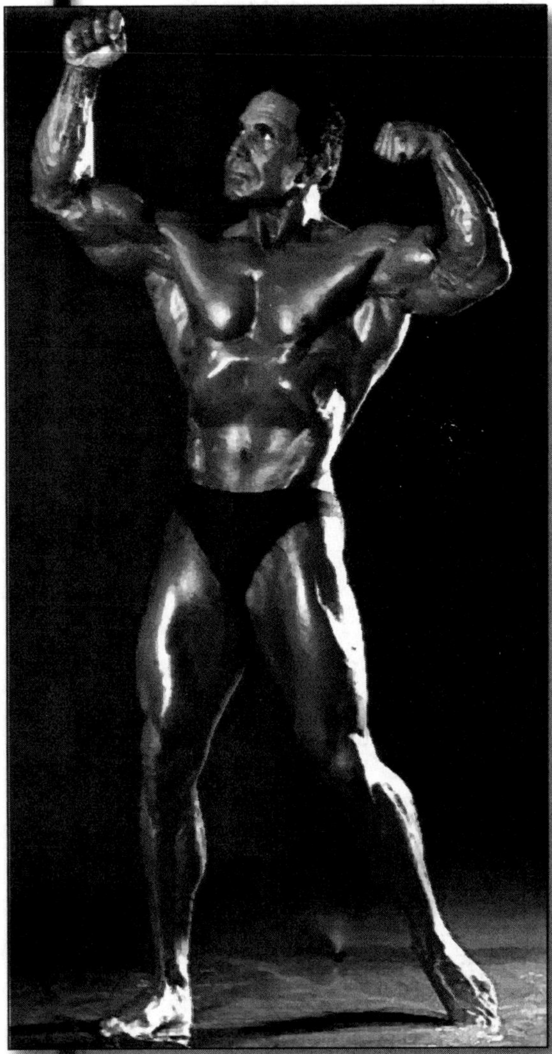

Bill Pearl at age 56: The Old Lion was talked into doing a guest posing routine at the 1985 Mr. Olympia competition. Bill continually redefined our attitudes towards age and aging. He has served as an inspiration to all those who know him.

If you are interested in holding back the hands of time, his approach, combining weight training, cardiovascular training and precision nutrition – is the finest system of life-extension known to man. He points the way for how best to retard the aging process. As the Irish Philosopher Mae West once said, "It ain't the age, it's the mileage!" Bill related to me that in retrospect, he shouldn't have retired from making public appearances at age 66.

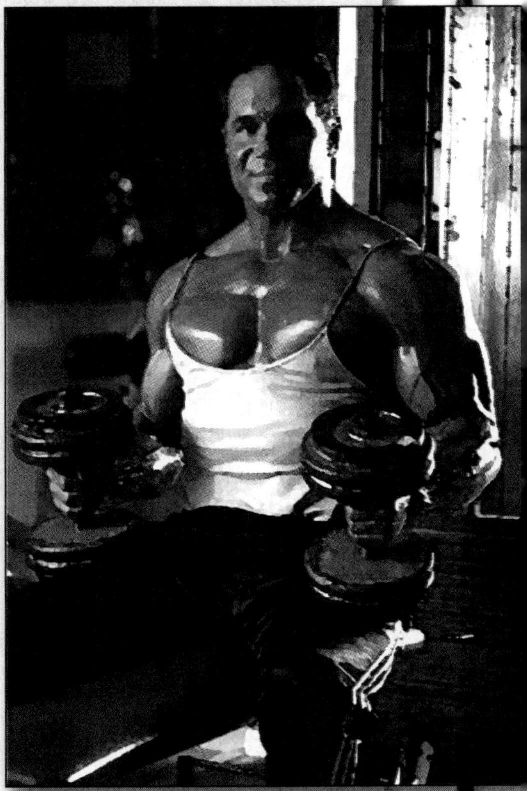

Bill at age 63... incredible don't you think? Insofar as I can determine, the rationale for the Pilates movement rests, in large part, on how good Joseph Pilates looked at age 58. If Joe P got an entire exercise movement and lifestyle founded on his late-in-life physique, perhaps we should create an entire religion based on Bill's.

How is this level of muscular development possible at such an advanced age? Nutrition is critical and Pearl is a Jedi Master on how best to manipulate lean muscularity. Maneuver the Energy Balance Equation to the breakeven point and use cardio-infused resistance training to create a fat-burning deficit. Elemental stuff. He began training at age 10. Now at 78 he has been training for 68 straight years! For decades Pearl has blazed a path for the rest of us to follow.

The Anti-Aging Role Model

"Curse ruthless time! Curse our mortality!
How cruelly short is the allotted time span for all which we must cram into it!"

—Winston Churchill

Bill Pearl is *still* important. Bill has been important for seven decades. Lately Bill is leading the charge in the battle against the ultimate foe: Father Time. Bill is 78 years old. And what makes him still so important is that Pearl is *still* stretching and expanding our preconceived notions about physical degeneration. Can the Grim Reaper be stiff-armed, held at arms length by a combination of weight training, diet, aerobics and stretching? Bill Pearl says yes, absolutely; and along with Jack LaLanne, he remains the age-defying posterboy.

Bill won the Mr. America title in 1955—when Dwight Eisenhower was President. That's a hell of a long time ago. Since 1955 Pearl has been the Alpha Male statesman for bodybuilding. He's now the ultimate tribal elder. Fifty five years ago the 23 year old Native American had just mustered out of the Navy. He entered and won the Mr. America title and proceeded to electrify the bodybuilding world. In the sixties he appeared to us mortals as the next step in the evolution of man. His girth seemed to be the next rung step up the ladder of physical perfection. Bill was thick yet symmetrical, bulky yet shapely, gargantuan yet graceful. Pearl, along with his European counterpart, Reg Park, set the philosophic tone for the sport.

The rise of Sergio Oliva and Arnold Schwarzenegger gave Bill Pearl a reason to return to the competitive battleground. In 1971 Pearl, Park and Oliva—along with Frank Zane and Dave Draper—all assembled at the N.A.A.B.A. Mr. Universe contest. Only Arnold was missing. Arnold had every intention of competing, but politics and financial commitments prevented this muscle showdown from being realized. At age 41, Pearl beat Park (past his prime) and the here-to-fore unbeatable Cuban superman, Sergio Oliva. Who would have won had Arnold entered? Pure conjecture, though in all fairness, the then 25 year old Austrian was a few years away from his all-time best condition, achieved at the South African Mr. Olympia contest. Pearl was at his physical zenith.

Pearl was on top of the World. At an age when most international level physique competitors had long since retired and were relating war stories about their glory days in smoky bars to bored bar flies, Pearl had reasserted his world dominance. He immediately retired from competition while on top. He dropped from sight, having moved from Los Angeles to Oregon.

Pearl might have dropped from sight, but he wasn't about to stop training. Every morning at 4 he famously rolls out of bed and by 4:30 is engaged in a 2 hour workout enduro. He is a lacto-vegetarian, totally eschewing meat, and is happily dependant on eggs, vegetables, dairy and fruit juice for his dietary needs. A competitive bicycle racer at one time, Pearl used to think nothing of jumping on his bike for a thirty mile jaunt. The latest Bill is *still* my role model. Like a twenty foot high neon sign he projects a simple message, one exemplified by vibrancy and youthfulness that seems to say, "Look at what can be accomplished with diligence, perseverance, tenacity and intelligence. Look at how the aging process can be retarded and held at bay. Look at what is *possible*!"

Never before in the history of civilization have men so old looked so young. Pearl demonstrates that a man can possess the body of a much younger man if they are willing to still practice the three interrelated arts. As long as the enthusiasm and fire in the gut remains, as long as you continue to train hard and eat with discipline, you are still in the game and can still live life to its fullest. Bill Pearl is showing us how to wring every last drop of vitality and essence out of life before life inevitably expires. Long may he roll!

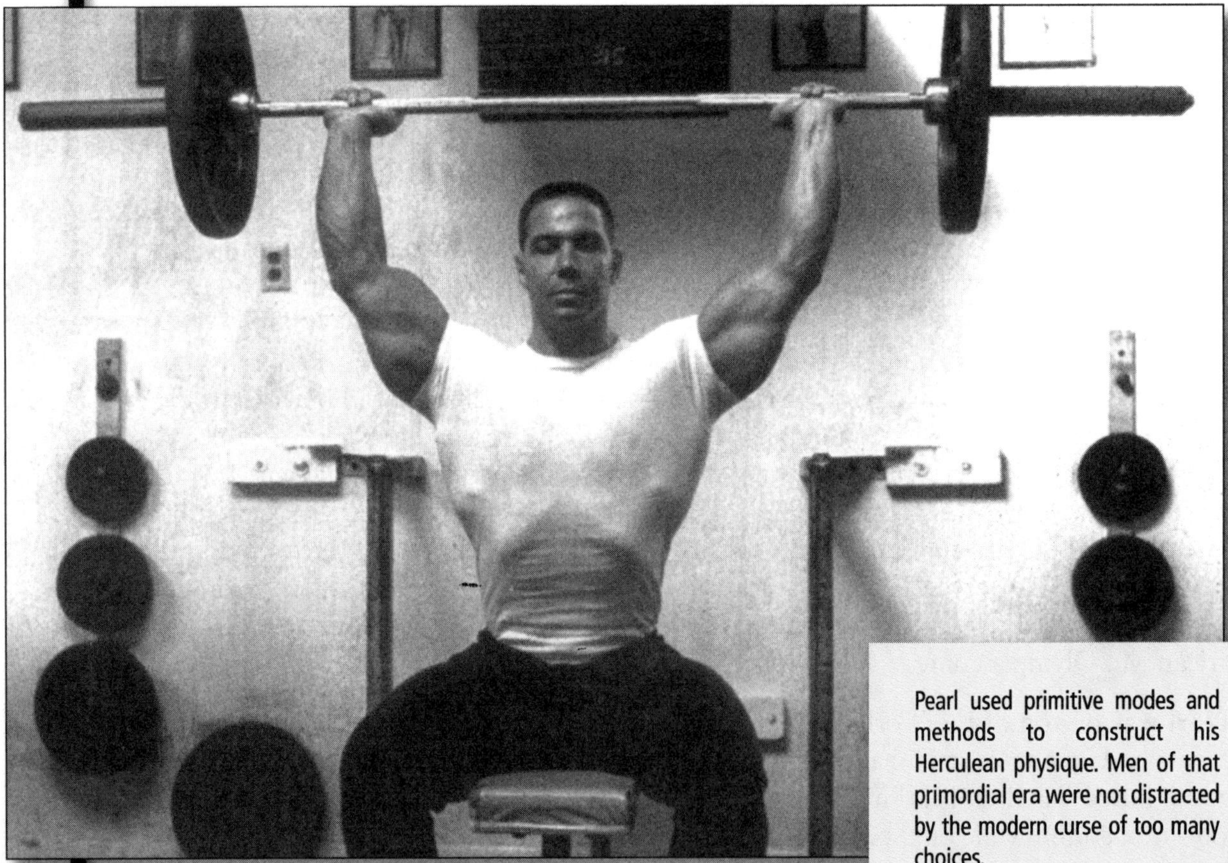

Pearl used primitive modes and methods to construct his Herculean physique. Men of that primordial era were not distracted by the modern curse of too many choices.

BOB BEDNARSKI

Iron Icarus

No athlete was ever as despised by the athletic establishment as Muhammad Ali. No athlete ever generated the venom and pure unadulterated hatred that Ali did. Even before Clay became Ali, even before he stuck his Black Muslim thumb into the collective eyeball of white America, Clay was vilified for his unrepentant braggadocio. His self-aggrandizing rhymes and poetry didn't sit well with the lockstep white men who wore the blue blazers and ran the Amateur Athletic Union with the brutal efficiency of a totalitarian dictatorship. As the dominant sport aristocracy, they ruled all of amateur sports in this country and it was, in many ways, a reign of terror; one that would have done Stalin proud. Imperious, regal, more important than the athletes, the slightest sass, real or perceived, and the offending athlete were hauled before a Star Chamber discipline committee. Act right, the officials said, or risk suspension or permanent banishment.

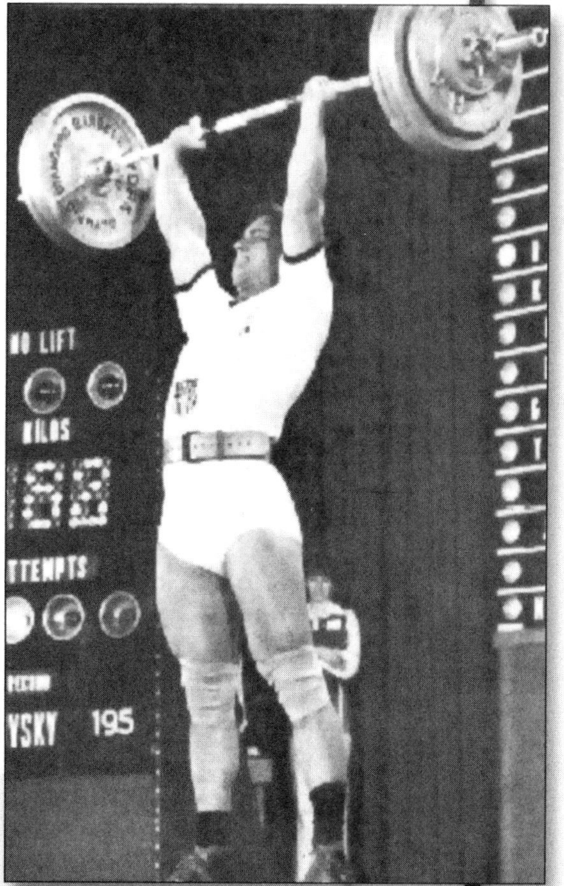

The Woonsocket Wonder: Bob Bednarski sets a World Press Record in the 242 pound class. He never again achieved the traction he had leading up to that incredible day in June 1968, when he broke the World Record for the press with a 456 pound effort and capped the day with perhaps the most dramatic lift ever made in any iron sport: his clean and jerk of 486 pounds. The jerk was the most weight ever lifted overhead.

His skyrocket trajectory seemed unstoppable. He was the odds on favorite to be the 1st man in history to lift 500 pounds overhead. He seemed poised to take over the world; he had rock star charisma, youth, talent and intelligence. He was on the fast track to immortality. Then it all went terribly wrong.

Clay/Ali became the antiestablishment sports hero. "Why can't he be a good example of his *race*; like that courteous Joe Lewis!" I heard one AAU official say. Worst of all, Clay/Ali began *infecting* other athletes. Bob Bednarski became infected. The Woonsocket Wonder crept out of Rhode Island. He'd been groomed to perfection by an amazing Olympic lift coach, Joe Mills. Bednarski commenced his rocket ride in 1963 and for five straight years he improved dramatically each and every year. He went from boy prodigy to National Champion to superstar in surreal succession.

Clash of the Titans: Barski goes to work for "The Man"

Few men were more establishment than Bob Hoffman, founder and 100% owner of the York Barbell Club. An egomaniacal multi-millionaire, Hoffman owned American Olympic lifting. He footed the bill for teams to travel overseas and his York Barbell Lifting Club was the eternal O-lift dominator. His money made him the big swinging dick of American Olympic lifting and everyone bowed and scraped to the uber-leader who signed the paychecks and picked up the various tabs.

Hoffman entered the sixties by bringing onboard heavyweight thinkers, men like Terry Todd, Tommy Suggs and Bill Starr. These men went to work for York in different capacities at *Strength & Health* magazine, the bible of American Olympic lifting. When Hoffman handed the editorial reigns over to Starr, the perfect Gonzo storm occurred: the emergence of a new breed of kid Olympic lifters coincided with a burgeoning use of both recreational and performance enhancing drugs. In order to secure the talent necessary to ensure that York maintained dominance, Big Daddy had to open his wallet even wider. If they were to entice the new breed to represent York, Daddy Hoffman and John Terpak, the fierce enforcer, would need to recruit counterculture athletes.

The Chicago Y under Bob Gajda's auspices was attracting talent and fast becoming the "anti-York." Bill March, Tony Garcy and Joe Puleo were a bit older and already in the York fold. Peter Rawluk, Jack Hill, Bob Hise, Tom Hirtz, Frank Capsouras, Enrique Hernandez, Phil Gripaldi, Rick Holbrook, Steve Zigman, Fred Lowe, Joe Dube, Ernie Pickett and Gerry Ferrelli were on the scene and available. The King of the youth movement was Bob Bednarski. He was simply the best of a great crop: he was the most talented and the most ambitious, he was the Sun God of the new breed. Bednarski dubbed himself the Ninth Wonder of the World. His shenanigans and Ali-like traits drove Hoffman and Terpak and all the York old timers to the brink of insanity. "Why can't he just shut his mouth and lift!" was the consensus amongst the white-bread establishment.

Bob Bednarski, the lifting Ali, worked for "The Man." And as good as he was in Rhode Island under Mills, when he moved to York and got on the corporate payroll, he got a whole lot better real fast. They assigned him various factory jobs and asinine tasks such as mixing protein powder and bottling suntan lotion. The immortal Bill March was also a York employee and pushed Bednarski mercilessly on the lifting platform. Plus there were Dr. Ziegler's magical little dianabol pills. Each week Bednarski grew bigger and better and stronger and faster and ever more self-assured, if that was possible.

I met Bednarski when he lifted at a competition at Gonzaga High School in 1968. Brother Don Dixon allowed me to train at Gonzaga with top local lifters like "Muscular Mickey" Collins. I became a fixture at Gonzaga. The meet turned out to be the start of Bednarski's rampage and run to greatness. At Gonzaga he set his first World Record besting Ernie Pickett's 446 World Record press with a 451 pound effort. I talked with him before the meet started and was awed and intimidated. I asked what he weighed and he said, "*250! How do I look?!*" He was obviously expecting flattery and being awestruck, I flattered until I was blue in the face. He seemed to beam. I hung out backstage, hovering on the periphery. He'd ask me to fetch him cokes. Bill March also lifted and I got to watch both men up close backstage and onstage. Because Bednarski allowed me to hover in his presence, I became a mindless lifelong groupie. I thought he was a God before I met him and after he talked to me, he walked on water as far as I was concerned. When a few months later "My Man" had his incredible lifting day in York, I was there. When he punched his 486 clean and jerk, I went into delirium tremors and almost fainted; I could not have been more affected had the Virgin Mary appeared or had Bednarski sprouted wings and suddenly started flying around the auditorium.

Training

I followed the ever-changing training strategies Bednarski rolled through over the years that marked his tenure at York. He was innovative and hard working and since he was a heavyweight, he sought to grow ever larger in order to move more poundage. In those days, any man who weighed more than 198 pounds was forced to lift as a heavyweight (how ridiculous) and the Soviet sports armada routinely sent 350 pound monsters to do battle. Here was Bednarski, lean, athletic, good looking, brash, cocky and suggestive; doing toe-to-toe battle with the biggest, ugliest monsters the Big Red Machine could cook up in their state-supported sports laboratories. At the zenith of his amazing career he used this training template....all the work sets, top sets listed are done after ample warm-ups. This approach allows for maximum concentration on a lift.

Bob Bednarski Training Template

Day	Exercise	Poundage/Reps
Monday	Clean & Press	350-385 x 3 (5 sets)
Tuesday	Snatch	305-315 x 3 (5 sets)
Wednesday	Squat	450-500 x 3 (2 sets)
Thursday	Clean & Jerk	405-435 x 1 (5 sets)
Friday	OFF	
Saturday	Total on 2-3 lifts	Work up to maximum single in 2 or 3 lifts
Sunday	Squat	450-500 x 3 (2 sets)

The High Water Mark of American Olympic Lifting – June, 1968

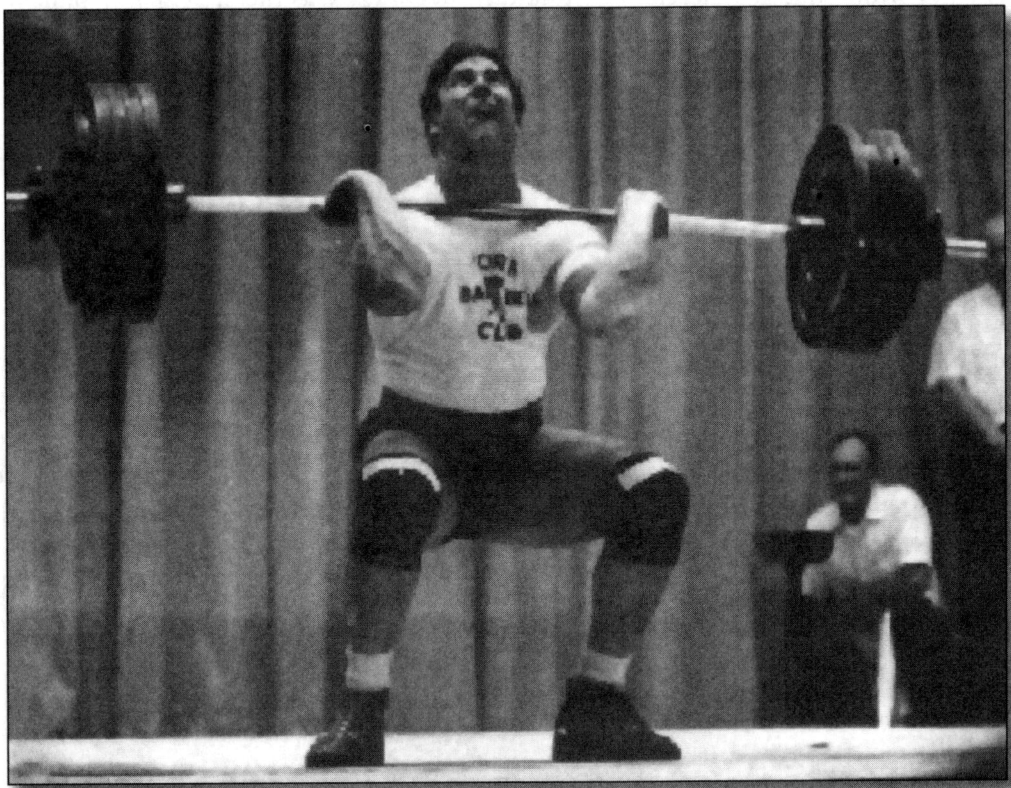

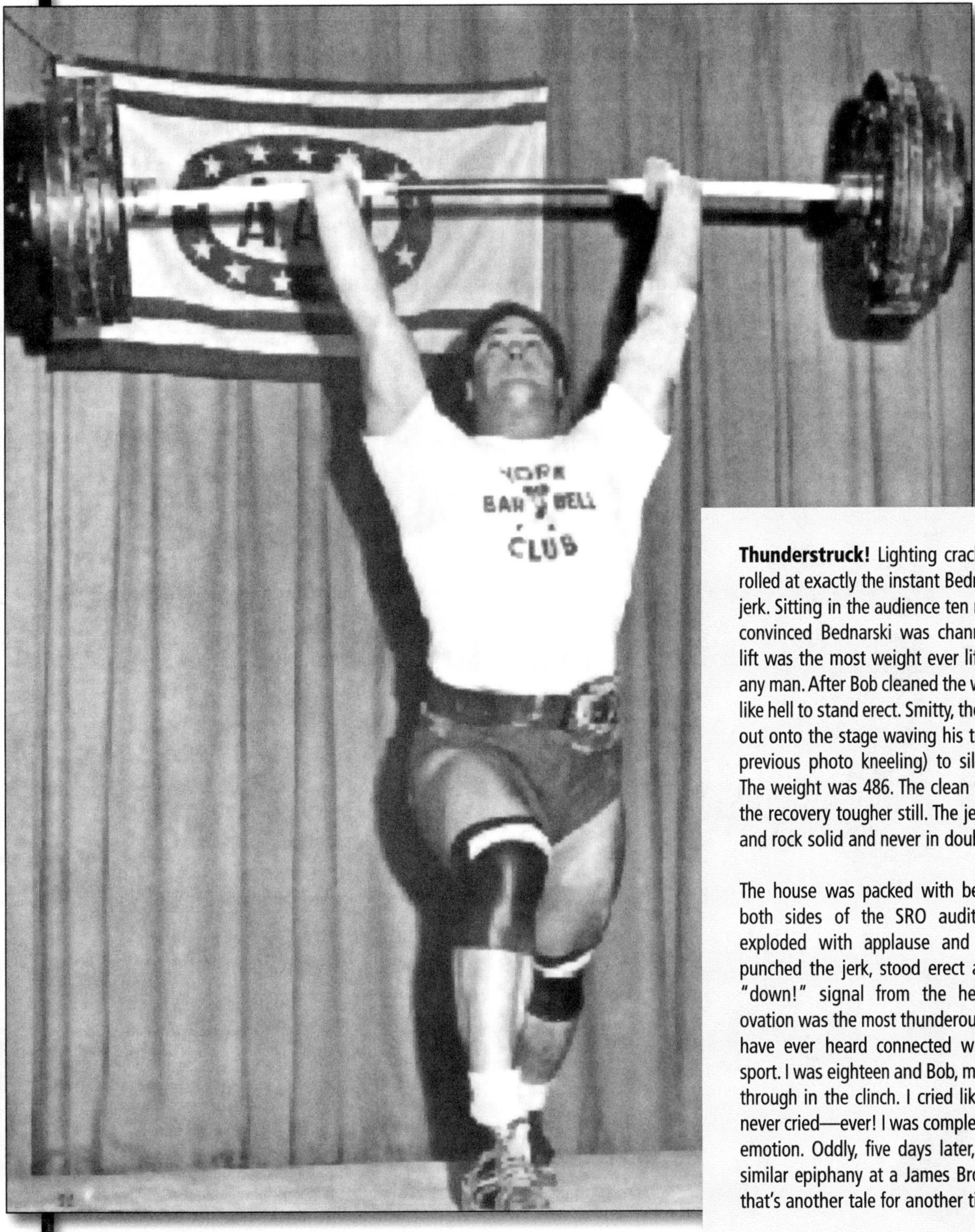

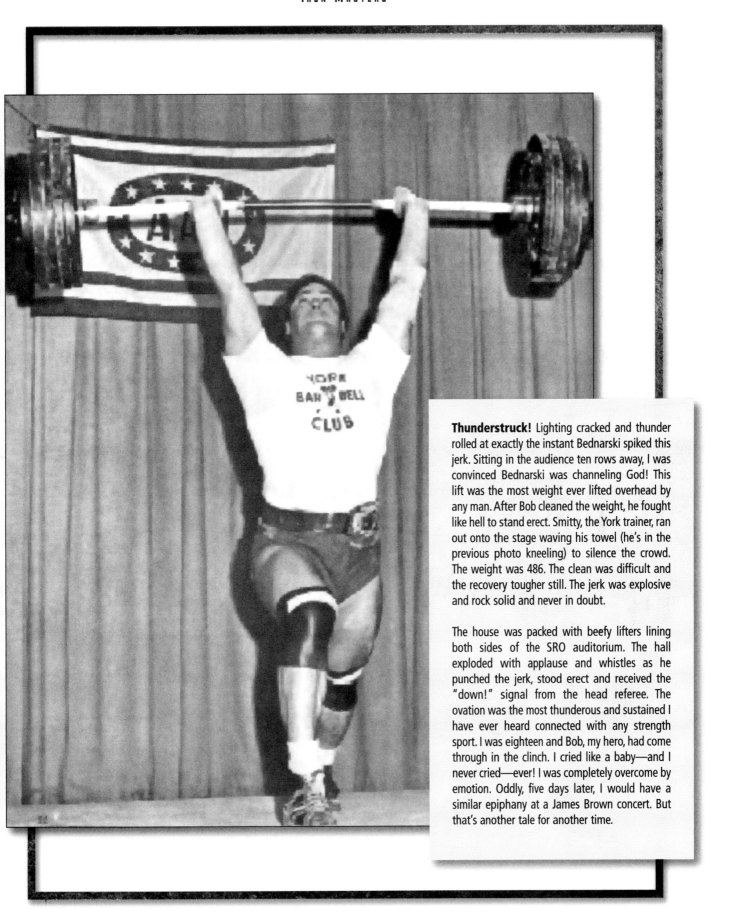

Thunderstruck! Lighting cracked and thunder rolled at exactly the instant Bednarski spiked this jerk. Sitting in the audience ten rows away, I was convinced Bednarski was channeling God! This lift was the most weight ever lifted overhead by any man. After Bob cleaned the weight, he fought like hell to stand erect. Smitty, the York trainer, ran out onto the stage waving his towel (he's in the previous photo kneeling) to silence the crowd. The weight was 486. The clean was difficult and the recovery tougher still. The jerk was explosive and rock solid and never in doubt.

The house was packed with beefy lifters lining both sides of the SRO auditorium. The hall exploded with applause and whistles as he punched the jerk, stood erect and received the "down!" signal from the head referee. The ovation was the most thunderous and sustained I have ever heard connected with any strength sport. I was eighteen and Bob, my hero, had come through in the clinch. I cried like a baby—and I never cried—ever! I was completely overcome by emotion. Oddly, five days later, I would have a similar epiphany at a James Brown concert. But that's another tale for another time.

Aftermath: The Iron Icarus melts his wings

Everything went to hell-in-a-hand basket after that glorious June day in 1968. Bednarski inexplicably didn't make the 1968 Olympic team when at the Olympic Trials he had an off day and Joe Dube and Ernie Pickett secured the two available spots. Big Daddy pushed through the 242 pound class in 1969 and Bednarski won over a beefed up Jan Talts of the Soviet Union. But wait! After making the winning clean and jerk, the lift was then taken away by a Red Bloc-loaded jury of appeals! What the hell!? Again, bitter disappointment was snatched from the jaws of sweet victory. Eventually, years later, the gold medal was returned, but Bednarski, once again, was left with ashes in his mouth.

He returned to York and competed at the National Championships, winning yet again. The following year he took bronze at the World Championships but it was apparent something was dreadfully wrong. He was fired from York after becoming embroiled in a scandal. The vibrancy and luster was off his rose. He had a few comebacks and went on to win a few more major titles. But his glory days were gone. It was spookily akin to Ali fighting too long. He was, as super-scribe Starr wrote, "a blazing comet." He died at age 60 of a heart attack. Barski etched a legacy that was impossible to ignore: 1969 World Champion, Silver in 1966, Bronze in 1970, no less than five National Championships, four in a row, fourteen World Records and numerous National Records. He was the Boy Sun King, the Iron Icarus that flew too close to the blazing orb, burned off his waxen wings and crashed to earth…it was one hell of a flight while he remained airborne and I shall never forget him.

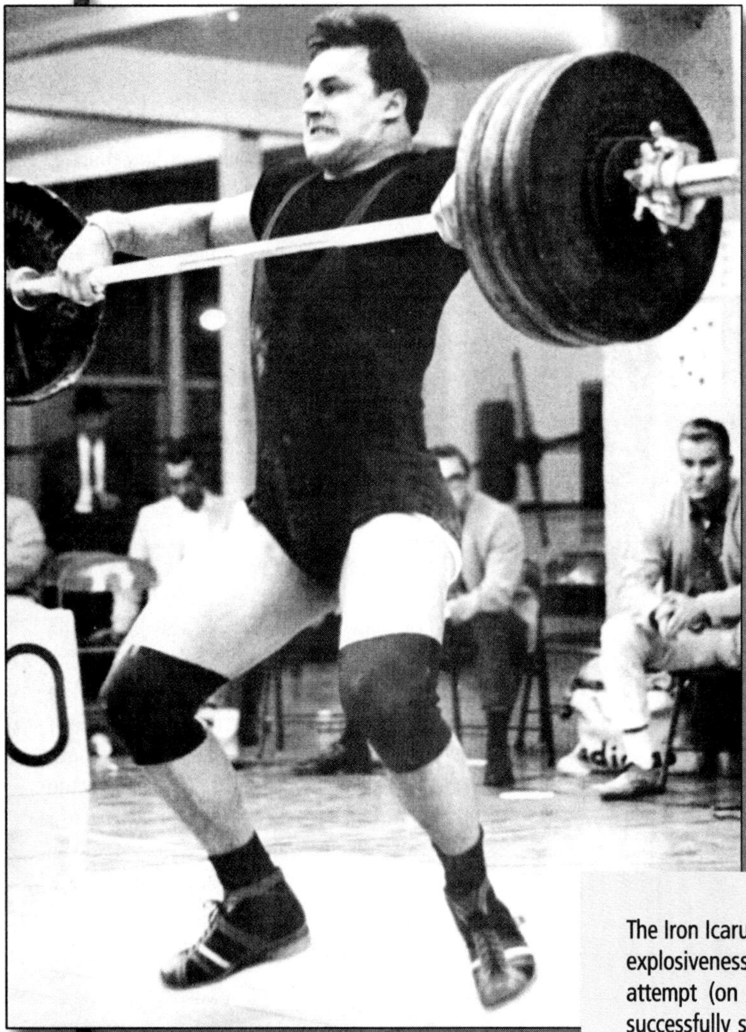

The Iron Icarus in full flight: Bob Bednarski exhibits his incredible explosiveness snatching 340 pounds. Had he not passed his 3rd attempt (on his record shattering day in June of 1968) and successfully snatched 360, he would have become the first man to break the 1300 pound total barrier.

Hugh Cassidy

Iron Master Renaissance Man

The first words Hugh Cassidy ever spoke to me were, "Hey Kid! I dig your squat style!" I was backstage at the first ever DCAAU Powerlifting Championships in 1968. I was 17 and taking my last warm-up. I knew Hugh was a pretty big deal in the then embryonic world of powerlifting. I ignominiously went on to bomb out, missing three squats with 500. I weighed 193 and insisted on starting with 500, though my best at the time was 510. I got bent forward and missed the lift on my opener. It felt heavy as hell and in those days if you missed and no one else took the same weight, you had three minutes before you had to lift it again: bip, bang, boom! Three strikes and Marty was out of the competition.

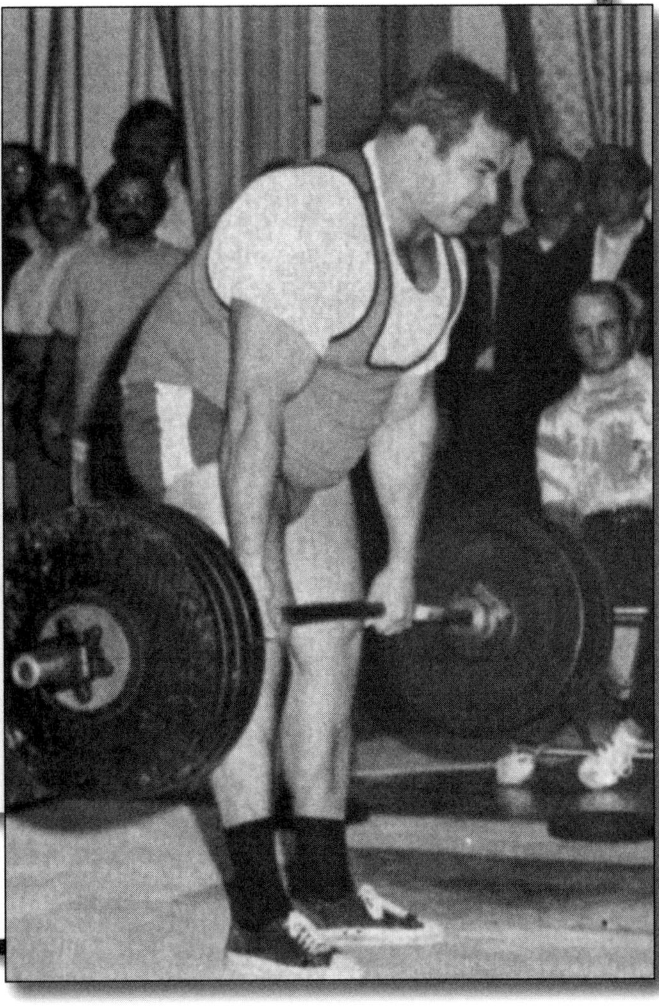

Cassidy pulls 790 to win the world championships in 1971. Tough freaking competition: Jim Williams and John Kuc! Hugh pushed his weight to 292 using sumo wrestler eating tactics and a bare bones approach to lifting that was rooted in intense work done in relatively infrequent sessions. We trained as little as twice a week under his tutelage—but oh were those sessions murderous! We needed 3-4 days of heavy eating and complete rest just to be able to walk normally.

Hugh pushed his bodyweight ever upward in order to keep the progress ball rolling. As a super heavyweight if he became stuck in the bench press at say 505x5 weighing 267, he knew that by pushing his weight to 277, 525x5 would go. "Eat your way through sticking points!" He used to say. I trained with Marshall Peck in Hugh's Fred Munster-like basement for years.

The next time I saw Hugh was on a road trip to the inaugural National Powerlifting Championships held in York, Pennsylvania in September of 1968. The trip was put together by a mutual friend, the gentlemanly Glenn Middleton. Glenn was an engineer with a huge international conglomerate and a strength aficionado who'd trained with the Schemansky brothers in Detroit. He would act as our tour director for road trips to York.

Glenn was a great lifting referee, tough and able. He was super strict and the lifters took to calling him "Dr. Red Light." He took a shine to me and always included me in the road trips he would organize to York for the Olympic and power competitions. Hugh once said of Glenn, "The guy is brilliant; so well rounded. He'll custom load bird shot, shoot a pheasant or brace of quail, then construct the perfect gourmet meal, cooking the birds to perfection"

Two carloads of local lifters left for York for the first ever National Powerlifting Championships; the York Picnic would be held the next day in a local park. At the competition I sat next to Hugh; he was a 242 pound lifter looking to move up to the heavyweight class. I was impressed with his methodical approach to eating. He was determined to push his weight to 300 and see what weights he would be capable of lifting. He carried a giant cooler into the auditorium. In it were a dozen sandwiches and two half gallons of milk. We sat and watched the lifting from great seats down front. Hugh would graze and munch, periodically eating a sandwich, washing it down with milk. We saw Peanuts West miss his squats and bomb out. Later, a triumphant George Frenn lifted and won at 242. During the trophy presentation Frenn physically wrested the microphone from MC Morris Weisbrott and proceeded to call forth a massively embarrassed Peanut from backstage. Frenn then launched into a fifteen minute Castro-like Peanut West soliloquy that no one in attendance will ever forget. At the time the number 1 hit on the radio was "Ode to Billy Joe." After Frenn's monologue, Hugh deadpanned, "Ode to Peanuts West." I was not to see Hugh again until 1979.

Eat Your Way Through Sticking Points!

Cassidy kept eating his sandwiches and drinking milk by the gallon. His sumo wrestler approach worked: at a height of 5'11" he eventually pushed his bodyweight to 290+ pounds and shocked the powerlifting world by upsetting both Big Jim Williams and John Kuc at the first World Powerlifting Championships in 1971. Hugh squatted 800, bench pressed 570 and deadlifted 790. He lifted equipment-less: no knee wraps, no supportive gear of any type, not even a lifting belt. He injured a knee the following year and retired from powerlifting.

Being a smart man, rather than stay gargantuan, as so many lifters do, Cassidy reduced from 295 to 195 and entered a few bodybuilding competitions. He continued to train on his little farmette located off Highbridge road in Bowie, Maryland. Hugh had many interests; he taught school and had a loving wife and four kids all within a few years of each other. He left powerlifting and never looked back. In the mid-seventies a young, promising lifter named Mark Dimiduk sought out Hugh and began training under Hugh's tutelage. Dimiduk eventually became a lifting terminator, winning the Junior Nationals, (beating Danny Wohleber) and then winning the National and World Championships. Mark began training on his own.

The hard lessons "The Duck" learned under Hugh formed the foundation for a fabulous powerlifting career. Mark squatted and deadlifted 800 and bench pressed 500 while weighing a lean and shredded 219. In 1978 I decided to begin weight training after a six year hiatus. During that time I had gotten into martial arts and trained at a facility with competitive fighters. I was bitten by the iron bug once again. After a year of generalized training, I saw an announcement in the "coming events" section of the Washington Post, Hugh Cassidy would be putting on a seminar in College Park. I attended and afterwards reintroduced myself. He remembered me. We hit it off and he invited me to train at his home gym. I stayed for many years and made fabulous progress.

All Aboard the Pain Train!

Hugh Cassidy's basement gym looked like something from the TV show "The Munsters." Homemade equipment (Hugh was an expert welder) was crammed and stuffed into every nook and cranny. The basement of his funky, homey, artist house had a ceiling only seven feet in height, so no standing overhead lifting was possible.

Hugh introduced me to Marshall "Doc" Peck, a semi-pro baseball pitcher who began having arm problems and switched from baseball to powerlifting. Peck eventually squatted 790, benched 530 and pulled 710 weighing 218. Hugh was training with Marshall and asked if I would like to become their third training partner. I accepted immediately.

I found Cassidy a riddle wrapped in an enigma tucked inside a paradox. He was an artist of the highest order, an excellent musician who played great guitar and exceptional bass. He worked in various bands, but opted out of the night club scene on account of his acute susceptibility to cigarette smoke. Hugh was a metal sculpture artist. He started off with simple one-dimensional wall relief tubing pieces, worked through an industrial glass table-top phase before developing refined welding techniques used on his three-dimensional nightmare creatures. Some of his devils and demons were so lifelike that they appeared ready to spring to life. As the ever eloquent Agro-American Peck once quipped, "Freaking Hugh's monsters give me the hee-bee jee-bees!"

Cassidy might be found in his ample truck garden, grafting pear branches onto apple trees, reading classical literature or welding art. He taught special needs children and had more mental horsepower and artistic creativity than any athlete I ever met, before or since. He was directly responsible for starting me off on my writing career when he graciously consented to co-author some powerlifting pieces. He was tough on me and had trouble with my "bombastic" style. He was on us hard in the weight room. We trained twice a week and slammed down calories to speed recovery on the in between days. Hugh's approach could be summarized thusly: train like a psycho, eat everything in sight, rest up and grow gargantuan. For young testosterone-laden men seeking size, strength and power his minimalist approach was magical.

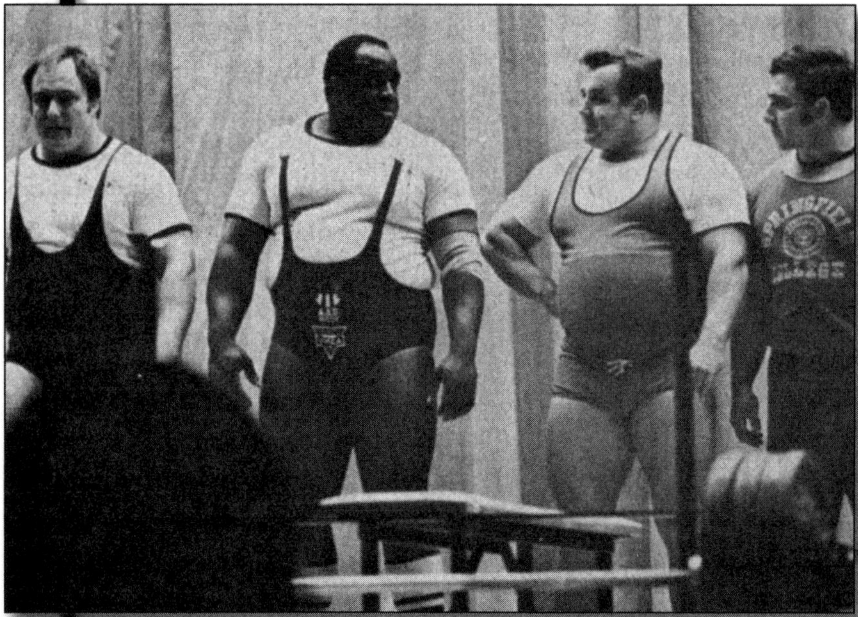

The introductions at the 1971 world powerlifting championships: On the left, a very young 340 pound John Kuc, then Big Jim Williams, the greatest bench presser in history (700 raw) and Hugh, who is no doubt wryly saying "Take it easy on me Big Jim!" Big Jim is no doubt saying back, "Don't try and jive me HUGE." They called Hugh, "Huge." Carlton Snitken leans in on the right to hear the banter.

Hugh Cassidy Training Split

Day	Exercise	Sets/Reps
Saturday	Squat	Top set of 8 reps, then 3 "back off" sets of 10 reps
		Top set of 5 reps, then 3 "back off" sets of 8 reps
		Top set of 3 reps, then 3 "back off" sets of 5 reps
		4 weeks for each rep range: 12 week cycle.
	Bench Press	Same as squat cycle
	Deadlift	Same as squat cycle
	Heaves	Heavy high pulls, 2-3 sets done explosively for 6-8 reps
	Biceps Curls	3-4 sets of 6-8 reps
	Triceps Work	3-4 sets of 6-8 reps
Tuesday		**Repeat Everything**

Lift Big, Eat Big, Rest Big, Grow Big!

We would start our Saturday enduro with squats and work up to a top set. Depending on what phase of the overall training 'cycle' we were in, the top set could be 8 reps, 5 reps or 3 reps. 8 rep sets were done for four straight weeks, starting 12 weeks prior to competing. Eight weeks out we'd shift to 5 rep sets. For the final four weeks leading up to the competition, the top sets were dropped to triples or doubles. Ditto for the all important back-off sets: these were done with lighter poundage.

Peck and I would wear knee wraps and a belt working up to the top set. Then take off the wraps and belt for the three back-off sets of 10 reps, 8 reps or 5 reps. The back-off sets were done with a considerably lighter weight than the belt/wrap top set. Pumped to the max after the squat back-offs, we would shift to bench pressing and repeat the same procedure: work up to a top set of 8, 5 or 3, then three sets of back-offs. After benching, our legs and lower back were somewhat recovered, so it was on to deadlifts. Again, work up to a top set, then three sets of back-offs. Hugh would have us do 'stiff leg deadlifts' on the back-off sets. Then for desert 3-6 sets of "arms" usually super-setting curls with triceps presses or pushdowns.

For a while Hugh got on a "heave" kick, which was sort of a massive high pull done with a lot of weight while trying to generate momentum at the top. When he'd insert these after deadlifts we'd groan. We would repeat the whole deal 3-4 days later. It would take us hours to get though this workout. Often I'd have to lie down before I had the strength to drive home. Peck and I would stop at the 7-11, buy a half gallon of ice cold whole milk (each) to drink on the ride home. Milk never tasted as good as it did after an August training session in the dungeon with only a single plastic fan to keep us from keeling over. Hugh would tell us when we complained of tiredness to fire down more calories. "Eat your way through sticking points!" He'd say. If the poundage was feeling heavy on Saturday weighing 216, push your bodyweight to 220 by Wednesday and make those weights seem light. This was a man-killer approach: train till you begin hallucinating, eat tons of food, drink four quarts or more of milk daily then rest until the 2nd weekly slaughter fest. This approach worked wonders for aggressive young men intent on becoming massively muscled competitive powerlifters. Hugh was a 'psyche up' master and could visibly manifest his internal psyche by the use of what he called "cooling breaths." He was able to make this happen at will.

> ***"I cannot explain it psychologically, but I have found that if I expel my breath in sharp gasps I get goose pimples all over my body. In this condition I lift far more in meets than in training, averaging 40 pounds above my best training effort for both the squat and deadlift."***

Cassidy was one of a kind: brilliant, moody, insightful, soulful, introverted and sensitive. My time with him laid a foundation of hardcore training that has served me well ever since. Never was the adage, "hard work pays off" more apparent then in his take-no-prisoners, ultra-simplistic, Purposefully Primitive approach that he exemplified and taught. Nowadays most lifters under-eat and under-train: many are vain surface-skimmers with low pain tolerance and lots of self-esteem. The Old School approach of train-till-you-drop is politically incorrect and even suggesting it to the new breed is a waste of breath. I have often thought that if I ever wanted to train a kid powerlifter to become a world beater, I would draft one of those X-Game skateboarders or motocross kids that do those death-defying jumps. I think that powerlifters and lifters of my generation had that same crazed mindset. Nowadays fanatical types participate in other sports.

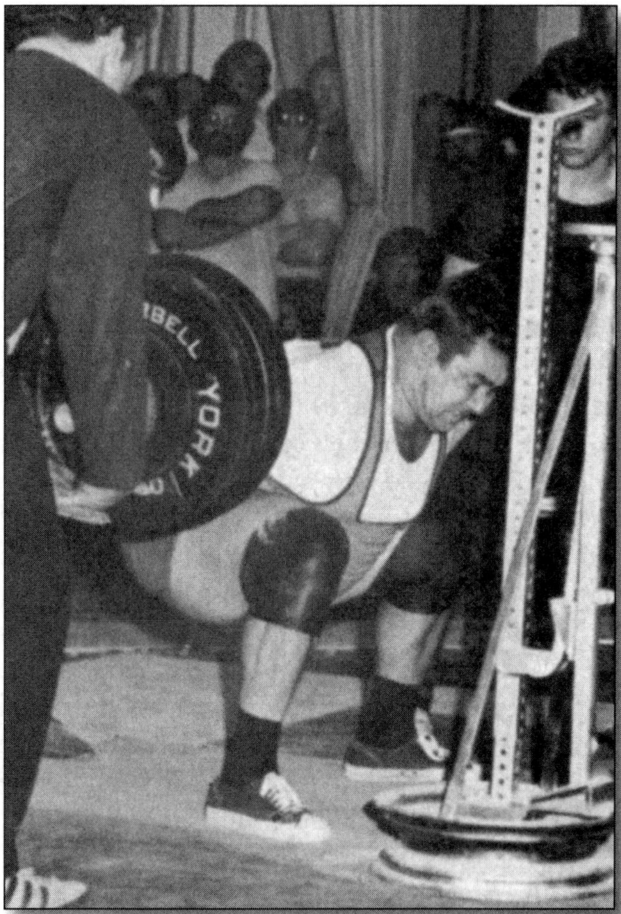

Hugh Says: "My squat routines are simple and basic and use no assistance exercises; squats alone twice a week work well for me. The following is a routine I use most of the time, with an emphasis on the 3 sets of 5 reps, which I believe are the hallmark of the routine.

The multiple sets force power as well as muscle growth to take place. And as your fives go up, so of course, do your max double or triple. Thus I warm-up with 275x8, 435x5, 535x5, 625x3 then 700x2...{then the 'back off' sets} 610x5, 625x5 and 640x5—I seldom do more than eight sets of squats regardless the routine. As the meet draws near, with about six workouts to go, I continue to go up to a max double or triple. I changed the back-off sets from fives to threes...prior to the {1971} World Championships in my last workout my back-off sets were 700x3 and 725x3. I was too tired to attempt a third back-off set of three. The 800x1 {photo left} made at the World Championships was easy—I wish I had taken more that day."

MARK CHAILLET

Powerlifting Ultra Minimalist

Going from training with Hugh Cassidy to training with Mark Chaillet was like being paroled from a Georgia chain gang to go live in a luxury spa. Not that training with Mark was easy or breezy, but Chaillet's Gym was a terrific facility, easily the best gym I've ever belonged to. The people were incredible and the place was heated and air conditioned. I made Mark's gym my second home for six straight years.

Marshall Peck and I were training with Hugh when we got wind that Mark Chaillet, already a power legend, would be relocating back to Temple Hills, where he was from originally. He would be opening a new gym dedicated to power and strength. Marshall and I were ecstatic. We had Hugh's blessing; we both had worked hard, made great progress on every front in every way, but Hugh agreed: our strength levels were making it apparent that it was time for a change. At Hugh's we used a 6' exercise bar and had taken to hanging dumbbells attached with coat hangers on each end of the bar to get over 600 for squats.

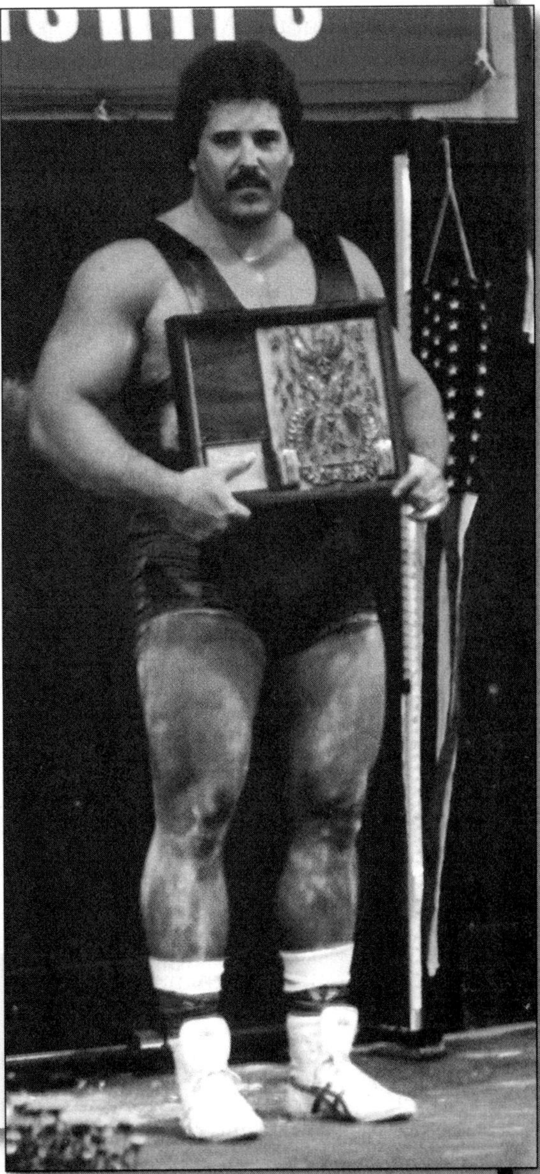

Mark in Maui after winning the APF World Championships. He weighed 279 and had just deadlifted 850+ minutes before this shot was taken.

Chaillet had been working for power God, Larry Pacifico, in Dayton for the several years. Larry "drafted" the finest young powerlifters from around the country to help him staff his empire of gyms and spas. At different times Larry had Mike Bridges, Mark, Joe Ladiner, John Topsoglu, and a whole host of other young power prodigies working for him. Mark decided to move back home and open a gym. He found a space overtop of an auto parts store. Mark's dad, Buck, a salty ex-DC cop, helped Mark build out the space and run the gym.

Buck didn't like too many people but he took a shine to me. I hit it off with the whole family, Mark's mom, his brother Ray, his sister, his wife Ellen, these were great people, my second family. Mark became as close to me as a brother and I cut my big league coaching teeth handling Mark at National and World Championships. Marshall and I moved to Mark's and joined up with the most amazing assortment of power athletes I've ever had the pleasure of training with, before or since.

Everyone made progress fast training at Chaillet's Gym. A communal strength synergy took hold and each week we all seemed to get bigger and stronger. Seeing guys routinely squat 900, deadlift 800 and bench press 600 raises your game. Being a big fish in a small pond is illusory and stunting. Chaillet's was a powerlift reality gut-check: a big pond full of big powerful fish.

How Little can you do and still get Super Strong?

It always seemed to me that Mark Chaillet really didn't like training all that much. Or perhaps to put a finer point on it, Mark didn't seem to like training in any way other than one way. He stuck with his particular, peculiar style of training for the six years I was his training partner. In a nutshell, twice a week he would have a mini-powerlifting competition. Mark would work up to a single, all out repetition in each of the three lifts wearing all his power gear. That was it. Monday at 4pm was squat and bench press day. Thursday at 4pm was deadlift day. I can count on the fingers of one hand the number of times over the years I saw him do any lift or exercise other than the three powerlifts. Every once in a blue moon I might see him perform a set of curls, or do a set of stiff leg deadlifts, but nothing consistent other than the big three.

Typically at the appointed time on Monday and Thursday, a crowd of lifters would show up to train either the squat/bench or deadlift. By crowd, I mean a crowd! Three platforms or benches would all be going at once. Mike Benardon, Don Mills, Joe Ferry, Bob Brandon, Marshall Peck, Jeff Bobalouch, Kirk Karwoski, Frank Hottendorf, Mark Dimiduk, Ray

Evans, Ray Chaillet, Bob Bradley, Big John Studd, Graham Bartholomew, Ray Hager, Big Buddy, Noah Stern, Larry Christ, Elliot Smith, Bob Snell, Greg Tayman...on and on... on one Thursday I counted thirteen men in the room, all of whom had deadlifted 700 pounds or more.

The procedure would be as follows: on squat day, the power rack that faced the rear wall would be used by Mark and the four other heaviest squatters in the room. This group would be the 750+ guys. On the second set of squat racks, facing the deadlift platform, the 600 to 750 pound men would set up shop. On a third set of racks, facing the wall adjacent to the bathroom entrance, the smaller guys, the 400 to 600 pound club, would squat. After squats, three benches would be set up, each handling a certain poundage range. On Thursday, deadlift day, the 700 plus guys lifted on the elevated main deadlift platform. The 600 to 700 range men would lift on the adjacent floor area and the up to 600 men would lift in the area by the bathroom. It was the most simplistic power and strength program I've ever been exposed to, before or since.

In mainstream powerlifting orthodoxy, making the single repetition the backbone of a training strategy is viewed as insanity. At Chaillet's the single rep was a religion.

Mark Chaillet's Super Simplistic System

Day	Exercise	Sets/Reps
Monday	Squat	Squat suit/power belt/wraps – work up to an all out single rep
	Bench Press	Bench shirt – work up to an all out single rep
Thursday	Deadlift	Work up to an all out single rep

Competition Training Cycle

Mark used the classical 12 week periodization cycle that was so in vogue back in the 80's and so out of vogue today. Typically Mark would take about four weeks to ramp things up. Eight weeks before the National Championships he would get real serious and the weights would start to fly. I was intimately involved in helping him plot out the cycle and in making any in-flight corrections as circumstance warranted. I am going to do this from memory so it might not be exact, but will give the reader a real sense of how a stud like Chaillet would peak his mind and body leading up to a championship. The real work would begin after four weeks of getting into decent shape.

8 Week Periodization Cycle

Week	Squat (Lbs)	Bench (Lbs)	Deadlift (Lbs)
1	800	415	740
2	820	430	760
3	840	445	780
4	860	460	800
5	880	475	820
6	900	490	840
7	920	505	860
8	940	520	880
	Off for 14 days	*Off for 10 days*	*Off for 14 days*
Competition	**960**	**520**	**880**

Mark might start the 8 week cycle off weighing a soft 255 and by the competition he'd weigh a rock hard 280 and lift weighing 275. He was a tremendous competition lifter who routinely would come back after being behind 100 or 200 pounds at the sub-total (the combination of a man's top squat and top bench press poundage) before decimating the competition. He would take a token opener in the deadlift of say 760 then turn to me and say, "Add it up—how much do we need—can we win?" If it was anything up to 860, the leader was dead.

He was the greatest conventional deadlifter I've ever had the pleasure of training with. Mark pulled 880 and had 900 within three inches of lock-out. He consistently could deadlift 840 to 860. Mark occasionally would do some stiff-legged deadlifts using 800. One afternoon, I saw him pull 835 standing atop a 100 pound barbell plate laid flat. His minimalist approach worked phenomenally well for him for almost a decade. I think that those who dismiss his approach are short-sighted. Plus, I don't see very many 269 pound men deadlifting 880 nowadays. Mark squatted an IPF legal depth 1000 in training. By legal I mean *deep*. I called him up on the depth on that very lift. He officially hit 940 wearing one of those old Zangas Supersuits, no briefs and legal length wraps. When it came to leg and (especially) back power, Mark Chaillet was "cock strong."

Stopping Machine Gun Sales at Chaillet's "House of Pain"

They'll be saints and sinners,
Losers and winners,
All kinds of people you ain't never seen

—The Band

The stories about Chaillet's Gym are so outrageous that they have taken on mythical proportions. I called Mark's gym "The House of Pain" in a Powerlifting USA article and for good reason; at Chaillet's I've seen beat-downs and sex between patrons, I've seen illegal activity and acts of heroism—sometimes all on the same afternoon. I will recount a few that come to mind. The names have been changed to protect the guilty.

685 pounds on the bar: Ray Evans has pulled, Pat Brooks readies, Mark and Marshall await their turn. I am working the camera and lifting.

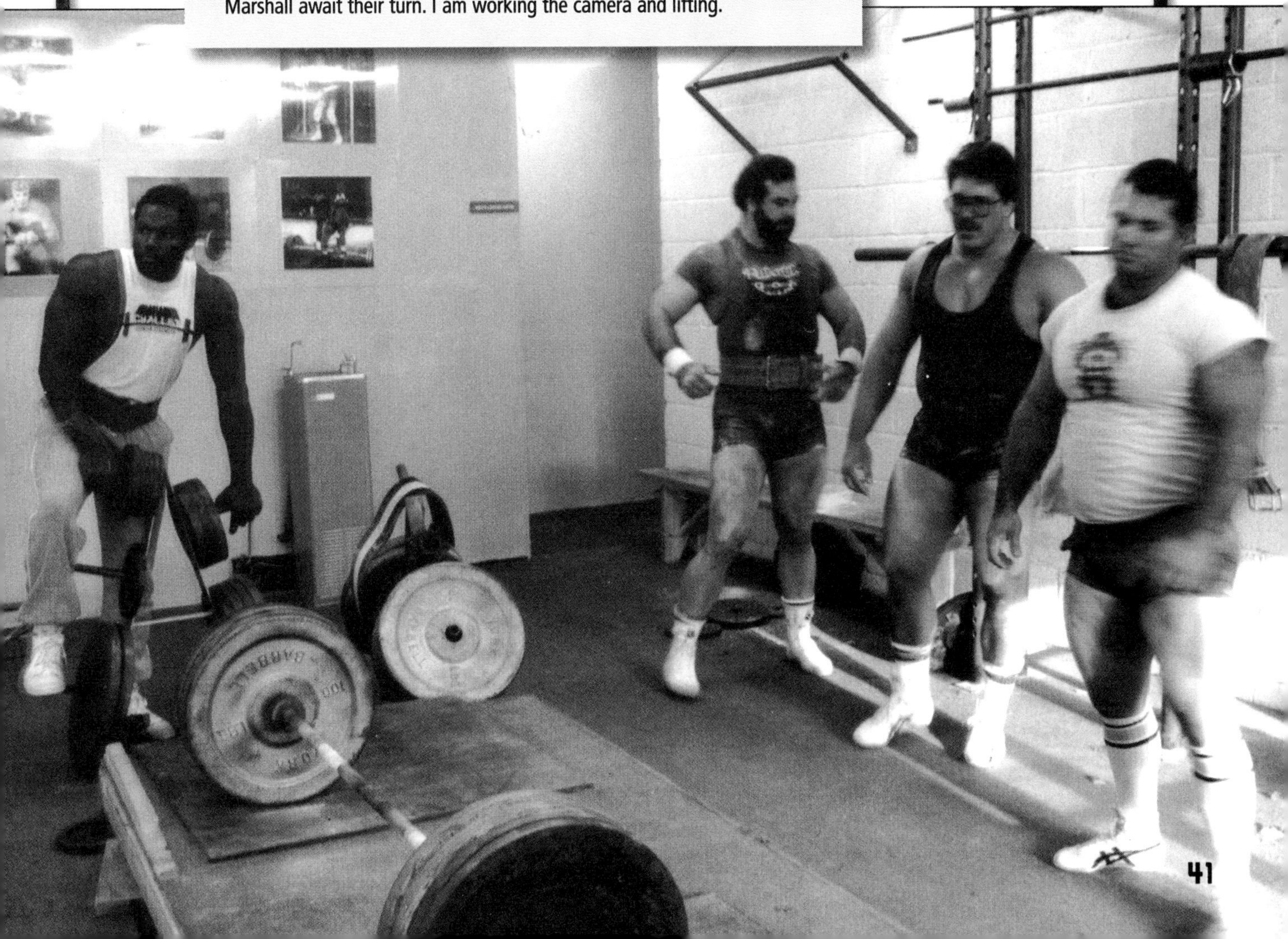

The gym had a gun bin and clients were required to pass weaponry across the front desk to either Mark or Buck—no questions asked. A towel was draped over the firearm as it was passed. Serious powerlifting, competitive powerlifting, at least in the 1980s, attracted a large contingent of both police officers and career criminals. Mark's gym bumped up against a bad section of the city and the cocaine trade was keeping both cops and crooks active. One afternoon, one of the best training partners I ever had, a deep cover narcotics officer, nudged me and gestured towards a good looking young fellow spotting a monstrous man with jail tattoos bench pressing 500 for reps. "That's ______ _______. He controls the coke trade in all of Southeast DC."

Interestingly, my cop pal, the coke kingpin, and his muscleman protector/bodyguard, were super cordial to each other. My man explained. "His sources have fingered me. So since he knows I'm a narc, he wants to make nice out of professional courtesy." A few years later the DEA arrested the young King Pin and found close to three million in cash. He had two money counting machines in his luxury condo. They sent his whole family up the river including his grandmother.

Bye! Bye! 880! Mark lifts alone. Big Buddy watches. I took the photo. Ray and a few others watch from the back room. Mark was the greatest conventional deadlifter I ever had the pleasure of training with. We were training partners for six years. He weighed 269 in this photo. The following week he pulled 900 to within three inches of lockout. Note his narrow foot stance and grip width: he taught me his deadlift style which I use to this day. He had the widest shoulders I've ever seen on man his height. His hands were gargantuan. Always a great deadlifter, over time he built an incredible squat.

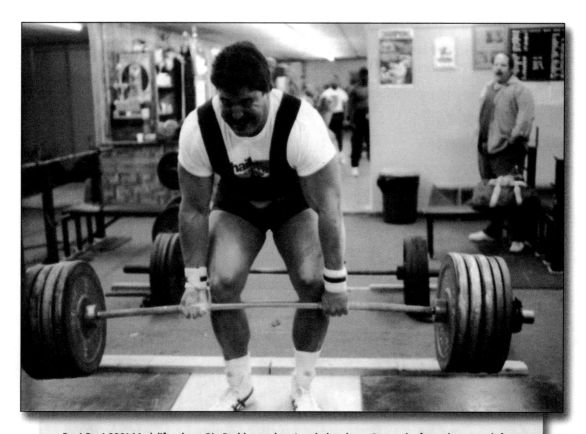

Chaillet's Gym was like Ric's Café in Casblanca: beefs and vendettas were usually left at the front door. Once you walked up the stairs and turned in your Glock or Berretta, you were no longer a lawman or lawbreaker, you were a powerlifter. During one period I trained with a DC undercover cop and a Baltimore cocaine ring enforcer who later went into witness protection. Neither knew the others man's trade. No one asked personal stuff. I overheard the coke enforcer mention he had some fully automatic AR-style machine guns for sale. The undercover cop wasn't interested in busting the guy; he wanted the rife for his own private collection and didn't want to go through the legal paperwork. The coke enforcer said he happened to have one in the trunk of his Cadillac and after the workout he'd "front it" to my cop pal and, "since you're a friend of Marty, you can pay me later." I stepped in and told each (separately) that this was a real bad idea. Ironically both men eventually landed in jail for long stretches: 20 years apiece.

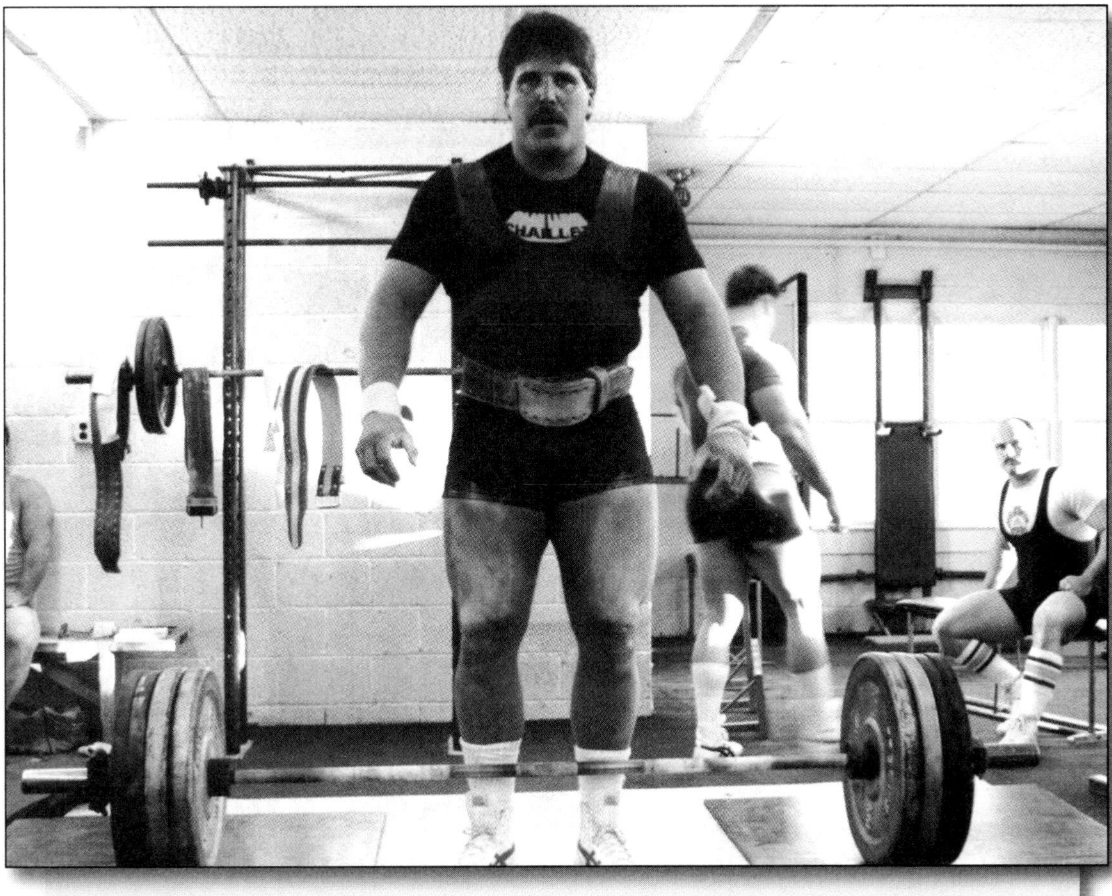

The Big Man warms up with 700: Note the lifting platform; a wooden sandwich ingeniously sat atop a half dozen auto tires. It absorbed the energy of the barbell being replaced or dropped. Note Mark's narrow foot stance: one "fist-width" between the heels. Chaillet had a terrific psyche-up routine that routinely added 10% to his efforts. His mental approach was formalized: three snorts on an ammonia popper and three successively louder stentorian bellows. At the National or World Championships his last-ditch deadlift histrionics were legendary. Many a great lifter was laid low when Chaillet would go from 9th to 1st after the dust settled in the deadlifts.

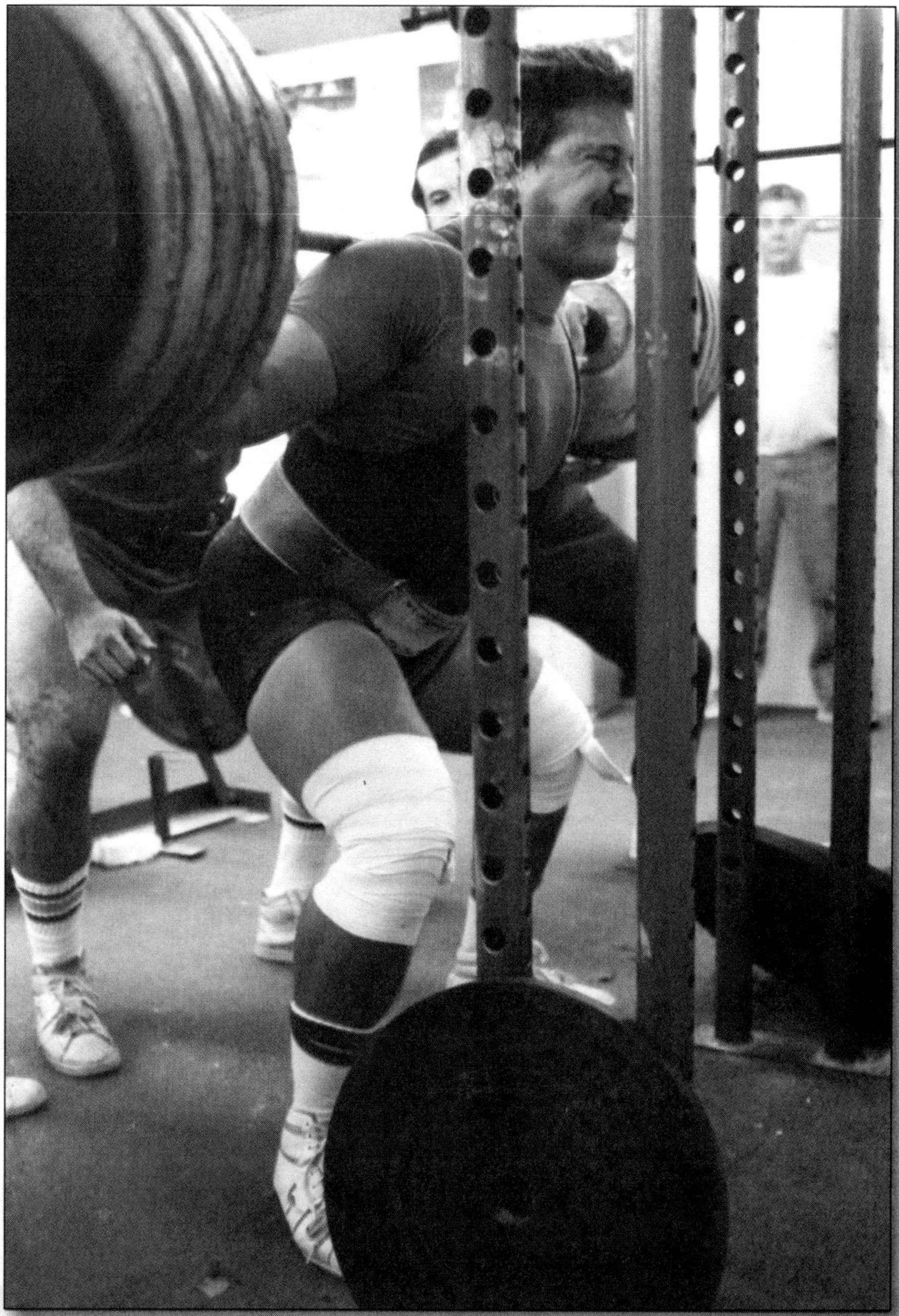

Mark maintains perfect push position with 1,000 pounds as Buck Chaillet watches the depth while leaning against the locker room wall. I knelt and took this shot while simultaneously giving him the "UP!" signal after he reached legal, IPF, below parallel depth. We worked very hard on dropping his depth down to below parallel. It took two years.

He was an amazing parallel squatter, but in the old, single organization USPF/IPF, unless the squat was unquestionably below parallel, the squat was failed. No monolift, Mark never had any problems setting up massive poundage. He weighed 279 in this picture. His minimalist approach worked fabulously for him.

DOUG FURNAS

The Athlete's Athlete

Doug Furnas was above all else an athlete. He was one of the true strength giants of our time, but being a hall of fame powerlifter was just one aspect of the Ice Man's extensive athletic career. He had a steely competitive demeanor, a savage work ethic and tremendous genetic gifts. He was successful in every athletic undertaking. Doug never reached his full potential in any one athletic arena because he would periodically spin off in another direction: from rodeo to

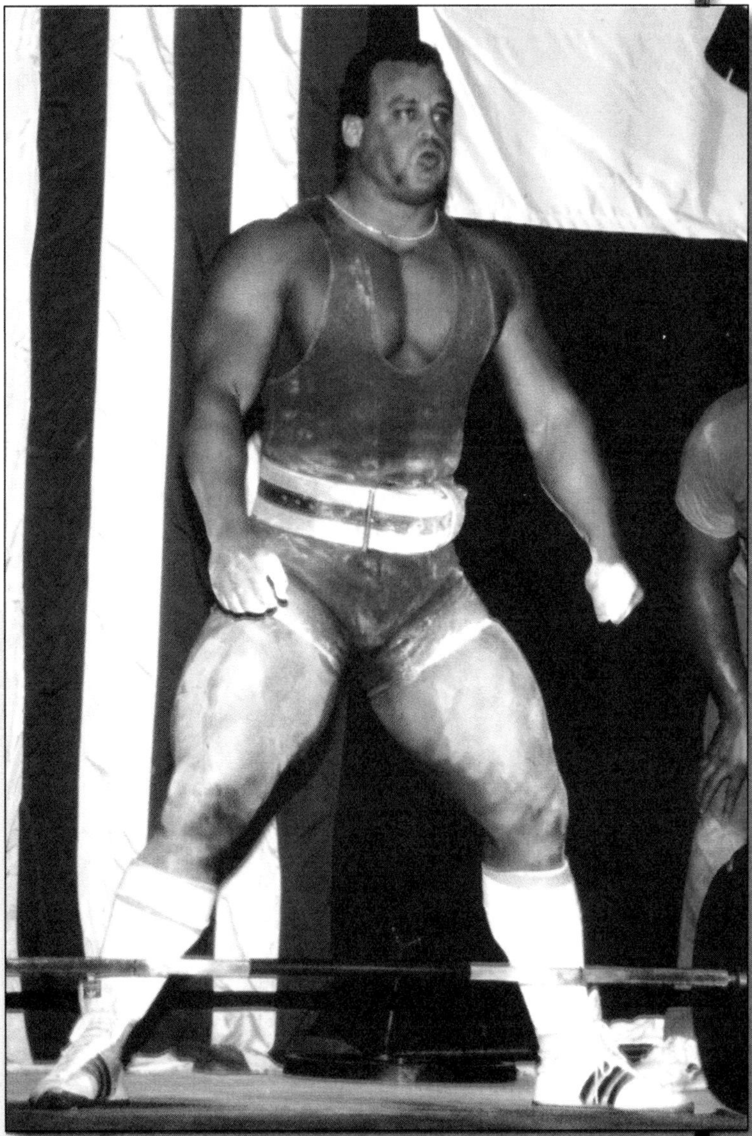

Man amongst Men: The Oklahoma Stud at his power peak: I took the shot in Minnesota 1985. I was coaching Doug, Ed Coan and Mark Chaillet all at the same time at this meet—plus running to the front of the stage with my Nikon to shoot photos.

At 5'10" and 275 pounds, Doug Furnas readies to pull 826. This lift would make him the first man in history to total 2,400 pounds twice. Despite his freaky physique he was loose and limber. He stretched prior to lifting and would routinely do the full splits. His thighs were 34 inches and calves 21 inches in this picture.

football to powerlifting to strongman to professional wrestling… he was an athletic Ronin Samurai warrior. "This gun for hire." He could have gone professional as a teen rodeo rider; he was starting fullback for a high school team that played in the State Championships; he played for the National Champion junior college football team before becoming a starting fullback for Tennessee on a team that included pro football immortal Reggie White. He played in the Peach Bowl. He played pro football for Denver with John Elway before taking up powerlifting.

He set his first World Record within nine months of dedicating himself exclusively to the sport. He ripped across the power skyline for four years before becoming a professional wrestler. He was a veritable wrestling God in Japan. During the late 1980's he was recognized everywhere he went in Japan and mobbed on the streets like a rock star. He wrestled in the WWF before an auto accident ended his athletic career. Doug was unquestionably one of the most innovative resistance trainers of the modern era. I am proud to call him a friend.

Doug Furnas was sophisticated in his strength philosophies and put theory into practice with incredible results. He had the good powerlift luck to stand on the shoulders of another iron giant, Dennis Wright. At a critical juncture in his multidimensional athletic career, Doug studied powerlifting under Dennis like Luke studied under Obi Wan. When Dennis slipped the leash, Doug squatted 881 weighing 238, using the most awesome squat technique ever seen. His squats were like Raphael paintings, as athletically exquisite as a Tiger Woods golf swing or a Michael Jordon leap-and-dunk. Doug had great mentors at various times in his athletic career, but none were more accomplished than Dennis.

Furnas excelled at every athletic activity to which he turned his full attention. He competed at stratospheric levels in every sport: starting off with rodeo as a man-child, then football, powerlifting and finally professional wrestling. He and wrestling partner Phil LaFon were five time tag team champions in the All Japan Professional Wrestling federation. Later he and tag team partner Don Keffutt captured the ECW World Tag Team title.

Doug's only athletic disappointment occurred when a hamstring injury prematurely ended his professional football career with Denver. The injury effectively strangled his pro ball career in its crib. He became disillusioned and was relegated to the Bronco taxi squad. For the first time in his life, he was not a starter or a star. His hamstring injury became a chronic injury and he became embroiled in irresolvable conflicts with Denver head coach Dan Reeves. He was trapped in athletic limbo: good enough to be kept on the payroll, never healed enough to demonstrate his wares, increasingly frustrated and disgusted, he headed home to the family farm to reconsider his future and athletically recalibrate. Football's loss became powerlifting's gain.

Near Death Experience Leads to Iron Introduction

Doug's love affair with a barbell commenced after he was nearly killed in a horrific auto accident. The Furnas family was returning home from a rodeo competition when their car was run into head on as they crested a hill by a drunk driver speeding down the wrong side of the road. Doug was 16 at the time. His body was completely shattered. Both his legs were broken, his shoulder was destroyed and his spleen exploded upon impact. Doug's father broke his neck. His girlfriend (who he later married) broke her back. Doug's mother broke both ankles.

It took him almost two years to heal. Lifting weights became a big part of his recovery and he developed a deep taste for weight training. He recovered enough to go back to school. His younger brother Mike and he were now in the same grade. All through junior high school, high school, junior college and college the two played together on championship football teams. The brothers played on a high school team that went to the Oklahoma High School State Championships. Both were selected as Oklahoma high school all-stars and played against the Texas all-stars in the Oil Bowl. Both played for Northeastern Oklahoma A&M, a junior college squad that won the Junior College National Championship.

That brought dozens of offers from Division I teams. The brothers decided on Tennessee because both were offered scholarships and they could continue to play together. Tennessee won the conference title and went to the Peach Bowl. On New Year's Day in front of 60,000 people, while millions more watched on TV, Tennessee lost by two points to Iowa 26 to 24 in the last 60 seconds of the game. Though he didn't know it at the time, that exciting loss would be both the high point and the tragic foreshadowing that the football high times had peaked and things were about to sour. Doug ended up with the Denver Broncos and after a hamstring injury became chronic, he voluntarily opted out. Doug was now free to immerse himself in powerlifting. He had followed the iron sport since his auto accident and dreamed of a time when he could focus on it exclusively. That time was now.

For the first time since third grade, Doug wasn't participating in a team sport. With powerlifting it was just him and the barbell and the aloneness appealed to him mightily. Now he didn't have to schedule his life around someone else's practice schedule. Now he could concentrate 100% of his energies on an individual sport. He would settle in and concentrate on becoming the best powerlifter he could be. His brother joined him. Now they would both commence on the powerlifting path, together once again.

He had followed the sport of powerlifting all through high school and college. He was particularly taken by another amazing athlete turned powerlifter, John Gamble. The monstrous Gamble had it all: massive and lean, John had a ferocious competitive attitude. Gamble was a balanced lifter who at his peak was untouchable. Gamble had an incredible physique and his sheer physical dominance provided Doug with a power role model, someone he aspired to emulate.

Doug compounded his physical and psychological assets with clean living habits; he neither smoked nor drank nor partied. He had a stern, collected, Ice Man demeanor. He seemed aloof because he was aloof. If you were in his inner circle he could be quite open and humorous. He was well spoken, but soft spoken and you would find yourself leaning forward to hear him better in conversations. From a distance he appeared humorless; he was the kind of guy if you were competing against you hated, but he was exactly the type of man you would want in a foxhole next to you. It was easy to envision him as a squadron commander leading a mass assault of M-1 Abram tanks across some desert landscape. After the extreme regimentation of football, dealing with coaches who held scholarships or money over his head, Doug was glad to be free of the smothering, all-consuming commitments of big time football.

He sought to maximize his abilities as a lifter. As a teen he had apprenticed under Okie powerlifting legend, Dennis Wright. Both men lived in the same neck of the woods in rural Oklahoma and it was only natural that Doug and Mike and Dennis begin working out together. Dennis would power through his own sessions and Doug and his brother would "ghost Dennis," following right behind, performing whatever exercises, set and rep selections Dennis decided upon. Doug and Mike would tackle whatever Wright set in front of them, no questions asked.

In the early days, Doug and Mike would powerlift between football seasons. After pro football, powerlifting was given undivided attention. It was the beginning of a legendary run of the table. Furnas' power career lasted four short years, but during that time he was a meteor streaking across the dark sky of powerlifting. He redefined the athletic possibilities. He campaigned for a season in the 242 pound class and set his first world squat record, 881 pounds, weighing 239. Standing 5'10" he was actually too tall for that class and really hit his stride when he moved up to the 275 pound class. He had played football weighing a leaned-out, trimmed to the max 225 pounds carrying a 6% body fat percentile. He was a blocking fullback who ran a 4.5 forty and had a 40 inch vertical leap. Adding 50 pounds of muscle caused him to come on strong and fast.

Furnas was the powerlifting equivalent of the perfect storm: great genetics combined with a great work ethic, a high pain tolerance and a hall-of-fame coach. Wright pointed out all the shortcuts and dead-ends ahead of time. Wright's primordial approach, lots of volume, lots of poundage, lots of sets and long sessions, was Old School all the way. No-mercy power training for those who could hang. The Wright/Furnas brother training sessions were legendary. The Furnas boys had highly developed pain tolerances from all those rodeo bumps and bruises, all those football practices, and before all of it, from the hard farm labor they were required to do as youngsters. Doug and Mike were subjected to the hardening effects of intense manual labor as children.

The family owned a 270 acre ranch and the boys were required to work and work hard. Mike was a year younger than Doug and just as athletic and just as combative. Doug related that as children the brothers were expected to "pull their weight" insofar as chores. When they were youngsters the duo were assigned to work together. The duo was expected to perform the work of a single adult male farmhand. Together they formed a "unit." Together the two little boys would run along in open farm fields, behind a moving truck, together dragging 100 pound hay bails up to a moving flatbed. They would routinely carry heavy water and heavy feed buckets. They worked long hours at physically demanding tasks. Meanwhile, Doug noted, that "while Mike and I were wrestling steers and each other, the town kids were out playing T-ball."

The brothers became "real physical" and when the twosome started playing high school football they were way ahead of their teammates. Football, however, was not the first sport young Doug excelled at: the entire Furnas family competed on the competitive rodeo circuit. They paid substantial entry fees to compete for cash prizes. Mom, dad, brother, sister, all rode and roped, competing for money. Hardcore rodeo taught Doug how to fall, how to get thrown and not get hurt; how to get up after being thrown, how to dust yourself off and shake off the pain. He gave serious thought to becoming a bull riding professional; his childhood rodeo contemporaries founded the Professional Rodeo circuit.

Forced to make a choice, Doug choose football. He ended up as a teammate of NFL all-pro and World Champion sprinter Willie Gault. Also on the Tennessee team was future Super Bowl MVP, NFL Defensive Player of the year and Hall of Fame immortal Reggie White. Doug and Mike Furnas effortlessly operated at the highest athletic levels.

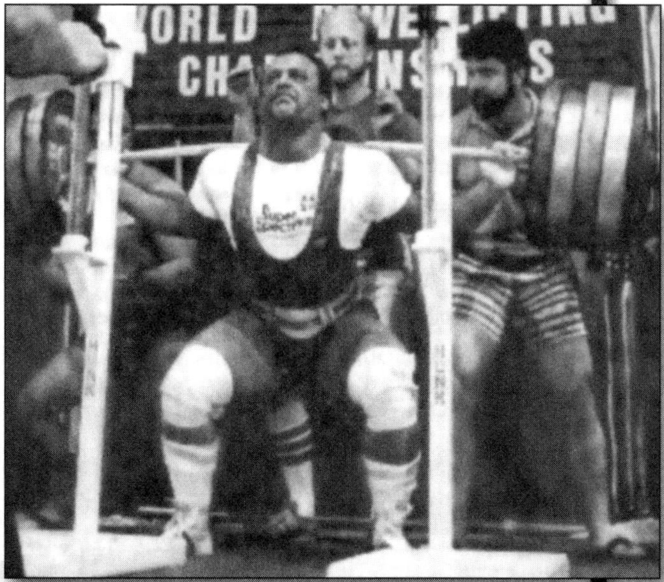

Squat Clinic: Here is Doug 2/3rd of the way erect with 985 pounds. Note his erect torso and how he is keeping his knees over his ankles. His head is thrown back to keep everything in proper structural push alignment. After the speed and ease with which he handled this weight, I suggested he take a 4th attempt with 1,020. Without a seconds hesitation he demurred "I want to save it {my strength} for the other lifts." He posted his first 2,400 pound total but never posted an official 1,000 pound squat. I often wondered if he had any regrets about not uncorking a grand on this particular day.

Dennis Wright: "Simplistic Genius"

Dennis Wright was a hall-of-fame powerlifter who got better as he got older. Dennis started off in the 70's as a gangly, yet surprisingly powerful 165 pound lifter. I saw him lift at age 50 and weighing 198 pounds. Dennis squatted 800 pounds, quadruple bodyweight, in exquisite fashion. He backed up the squat with a 475 pound bench press. The 800 pound squat was pure technical perfection. After a slow, controlled descent that ended in a precision turn-around, two inches below parallel, the ascent was explosive and crisp. Watching Wright's lifts that day, I was struck that every squat he took was an *identical* copy of the previous one or the subsequent one. I was seeing a Samurai master handle an *o-dachi* long sword.

Doug related that he and his brother always made it a point to arrive for training sessions with Dennis 15 minutes early. They would sit curbside in the car until the appointed training time, drinking coffee. The brothers would fire each other up as they sat, talking themselves into a quiet frenzy, getting psyched for the workout. I asked, why they didn't just go in early, or arrive on time. Why arrive early? I asked. "We were showing Dennis respect. We made it a point to arrive early in order to show our eagerness and gratitude. Going in early would have been disrespectful."

Dennis Wright would work the hell out the brothers during a session. A typical weekly squat week would find the men performing four sets of 5 reps on Tuesday with a "static" poundage. On Saturday they would work up to a heavy 5 rep set, then a heavy 4 rep set, then a triple, then a double and finally a single. Not done they would "back down," i.e., reduce the poundage, and hit sets of either 5 or 7 second pause squats. "Dennis was a simplistic genius. Everything I have ever done was a result of what I learned from him." More Furnasian deference.

When Doug began concentrating on powerlifting his poundage began to soar and he dropped the twice-a-week squat template. "I wasn't recovering session to session. I played with a second "light" squat day, but that seemed like a waste of time. Eventually I dropped the second weekly squat day—and that's when my lifting took off."

In each session they would strive to equal or exceed previous personal records, though capacity might take differing forms. As a result of all the Old School squatting and pause squatting, done Dennis Wright style, (lots of volume, lots of intensity, lots of poundage) Doug grew gargantuan legs. It was said that his thighs measured 34 inches while his waist size was 34. He refused all inquiries into his girth measurements. Eventually, he weighed 275 pounds, yet was ripped and shredded. Even at his heaviest bodyweight he was always lean and athletic. He bench pressed 620 in training and 600 officially, this while wearing a loose, size 60 inch 1st generation Inzer power shirt. His shirts were so loose I asked why he bothered wearing them at all; he could put the shirt on himself. "I like the way it keeps my torso warm."

Dennis Wright was a great bench presser and gave the Furnas Brothers a template that mined the same training vein as the squat: work up to the target poundage, always stressing perfect technique. They would perform bench press "assistance work" and followed an axiom Hugh Cassidy passed along to me: the best assistance exercise for a particular lift is an assistance exercise that *most closely resembles* the lift itself. Therefore the best assistance exercise for the flat bench press would be more flat bench presses using a wider or narrower grip. Dennis passed onto Doug a bench system that Doug modified and eventually perfected.

A typical Furnas bench workout might find him working up to a top set, before cutting the weight and performing two sets of wide grip bench presses using a pause on the chest. Then he would drop the poundage and hit two sets of flat bench presses using a narrow grip. Narrow grip bench presses would also be paused. With narrow grip benches the sticking point occurs as the bar approaches lock-out and concentrated use of narrow grips improves lockout ability. Wide-grip bench presses were purposefully paused to build "starting power." Triceps would be worked hard after benching.

Doug used a sumo deadlift technique and tried to harness his amazing leg strength in his pulling. He viewed the deadlift as a "reverse squat." He used a wide stance in both lifts and maintained a bolt upright torso. He never let his hips rise to get the deadlift started and eventually pulled 826. His deadlift limitation was his grip. He had violent allergic reactions to magnesium carbonate, lifting chalk, and this meant he had to pull without it. Doug found that if he successfully pushed his squat upward, his deadlift would tag along. There was a consistent ratio between the two lifts and as he approached 1,000 in the squat, his deadlift rose proportionally.

Incredible Eddy Coan shared training ideas with Doug on a regular basis. The two saw eye to eye on so many areas that they arrived eventually at a power training consensus. Their template was adopted by many of their contemporaries and changed the power thinking of the day. It was an amalgamation, a blending of strategies that amplified results. In person they were impressive: Doug's persona, quiet intensity, made an interesting contrast to Ed's Irish fierceness and fire. Like Mick and Keith, John and Paul, Butch and Sundance, they became Iron partners. There was a period of time when the two were inseparable at National and World competitions.

After retiring from powerlifting, Doug kept his hand in the game by coming to the Nationals to work with Ed Coan. I had the pleasure of coaching each man at National and

World Championships. It was a white-knuckle, hair raising experience to work with these guys. It was terrifying to handle Doug, Ed and Mark Chaillet—all at the same time! Any mess up and months of work could be destroyed.

Coaching Coan, Furnas and Chaillet Simultaneously

What a trio: each man needed special handling. With six months of preparatory blood, sweat, tears and training preparation on the line, coaching these men on report card day was no freaking joke! These guys were all business on game day. They only competed twice a year—at the National Championships and at the World Championships—so there was a helluva a lot at stake. When these big guns, the biggest stars in the sport, were rolled out together, world record smashing was expected and demanded.

My job was akin to that of a NASCAR pit crew chief handing three racecars at once: it was up to me to time the process, ensure that all warm-up attempts were done in a timely fashion, make sure the backstage warm-up poundage was loaded correctly, that spotters were in place and alert. Gear needed to be put on at just the right time: wrap a man's knees too early and kiss the lift goodbye. The wrap tension will cut off blood circulation and turn a man's legs blue. Start the knee wrapping procedure too late and the lifter is rushed and hustled onto the platform, deprived of his critical pre-lift psyche-up. At worst, late wrapping causes the lifter to be "timed out," disqualified from lifting that attempt because he was not on the platform within the allotted time. In addition, there were spectators and well-wishers that needed to be kept at bay during the warm-up procedure. Each man needed to remain psyched, centered and concentrated; a casual backslap or civilian intrusion at the wrong moment could shatter a carefully constructed psyche. It was intimidating and invigorating all at the same time...I would experience pure fear before every attempt; this was inevitably followed by ecstatic elation after some amazing lift.

These guys nearly always made their lifts and they were spectacular to watch, truly electrifying. They routinely shattered world records, one after another, and did so with predictable regularity. I was the crew chief when each of these hall-of-fame men achieved their respective best all-time power performances. Doug was the first man to total 2400 pounds twice and was by far the lightest ever to hit 2400 at the time—until his partner, Ed Coan, cracked 2400 weighing a mere 219 pounds, a few years later. Chaillet was walking drama: with his blunderbuss deadlift he would usually end up the last man left to deadlift, the man who can and did snatch victory from the jaws of defeat repeatedly. He was the definition of nerve wracking.

Then Doug was gone. He quit powerlifting at the absolute zenith of his career. He simply walked away. He had won national and world championships, he had set numerous world records and to continue onward would be mere repetition, improving upon that which he had already accomplished. He turned his thoughts towards making a living and decided to enter the lucrative yet intensely competitive world of professional wrestling. He was accepted immediately and worked his way through the national and international circuit until he was summoned to the highest level of pro wrestling ranks: the WWF. His lack of flamboyance prevented him from becoming a comic-book superstar, yet his amazing athletic ability assured him a place at the table.

In a dreadful dose of Shakespearian irony, yet another horrid auto accident ended his athletic career. A van full of professional wrestlers were driving from one show to another when the driver fell asleep and drove off the road, plunging into a ravine deep in the Canadian wilderness. Doug's body was shattered yet again. Auto tragedy commenced his iron journey decades before and decades later another auto tragedy ended it; a gruesome set of chronological bookends denoting the beginnings and ending of an amazingly versatile athlete's amazing athletic career.

How did Doug train?

Both Doug Furnas and Ed Coan followed a similar training template: we list their collaborative protocol in the section on Coan.

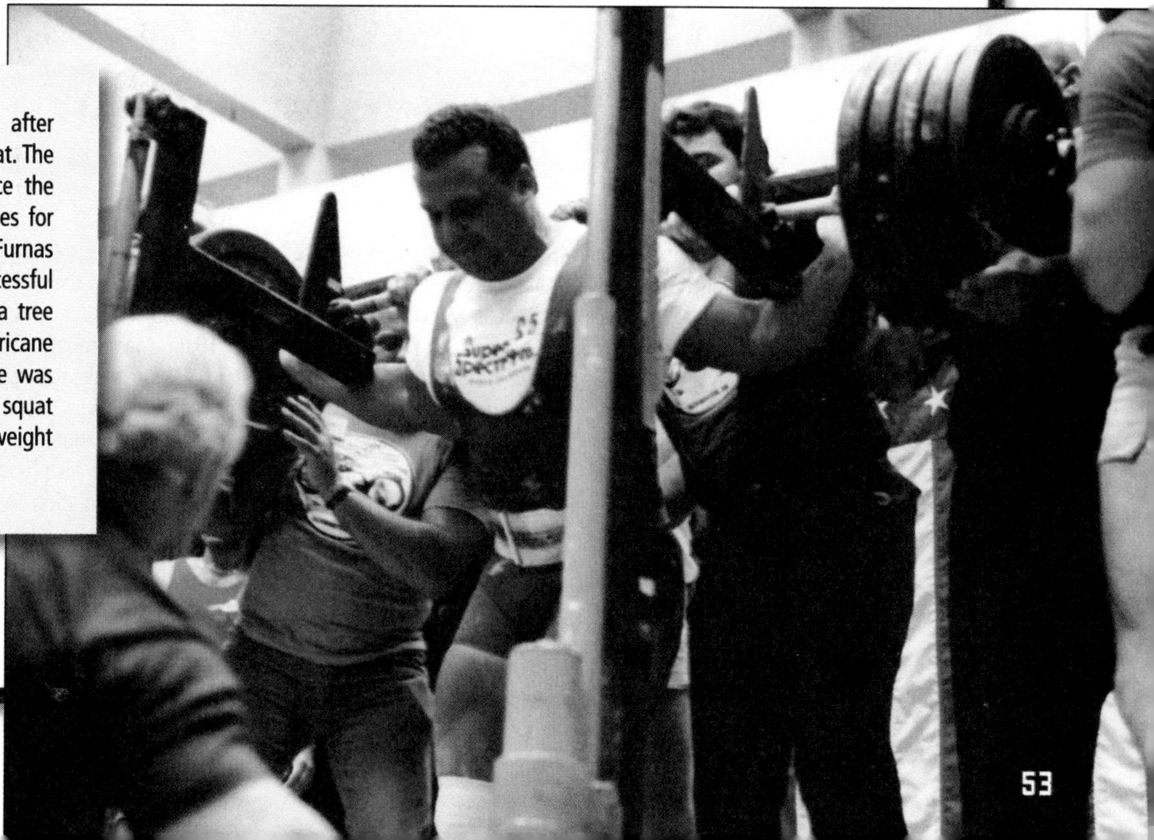

Minnesota Triumph: Furnas after completing a 970 pound squat. The boys are helping him replace the barbell as Ernie Frantz reaches for the white lights. I never saw Furnas get a red light on a successful squat. He would shake like a tree full of dead leaves in a hurricane trying to get set up: once he was able to establish his wide squat stance, he would squat the weight like it was 135 pounds.

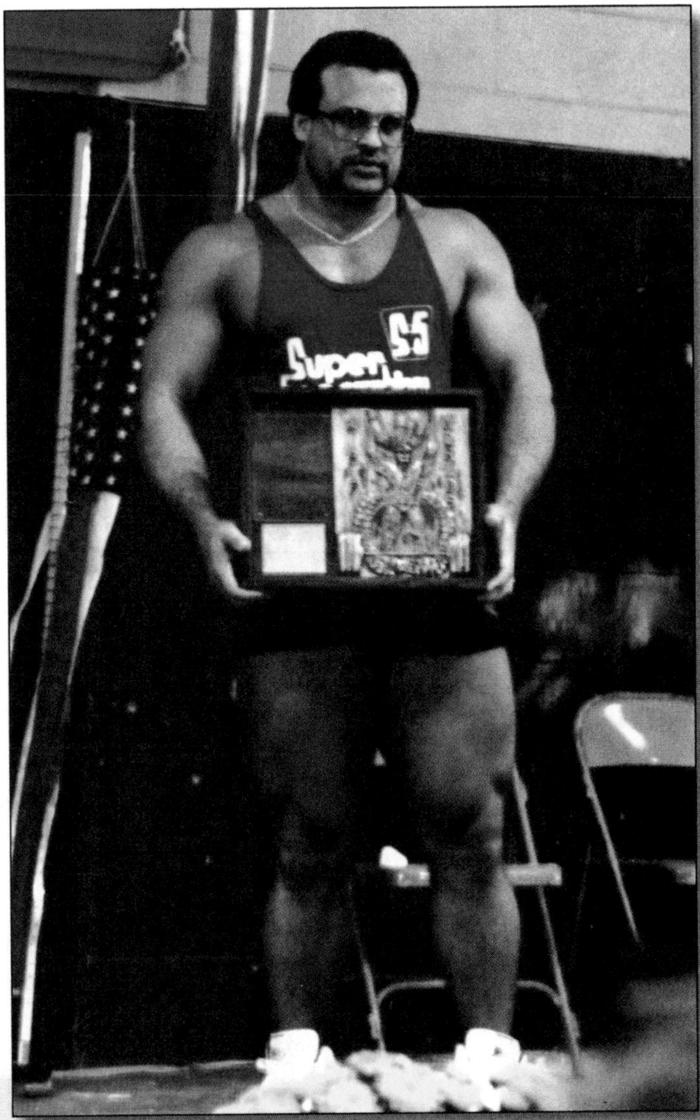

Doug in Maui after becoming the first 275 pound lifter to total 2400. I was there coaching Mark Chaillet to his first world title. That morning the Chaillet posse went to breakfast with Ed Coan, Doug Furnas and their respective crews. We ate at Moose McGillicudys second floor walk-up restaurant in Lahania. As we ate I kept glancing at my watch. Lifting was scheduled to start at 10am. Mark caught my concern and addressed the table, "Hey, maybe we better get going it's almost 8:30!" Doug, stoic, soft spoken, steely, looked up between bites of scrambled eggs and said, "Don't worry Mark, they won't start without us." Chaillet laughed and I laughed (nervously) and we continued eating. Furnas didn't laugh. He was right, they waited until we arrived. His techniques were impeccable and his styles played to his physical strengths. Doug had short arms: this helped his bench press and hurt his deadlift. The solution was clever and effective: pull in such a way as to create a "reverse squat."

ED COAN

The Greatest Powerlifter Of All Time...

Without a doubt the greatest athlete I've ever had the pleasure of working with is Ed Coan. Incredible Eddy is the Jim Brown/Michael Jordan/Muhammad Ali of powerlifting and his exploits are simply astounding when viewed from any athletic angle, be it peak performances or longevity.

Coan's friend and compatriot, Doug Furnas, was a powerlifting comet: a man who tore through our sport after rodeo, after big time college and pro football and before pro wrestling. Powerlifting, for Doug, was just another whistle

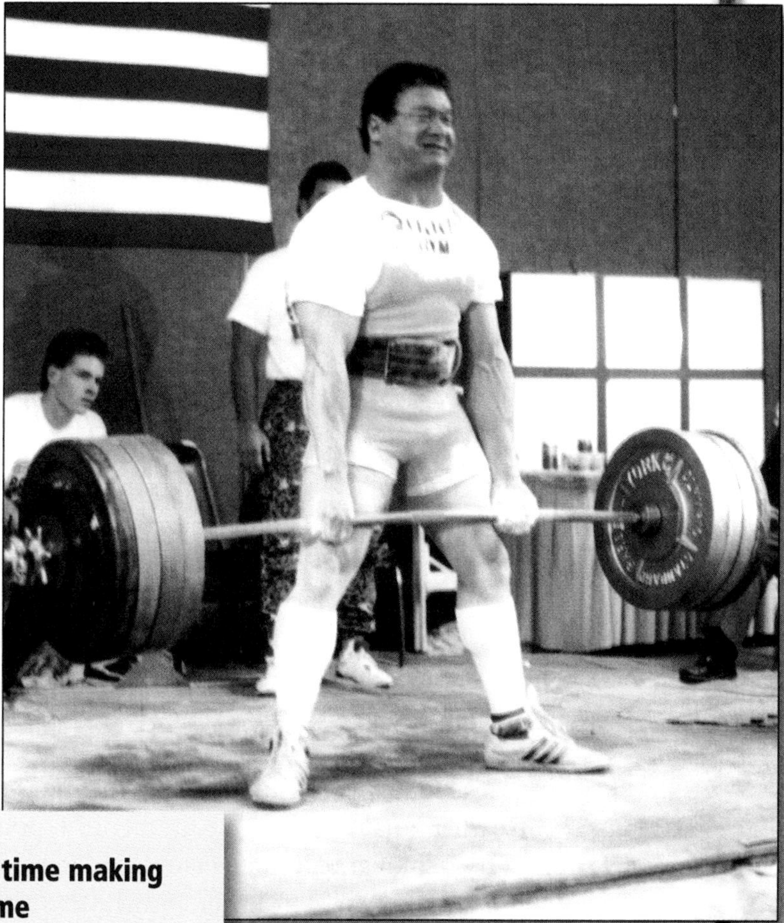

The greatest powerlifter of all time making the greatest powerlift of all time

This is Ed's historic 901 pound deadlift weighing 219. I coached Ed on this day. He actually missed two lifts on his way to posting a 2,400 pound total; he missed a 986 pound 3rd attempt squat and a mind-blowing 920 third attempt deadlift. He had doubled a 900 pound deadlift in training prior to this competition! The 900x2 training lift was paused between reps.

stop, an athletic interlude before commencing his decade long journey as a professional wrestler. Doug passed through the strength universe for a few brief years, leaving an indelible mark, before exiting our sphere and heading onto other athletic worlds to conquer.

Ed landed on planet power in 1981 and as this is being written, Incredible Ed has not been beaten in head to head competition since July of 1983 when he took second place at the National Championships to the power dominator of the previous decade, Mike Bridges. When Ed took second place to Mike, in their one and only meeting, it was symbolic: a handing off of the strength torch from the greatest lifter of the 70's and 80's to the greatest lifter from that point forward. It was Bridge's last competition and marked the start of Coan's utter and complete domination, a reign that is unmatched in any sport.

It is actually difficult to come up with appropriate frame of reference when attempting to relate to outsiders what a phenomenon Ed Coan actually is. In my book on Ed, *Coan: The Man, The Myth, The Method*, I made some mathematical analogies that bear repeating. At one point in time, 1991, Ed Coan was mathematically 14.5% better than the rest of the world's top powerlifters in the 220 pound class. The second best 220 pound World Total was 2,100 pounds; a great total considering that the inflationary gear and equipment "revolution" had not hit powerlifting. The Monolift had yet to be invented and bench shirts of the time added 30-40 pounds to a lifter's bench press, not 40% to 60% to the lift.

To duplicate Coan's degree of separation from the rest of the field, a sprinter would need to shatter Asafa Powell's current 100 meter yard dash record of 9.77 seconds by posting an 8.35 time. Michael Johnson's current 200 meter World Record of 19.32 seconds would have to be bettered with a 16.52 time. The Cuban Sotomayer's World High Jump Record of 8' ¼" would require someone to leap 9'2" and Randy Barnes' 75'10" World Record in the shot put would need to be blasted to smithereens by someone tossing the 16 pound iron ball 86 feet. That was how far in front of the rest of the strength world Ed Coan was at one marvelous point in time.

Insofar as his longevity: consider the fact that he is riding a 24 year unbeaten streak. I will repeat an earlier analogy: imagine if the 154 pound boxer Ray Leonard fought and defeated every ranking *heavyweight* contender to miraculously secure the Heavyweight Championship of the World in 1983. Now further suppose that Ray remained a 154 pound fighter and fought for the next 24 years and never lost a single bout. That is the greatness of Incredible Eddy Coan.

Irish Ed is no genetic freak. It would be too cheap and too easy to write off his accomplishments as the result of some sort of accident on the part of nature. Ed is an extremely intelligent and conservative individual who was methodical yet innovative. To those who knew him, Coan was regimented and steadfast. He had an amazing competitive psyche that was so fierce it was frightening—but it wasn't outward and demonstrative. You had to be fairly close in order to appreciate his internal fire. They say "the eyes are the windows into a man's soul" and Ed's eyes could burn holes in wooden walls and start fires prior to a world record attempt. If you stood within three feet of him prior to a big attempt, he literally generated intense body heat. I repeatedly felt the air temperature around his body rise appreciably prior to a gigantic lift. I suppose this was an outward manifestation of some unique internal psychological process.

"This boy will consign us all to oblivion!"
—Rival upon hearing Mozart for the first time.

"Well that's bad f___ ing news for the rest of us!"
—Nationally ranked lifter learning Ed was moving into his weight class.

I met Ed Coan and Doug Furnas in the mid-eighties while coaching Mark Chaillet at National and World Championships. Mark was a force to be reckoned with, and like Doug, moved up from the 242 pound class to the 275 pound weight class. I had shattered my leg in 1983 and was effectively finished as a lifter. I morphed into a coach and traveled with Mark and his ample posse to competitions, acting as his coach.

The most memorable powerlifting competitions of all time were the incredible Bacchanalian power festivals Larry Pacifico ran in Dayton. Ed and I ran into each other repeatedly at these meets and I was dumbstruck with his lifting. He was a 181 pound lifter when I first began seeing him lift up close and personal. One year at one of Larry's meets I was on my way to dinner at the Spaghetti Factory across the street from the Dayton Convention Center. I happened to cross the street as Ed and his crew was headed in the other direction. He waved me down and got right to the point. "Doug (Furnas) had a last minute emergency and cannot make it to the competition—can you coach me at the competition tomorrow?" Of course. I was flabbergasted and flattered.

So began a long association that allowed me to coach and assist Ed in those competitions where he performed the greatest powerlifting exploits of all time. I coached him when he posted his greatest ever totals and when he lifted his heaviest ever individual lifts. It was a heady and remarkable time. Describing those golden days of yore to younger lifters is odd. The modern powerlifter only knows of powerlifting since "The Great Disintegration and Scattering." When I speak of the heights powerlifting once attained before the splintering, these lifters gaze at me as Dark Ages men would if I were describing Rome before the Huns sacked and burned the city to the ground....

"...Imagine a time in the obscure town of Dayton, Ohio when, for a brief sliver of time, everyone who powerlifted competed in a single federation. Those who attended these unified National and World Championships, run under the direction of power impresario Larry Pacifico and his brother Dick, saw the very best, all lifting together, using the same rules, before sold-out convention center audiences. We honestly believed that mainstream acceptance of powerlifting lay just around the next corner.

Imagine a powerlifting competition where all the top lifters in the country competed in a single place at the same time. Imagine a promotional genius who had the wisdom and foresight to hold championship power competitions in the same town, Dayton, Ohio, at the same time, year after year.

As a result of keeping the competitions consistent, over time an audience, an educated audience, grew to love and anticipate the Powerlifting Championships. Year after year, locals and visitors would descend on Dayton to attend these power extravaganzas. Eventually, thousands of people would fill the Dayton Convention Center. People would actually scalp tickets to see the heavyweight finale.

A packed house would sit in air conditioned comfort and watch the greatest lifters in the World ply their trade in front of strict judges in a competition run with the smooth efficiency of a Swiss Watch. Loud, vocal, bawdy, voracious fans hollered themselves hoarse when favorite lifters strode to the platform. Looking around the packed auditorium, the audience profile would be very similar to the type of crowd that attends the annual Sturgis Motorcycle festival each year. By keeping the competitions in Dayton at the same time each year, people were actually planning vacations around attending the Powerlifting Championships.

Returning champions had their airfare and hotel rooms paid for. Larry sent courtesy buses to the airport to pick up top lifters and whisk them back to the luxury hotel that adjoined the Convention Center, connected by a skyway. Each year Larry and Dick layered on another new and exciting twist or wrinkle. At its apogee, Larry flew in Klaus, the funky blind organ player from Germany, and between lifts or in dead spots, Klaus would get the crowd going by playing wild dance music.

Larry had a buffet steam table set up in the auditorium, 100 feet from the lifting, audience members could stroll over from their seats, purchase a hot meat loaf platter, perhaps some roast turkey with mashed potatoes, salads, pies, cakes, vegetables and (drum roll) a bottle of beer for a buck! Then walk back to their seat in time to see Hatfield squat 880 at 220 or Cash pull 832 to beat Fred and Larry. How about seeing Jacoby battle Ladiner? Back and forth these two battled, the lead changed hands something like six times. Joe pulled the winning deadlift of 800 only to be turned down in a 2 to 1 decision! Those were indeed the days.

I remember returning from the buffet line and telling my seatmate, Big Bob (an 800-pound raw squatter who had spent time in prison for manslaughter) "Bob, if we died and went to heaven—could it be any freaking better than this!" He shook his massive head clicked my beer bottle with his and said, "Amen to that Little Daddy!"

You might see John Gamble, Terry McCormick, Dave Shaw, Larry Kidney, Tom Henderson, Bob Dempsey, Mark Chaillet, Sam Samangeio and Steve Wilson all doing battle in the 275 pound class—along with a half dozen other heavy hitter lifters. How about watching Ed Coan deadlift or Lee Moran squat? Or the time Fred Hatfield did battle with Jim Cash and Larry P in the 220 class? You could see Lamar Gant pull 650+ weighing 132 pounds. I remember every time Iron Immortal Doyle Kenedy would stride out to lift, some crazed nut would stand up and yell over and over, "MOUNTAIN MAN! KILL THE WEIGHT MOUNTAIN MAN!"

The feeling of camaraderie among the lifters was palpable: I remember Larry Kidney make a terrific clutch deadlift with 780 and then giving John Gamble a heartfelt hi-five as John passed Larry on his way to the platform to pull the 800 pound poundage that would beat Larry—the enemy was the barbell, not each other. After the competitions it was bawdy, wild, beer-soaked reveries at the Spaghetti Factory or the magnificent Sunday lobster brunch in the meet hotel. It was a precious golden time—now gone forever!"

Nowadays you are lucky to get 100 hundred people to attend a power competition. Other than the lifters, their training partners, girlfriends or families, no one comes to watch powerlifting anymore. There are a dozen federations all holding "National and World Championships." The pre-scattering competitive environment spawned giants like Kaz, Larry, Coan, Ladiner, Bell, Lamar and Doug. As a result of his intense incubation in the undivided pre-scattering times, Ed Coan soared. If you plotted Incredible Ed's power progress on a chart, it would look like a bullet shot straight up in the air.

Body Weight	Year	Squat	Bench	Deadlift
181	1984	804	501	793
198	1985	859	483	859
219	1991	964	552	901
241	1999	1,003	573	887

He started off at a high level in the early eighties and just kept getting better and better and better…It was one of the most amazing runs in the history of sport. Statistically, the numbers speak for themselves…

Number of times totaling in excess of 2200	30
Number of 900 pound squats	42
Number of 1000 pound squats	1
Number of 500 pound bench presses	45
Number of 800 pound deadlifts	47
Number of 900 pound deadlifts	1
Official World records	22 IPF 27 APF/WPC 27 USPF
Unofficial World records	29
Official USPF National records	39

How the Greatest Powerlifter in History Trained

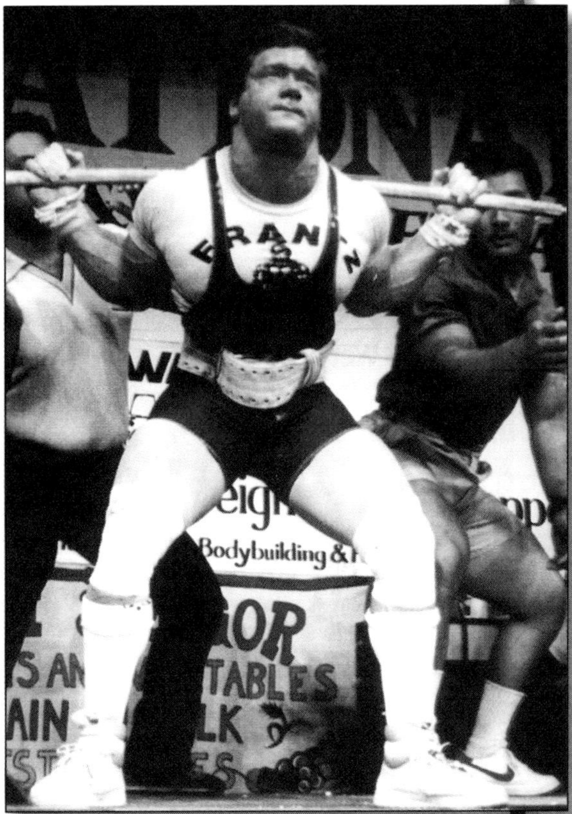

Ed and Doug Furnas took training cues from men like Dennis Wright and Bill Kazmaier. They designed a powerlifting training template that became the standardized training regimen for the great lifters of the eighties and early nineties.

Ed would spend the off-season getting as strong as possible in the three powerlifts, or their close exercise variations, wearing little or no equipment. Then, 14 weeks prior to a major competition, he would commence a powerlifting cycle broken into three, 4 week mesocycles. During each four week cycle, a specific rep sequence would be selected and practiced across the board. Rep reductions were coordinated with the addition of power gear: knee wraps, lifting belt, squat suit, and bench shirt.

Coan had a repertoire of assistance exercises he used religiously. His approach was Purposefully Primitive and simplistic: get as strong as possible in the off-season in a variety of lifts wearing no gear whatsoever, not even a lifting belt. Then, when commencing the powerlifting pre-competition cycle, he would add supportive gear, a bit at a time, every four weeks. This kept his off-season interesting. He was a realist: neither he nor Furnas (nor Karwoski at the end of his career) missed reps in training. This was a testament to Ed's realistic assessment of his abilities. Small incremental steps were systematically taken that eventually delivered him to the predetermined destination.

A typical Coan poundage jump in the squat during the final stages of the cycle would never exceed 20 pounds, a trifling 2% weekly increase for a 1,000 pound squatter. Coan and Furnas were stylistic masters, each developed exercise techniques that fit their respective limb/torso lengths and practiced continually at refining and honing their techniques. They took great pride in technical execution. By staying within the technical boundaries of a lift, by never overestimating their strength levels, by being conservative, both men stayed injury free. This is a classical Coan routine taken from when he was at his absolute zenith. The Furnas template would vary slightly.

Coan Trains

Day	Bodypart	Exercises	Sets/Reps
Monday	Legs	Squat	7-10 x 2-8
		Single leg press	2 x 10-12
		Single leg curl	2 x 10-12
		Leg extensions	2 x 10-12
		Seated calf raise	3 x 10-12
	Abs	Abs	3 x 20
Tuesday	OFF	OFF	OFF
Wednesday	Chest	Bench Press	7-10 x 2-8
		Close grip bench	2 x 2-8 (pauses)
		Incline Press	2 x 2-8
		Triceps extensions	2 x 2-8
	Abs	Abs	3 x 20
Thursday	Shoulders	Press behind the neck	5 x 2-8
		Front dumbbell laterals	3 x 10-12
		Sitting side lateral raises	3 x 10-12
Friday	Back	Deadlifts	8 x 2-8
		Stiff leg deadlift	2 x 8-10
		Bentover rows	2 x 8-10
		T-bar rows	2 x 8-10
		Chin ups	2 x 8-10
		Pulldowns	2 x 8-10
		Bent over dumbbell laterals	2 x 8-10
	Calves	Seated calf raises	1 x 20
	Abs	Abs	3 x 20
Saturday	Light Chest	Light wide grip bench press	3 x 8-10
		Dumbbell flys	2 x 10-15
		Weighted dips	1 x 15
	Arms	Triceps extensions	2 x 2-8
		Barbell curls	1 x 20

In 1999 Coan achieved the highest powerlifting total of all time, regardless of bodyweight, when, weighing 241 pounds, he posted a 2,463 total. This is his 1,003 pound squat. Note the depth and the fact that no monolift was used. I coached Ed at this competition and have always felt that the fact that Bill Kazmaier made the trip to personally watch Ed lift took his performance to another level. Despite handling Ed for years in competition, I had never seen Coan so fired up. When Kaz walked into the backstage warm-up area, I felt an electricity run round the room. It was, "Oh Hell, The Man is here to assess The Man." I felt that Kaz's presence lifted everyone to the next level. As we came off the platform and passed Kaz after the 1,003 squat, I saw Kaz watching from his vantage point, stage left. I asked him, "What did you think of that Kaz?" Big Kaz was ecstatic and said, "Wow! He took that squat so low!" It was the ultimate compliment from the ultimate authority. High praise from Caesar.

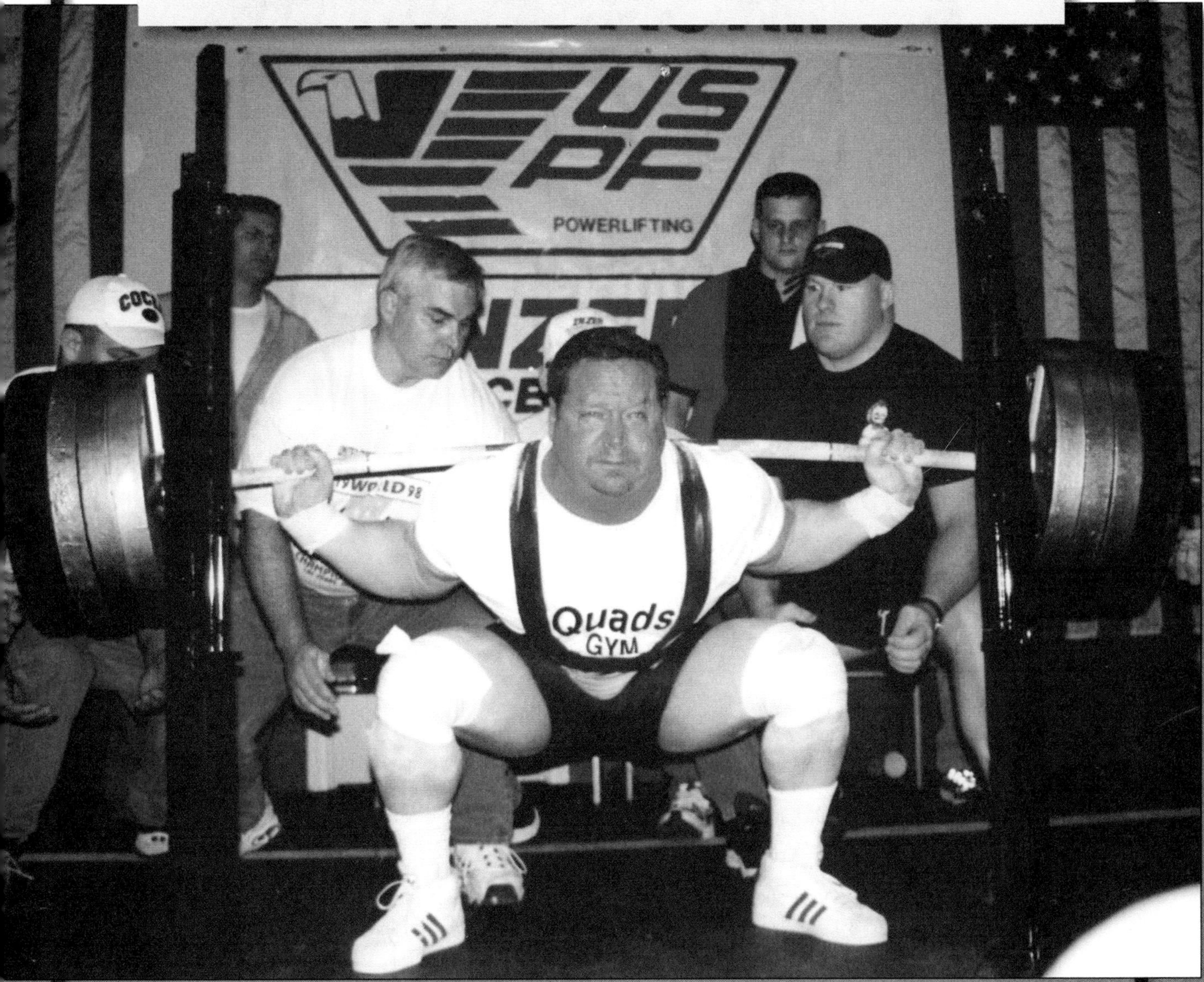

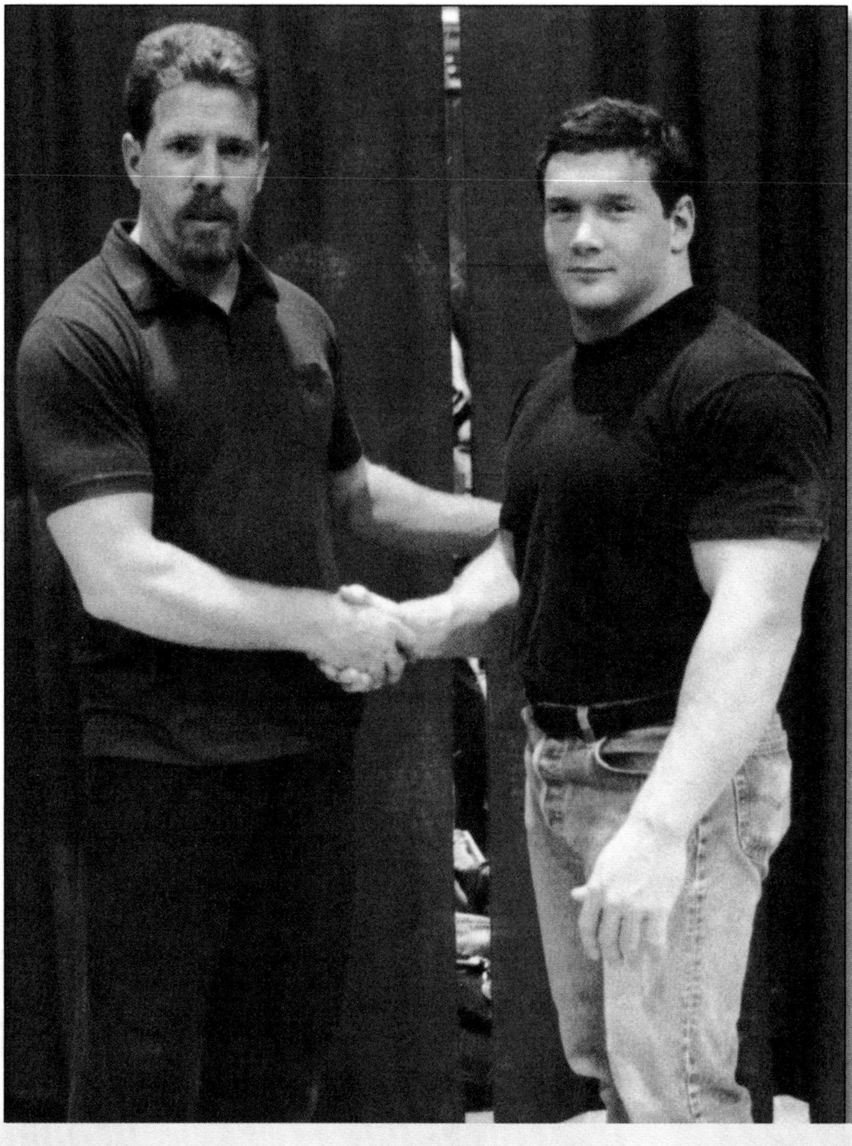

Ed and I after his historic 2400 pound total He weighed 219 pounds. I weighed 235. This gives a frame of reference to Coan's dense thickness and muscular compactness. Note how his huge hands swallow mine despite the fact that I'm five inches taller. How many guys 5-5 wear a size 11 shoe? I once sat behind Ed and Willie Bell at a Black's Gym team meeting. Ed and Willie sat side by side on identical height chairs. Willie was a stud having pulled 830+ at 242. Sitting behind them was eerie: though Willie was five inches taller, sitting down their torso height was identical, highlighting the shortness of Coan's legs. Ed was twice as wide and twice as thick as the heavily muscled Bell, a world champion in his own right. It was a lesson in body leverages and structural architecture that I will not forget.

KEN FANTANO

Power Theoretician

Ever see a man wearing a t-shirt bench press 625 pounds for two reps, each rep paused on the chest? Ever seen a man strict incline press a pair of 200 pound dumbbells, creating a 400 pound payload, for 6 reps, each rep paused on the chest? Ever seen a man bench press with such explosiveness that he snaps the rivets clean off a heavy duty powerbelt? The same guy also squatted 953 ass-on-heels for a double.

Kenny Fantano was unique in every way; like Mark Chaillet, Ken was a fabulous powerlifter who wasn't at all interested in powerlifting-related people, places and events. We spent countless hours in his gym playing cards on the glass-topped counter while a revolving cast of pirate characters would drop by, Fat Pat, Demented Danny, Mic, countless others would rotate in

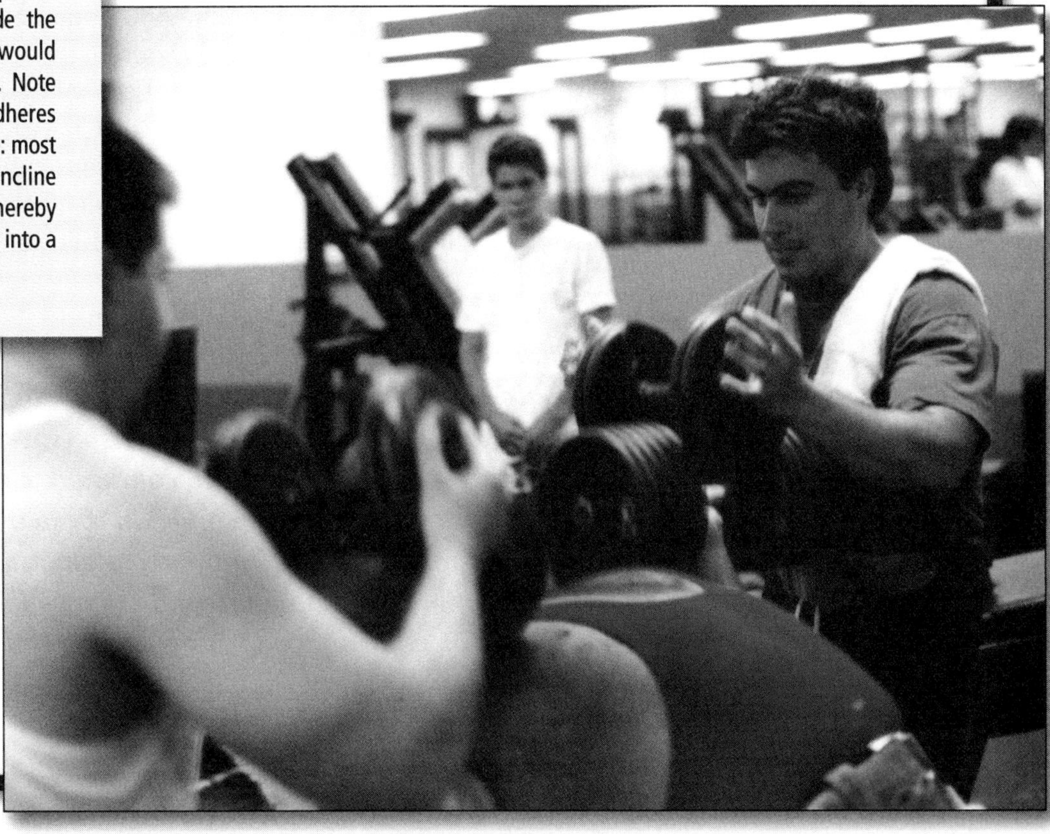

The boys balance a pair of 55's atop 145's to create a pair of 200 pound dumbbells in order to provide the requisite resistance. Ken would perform 6 strict paused reps. Note how his incline posture adheres tightly to the 45 degree bench: most men faced with max incline poundage arch upward thereby turning the incline bench press into a flat bench.

and out of the afternoon pinochle games. Amongst the card players the talk would range far and wide...sports, women, TV, movies, yet when the talk turned to powerlifting gossip Ken clammed up like a Mafioso being grilled in front of a Senate Subcommittee. While the rest of us would babble on about this or that power personality, place or event, Ken would study his cards and stay silent until another topic more to his liking arose. A great lifter, a formidable power theoretician, he was not the slightest bit interested in the politics, personalities or the minutiae of our weird fringe sport.

He stood 5'10" and weighed 365 pounds in top condition. His massive body was tight and taut with not an ounce of flab, his massive gut stretched hard against his skin. To poke or punch that gut was to poke or punch concrete. He was athletic, explosive, nimble and agile. Ken reminded me of the great athletic comedienne Jackie Gleason who could break into a frantic, incredible dance routine and at the end flip himself over. Ken had that same big man dancer-like athletic agility.

Every day when the weather was right, the Muscle Factory gym rats would head out back to the parking lot and play wiffle ball, the child's game, in savage Rollerball/Thunderdome-like fashion. Monstrous musclemen incongruously playing baseball with a plastic ball and bat, exhorting or damning each other, loudly, profanely, with a streak of taunting nastiness. Neighborhood kids would hear the swearing and commotion and flock to participate. It was a surreal blending of powerlift monsters, thugs and innocent kids, all playing wiffle ball with incredible intensity. Kenny batted "cow-handed." He was a lefty yet batted with his right hand overtop of his left from a left-handed stance. Once a 12 year old boy new to this game and oblivious as to how powerful an adult with a 600 pound bench press actually is, acted stupid. The kid was playing 3rd base and would continually crowd home plate in a batter-intimidating move. When Fantano came up to bat, Danny D yelled "BACK UP KID!" But the overly aggressive tweeny was looking to impress—CRACK! Too late! The kid ate a 200 mile per hour wiffle ball, a line drive blast right to his skull. He lay on the parking lot pavement, bleeding a little. No one rushed to his aide. Ken got a double out of it and as he stood on 2nd base he yelled at the prone youth, "THAT'LL TEACH YOU! YOU DUMB ASS KID!"

I moved to New England in 1988 to take a job running a warehouse in Milford, Connecticut. It was an 80,000 square foot steel warehouse that had an exclusive contract with the Irish Government to offload and store steel girders. They had continual employee problems with the crew of rough necks that worked in the warehouse. There was a liquor store across the street from the warehouse and at lunchtime half the warehouse workers would walk across the street and buy 40 ounce quarts of malt liquor or pints of Richard's Wild

Irish Rose. They would blatantly sit on the curb across from the warehouse in plain view and guzzle down the booze. After their liquid lunch, they would stagger back across the road to go back to work.

The drunks would move 5,000 pound steel beams using forklifts and overhead cranes. Ever seen a drunken warehouseman operate an overhead crane with a steel beam feebly attached? Quite frightening. The then warehouse supervisor was a politically-correct, politically-connected guy: his brother-in-law ran the largest port in the area. My boss had hired him as a favor. As a foreman, he was nice to a fault. He believed that "what the men do on their lunch hour, off property, was none of our business and beyond our control." His politically correct stance was heartfelt. He always "stood up" for the rights of "his men."

The whole enchilada exploded when a belligerent, drunken warehouseman half-ass hooked up a forty foot I-beam and while transporting the monster down one of the bays, had it bust loose and fall 25 feet. It crashed into one of the 50 rows of 12 foot high stacked steel and set off a domino effect that caused one row of girders to crash into the next...and the next...and the next...

No one was killed or injured, but an entire bay was shut down for a month as over 2,000 40 foot steel beams had to be picked up, sorted and restacked, one stinking beam at a time. It looked like a game of pic-up-stix with steel girders. The cleanup required three men working all day everyday. The foreman refused to fire the guy who caused it. "You can't accuse him of being drunk—you have no proof!" My boss had enough of this jailhouse lawyer and kicked him upstairs. Enter Marty G. and Biggie W. I was brought in along with "Biggie W," an infamous longshoreman enforcer known around the Baltimore docks as "one punch." We cleaned house. I got things squared away with Biggie W's help and now, with a big raise and time on my hands, I turned my attention back to training.

Powerlifting Architecture

For a guy who hated to talk about powerlifting gossip, Ken Fantano had sure as hell thought long and hard about powerlift biomechanics. His treatise on bench pressing was light years passed anything I'd ever encountered, before or since. He'd sit at the glass-topped counter of his funk-a-fied gym, The Muscle Factory in West Haven Connecticut, find a scrap of paper and a pencil and begin a detailed explanation on how and why he and his amigos bench pressed the way they did. He had bear paw mitts and looking at him you would have thought he'd be better suited to use crayons. When he picked up a sharpened pencil, he suddenly exhibited a deftness and neatness in his drawings that fairly screamed art student! Actually, his drawings owed more to structural engineering than art. He would produce a series of drawings, precise little bench press replications, each captured a different portion, a different point-in-time of the patented Fantano-style bench press. He would quickly and expertly sketch a stick figure lying on a bench and as he drew (left handed) he would verbally run down his approach.

His commentary was quiet, yet infused with insight and disconcertingly laced with the expert use of sailor profanity. It was spellbinding for those who understood bench pressing. "First mistake Mart: everyone lowers the barbell way too high on the chest. Way too close to the neck. We touch the bar low—way low—just above where the belly meets the sternum." He would abandon Stick Man Drawing Number I and start on stick man bencher Number II, this one with the bar halfway to the chest, "All kinds of things happen as the bar is lowered...the legs are progressively loaded with more and more tension; the leg tension maxes as the bar touches the chest. We purposefully let the bar sink into the chest. We pull the weight *into* the torso, pause the sunken weight and when we hear the referee yell, PRESS! BAM! It's on!" He zeroed in on the paused bar. "To commence the push, we jam the legs backwards *hard* towards the torso. The leg jolt continues into the torso, ending in the chest. We purposefully create a jolt. The jolt, timed right and executed with enough power and push, creates momentum where there was none." He drew my attention to the legs of stickman II.

"A correct leg drive starts at the feet. It travels through the legs and ends up entering the prone torso. This sends a *freaking shock wave* through the torso Mart. We time the bar push to start at that *exact instant* when the leg shockwave passes into the torso and up and under the barbell. When the shock wave arrives at the barbell, the chest/shoulder/arm muscles contract explosively. The jolt is combined with an expansion of the chest and waist. As the chest is expanded the muscles of the shoulders, pecs and triceps are contracted. It launches the barbell skyward like it's been shot out of a cannon Mart."

Ken had learned how to expand his chest/waist so dramatically and powerfully that he literally ripped the rivets off specially made reinforced powerlifting belts, tearing the monster steel buckle clean off the thick leather. "The leg drive and chest/waist expansion and muscle contractions get the bar moving upward." He was on to Phase III. "Now that we get the bar moving upward off the chest explosively—if you do it right Mart, the bar *leaps* off the chest. It all depends on the timing." He paused to check and see if I was on his wavelength. I was. It was akin to being an actor watching DiNiro on The Actor's Studio. Assured I was paying attention, he forged ahead. "As the bar leaves the chest and heads upward; we don't push straight up we use a rearward arc-pathway. We move the bar, started off low on the chest, up and back, in a slow curve."

Ken would draw a second barbell at lockout; this atop the drawing of the lifter with the barbell low on his chest at the start. He'd then draw a dotted arc line from the low-on-the-chest barbell at takeoff to the bar in the completed position. His explanation was genius to the informed. "The optimal arc should look like this..." He paused to sketch in the arc, "The arc means the angle of the upper arm doesn't change or straighten through the first 7/8ths of the push. The elbow angle stays intact until the last 1/8th of the push." Done with the written explanation he'd walk over to a bench and demonstrate. It all made perfect sense. Seeing him bench was pure poetry. His bench press nuances were subtle and teachable: his three training partners all had 600 pound bench presses.

Ken had equally iconic ideas about how to construct a long-range power training template. He took 20-24 weeks, training methodically to prepare for national competitions. Phase I took 12 weeks and was dedicated to elevating the athlete to the highest possible level of strength conditioning before embarking on the final pre-competition push known as Phase II. "We have Phase I goals and those goals are *more important* than Phase II goals. If you don't make the Phase I goals, no matter what you do later, it's *not* going to work. There's no trick in the world that if you fail in Phase I you're going shine at the meet."

Ken felt heavy incline bench pressing with dumbbells was where he gained "all my muscle and strength for competitive benching." The bench press, he felt, "is a technique lift. I built my bench press *power* using paused reps in the incline bench press." He felt heavy incline pressing needed to be done using a specific procedure: "In the off season, during Phase I, we incline bench press for four sets of six reps." In order to move poundage up, multiple sets with a top weight were required. "If you did four work sets using 100, 105, 110 and 115 pounds dumbbells for six reps in week 1, in week 2 you *don't* get to move up to a pair of 120 pound bells on the top set. You won't make it. Instead you go 105, 110 and *two* sets with the 115's. The following week push the 105 pound bell then do *three* sets of six paused reps with the 115's...NOW you're ready for 105, 110, 115 and 120 x 6. You need to make three sets with the top poundage before you're ready for the jump upward."

All of Fantano's flat benches and incline benches were paused on every rep of every set. Why? "If you don't pause all the reps, you're wasting your time. If you don't have strength from a dead stop, muscle tissue won't get thicker." In his Phase I cycle prior to squatting 953x2, Ken front squatted 700 x 6 using a cross-hand grip. This told him his raw leg strength "was there" and laid the groundwork for a successful Phase II squatting regimen. On four successive Sundays leading up to the 1989 APF Senior Nationals he squatted 881x3, 913x2, 931x2 and 953x2. At the actual competition his designs on a 963 squat were derailed when he broke a rotator cuff on his 942 second attempt squat. Severely injured he still bench pressed 606 less than an hour later. His shoulder surgeon later told him he had bench pressed six hundred pounds "using one arm."

"The Weight Don't Care; It Has Only One Friend: Gravity!"

Sunday Phase II training sessions could take four hours to complete. Fantano had specific ideas about rest periods between sets.

"We want to lift everything on a 'calm heart.' People don't realize that to be a super strong person you have to always work in the anaerobic zone. If you don't have nitrogen in your blood you don't have *nothing!* You might as well go home.

To work in the aerobic zone is a waste of time; you want to gas the oxygen out of your system. You want to force your system to burn the oxygen up and force it to store more nitrogen—that's why we hold our breath during an entire set.

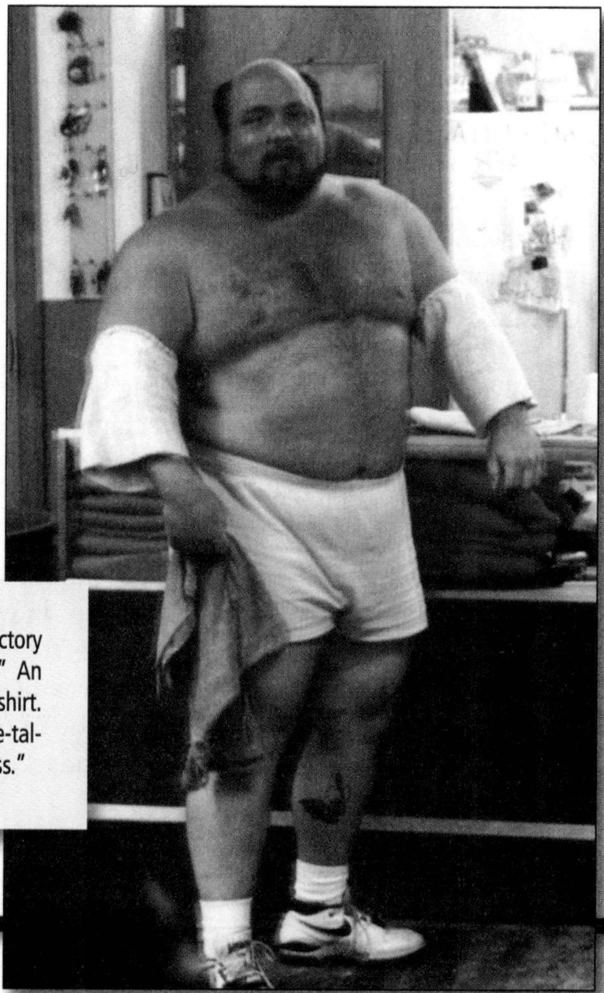

Ken Fantano stands in front of the Muscle Factory counter modeling his patented "elbow warmers." An hour later Ken bench pressed 640 without a bench shirt. Note how tight his physique is. I would call him "Eye-tal-eye-an Thick Bitch." He would call me "Irish wise ass."

Oxygen can't help you, anyway. Breathing during a set is just a panic device. You breathe because you are scared or nervous. New oxygen takes 20 seconds to get to a muscle: we hold our breath, let the oxygen burn off, we want to use the nitrogen."

When the nitrous oxide-infused Muscle Factory Boys rolled into their 8 to 12 week pre-competition Phase II cycle, the weights really started to fly. Prior to bench pressing 625x2 Ken finished his "light" Phase I benching cycle with 500 for 10 paused reps. He blasted up 565x6 paused reps on his heavy day. He was shooting for a 650 bench press at the competition and knew he would need to bench 625x2 in the gym. Normally a 625 double would convert into a 660 or 670x1 bench press; however having to squat 880, 940 and 965 at the meet prior to bench pressing would realistically knock 30 to 50 pounds off his competition bench press.

He started Phase II by bench pressing 500x6 using 5 second pauses between each rep. In successive weeks he pushed 510x6, 520x6, 530x6, 550x2, 575x2, 600x2 and 625x2. Immediately after bench pressing (on Wednesday) Ken performed "light" dumbbell inclines. He used a pair of 150's and hit 2-3 sets of 10. He would always drive the bells "up and together in order to get the muscle contraction I am looking for." After bench pressing and light inclines he would perform three sets of 3 reps in the close grip flat bench. He closed gripped 550 for three paused reps in the flat bench in the same workout he doubled 625. The Wednesday bench day workout would be concluded with 3-4 sets of 15-20 reps in the triceps pushdown: high rep, fast pace, complete lockout on each and every set. The Wednesday routine took 2-3 hours.

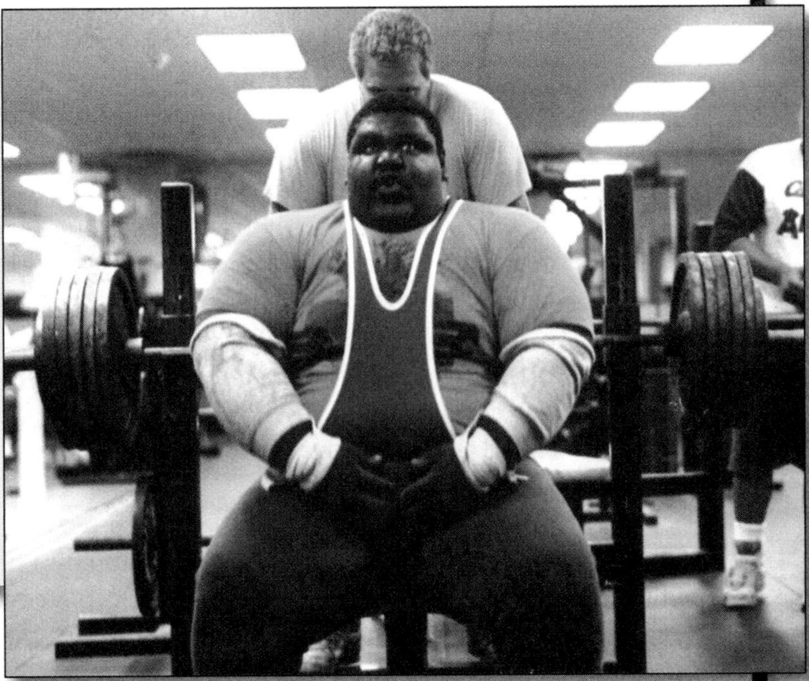

The boys benching at the Muscle Factory: 420 pound Jean Donat readies himself prior to bench pressing 555x5, all paused reps. Danny D leans forward to offer JD a secret psyche phrase. Note the elbow warmers and the lack of a bench shirt. Jean officially squatted 940. At 5'6" Jean could leap and run like a deer. Jean was a gentle giant and had been a star baseball catcher before taking up powerlifting. Danny had also come from a baseball background.

Jean Donat and Ken would stroll around the gym with their arm warmers looking like deranged street people. Soon Danny and others began wearing arm warmers. I just sat and drank beer and marveled at all the idiosyncratic anomalies. I'd seen a thousand weird things at Mark's gym and in Hugh's basement. Hugh once tried training using blue light bulbs for gym light after he'd read something in Scientific American about colored lights affecting athletic performance. I was witnessing New England flavored eccentricities.

Danny once yelled halfway through a bench session, "Hey Mart! Pick up the phone and order us a PIE from next door— that way it'll be ready as soon as were done." Mystified, I said, "A pie?! What kinda pie? Pecan? Apple? Banana Cream? The boys thought that was the funniest thing they'd ever heard. Pizza was called Pie in New York/New England. The boys thought I talked funny...which was odd because they talked exactly like the guys from the Sopranos, and this was 15 years before the Soprano's were invented. Powerlifters spend a lot of time with each other and develop group identities. This leads to group psychosis and mad antics. As Mad Irish I fit right in with the West Haven crew.

Power Enduro

Sunday was "Squat Day" at the Muscle Factory: the gym was closed to the public and entry was by invite only. The workouts were deadly simple and decidedly similar to what I had seen at Cassidy's and Chaillet's. The squat procedure was to take as many warm-ups as needed. Ken needed a lot: he had old knee and back injuries from athletics and he was guarded in his descents. He might take 10 warm-up sets before he would be ready for the three top squat work sets. The number of repetitions would be dependent on the nearness of the competition: never more than six reps, never fewer than two. The three work sets would be "poundage spaced" to replicate competitive condition.

If Ken, Jean or Dan were working up to 900x2 reps on a particular day, the three top sets might be 820x2, 860x1-2 and 900x2. This would roughly replicate a 1st, 2nd and 3rd attempt squat if they were hypothetically competing on that particular day. Like Ed Coan the Muscle Factory boys never did single reps in any lift. Ken and Jean didn't wear bench shirts. "Too much of a hassle Mart." Was Ken's curt reply when I asked him why he gave away needless pounds to other competitors. The discomfort and aggravation of wearing the shirt was not worth the 30-40 pound bump the bench shirts of the day provided. On Sunday it could take four hours to train.

There was a methodical pace to these enduro sessions. The men would plow through the work using a mechanical approach. They wanted to lift on calm hearts and it might take five minutes or more for 300-plus pound men to recover from a giant weight and achieve the completely revitalized state.

There would be a big crowd, at least 10 guys. The squats were followed by deadlifts. Again the procedure was super simple: work up to a series of top sets, usually 2-3 rep sets. Ken and Dan were in the 700 deadlift club, but Jean had hands the size of Mary Kate Olson and could not hang on to anything past 620. They were serious about improving this obvious weak point and they worked the deadlift hard. The Sunday session took forever and it was all solid work. All were athletic and they pushed each other mercilessly. It was a great core group and a great lifter auxiliary. Crazed Dan wore a suit, wraps, and a belt on every single squat set, 135, 255, 345, 455, 545, 655, 745, 835 and 900. Why? "'Cause I don't want to use a *single extra ounce* of my available strength until I get to 900+." Okay, but a 900 pound squat guy wearing knee wraps and squat suit on 135?! It smacked of psychological illness. Ken overheard me and said, "Don't bother trying to talk no sense to him Mart—he's got cement for brains."

Fantano Phase II Competition Training Template

Day	Exercise	Sets/Reps
Wednesday	Bench press	Three top sets, 40 lbs between each set
	Incline dumbbell press	Three top sets of 10 reps - static
	Narrow grip flat bench	Three top sets of 3 reps, 40 lbs between each set
	Triceps pushdowns	Three to four sets of 15-25 reps
Sunday	Squat	Three top sets, 40 lbs between each set
	Deadlift	Work up to top set of 2-3 reps
	Light bench press	Three sets 10 reps, 500 lbs paused

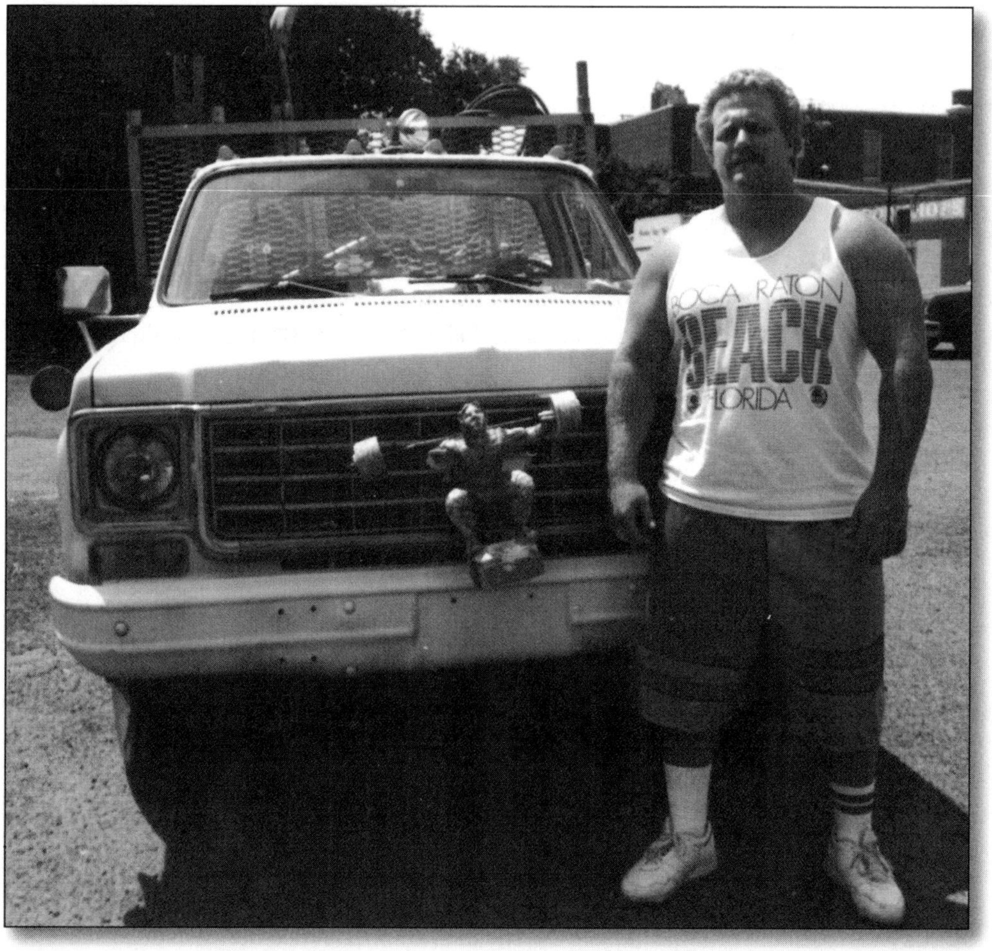

The infamous Danny D. had a 940 pound squat, a 600 pound bench press and a 720 pound deadlift weighing 270 at around 5'8". He worked 10-12 hour days as a fence installer and stands in the Muscle Factory parking lot in front of his fencing truck. Note the squat trophy lashed to the grill. Danny was quick tempered and mercurial: he had been a topflight baseball player in high school. He would fight at the drop of a hat. He once beat a guys' ass in a bar fight at a biker bar and then kept the loser in a headlock the rest of the evening. He held the guys' head and neck tight with one arm while he drank with the other. "HEY! Look at my hunting trophy!" He'd yell as he showed off his captive to newcomers. He held the guy this way for three hours and had to be stopped by other lifters from extracting a gold filling from the poor bastard's mouth.

DORIAN YATES

The Iron Monk

Dorian Yates marched to the beat of a profoundly different drummer. Aptly nicknamed, "The Diesel," Yates was iconoclastic in the truest sense. During his formative teenage years he was swept up by the street turmoil of the English punk rock scene. Fueled by reggae, The Clash and the youthful nihilism and disenfranchisement of the era, he became "a troubled youth" and was actually introduced to weight training in reform school. He was the embodiment of the classical English Hard Man and grew up wild; the archetypical alpha male, cruising the tough streets of Birmingham. He and his street mates might engage in soccer hooliganism or become embroiled in "dust-ups" with rivals or civilians that didn't demonstrate proper deference. As Elton wrote,

> *I'm the juvenile product*
> *Of the working class,*
> *Whose best friend*
> *Floats in the bottom*
> *of a glass...*

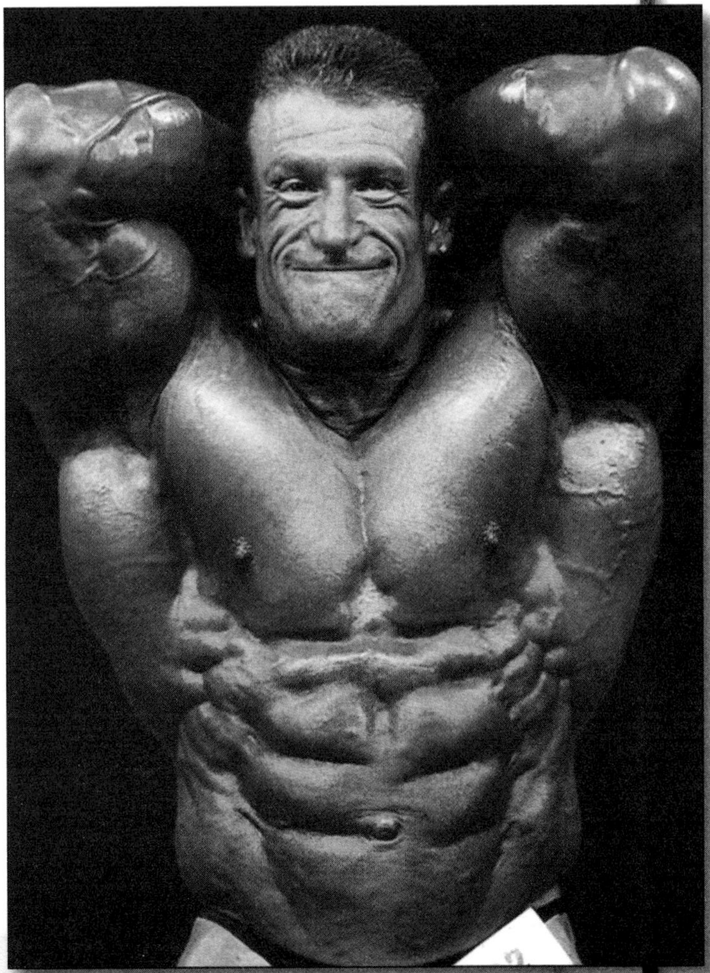

The Olympian Dominator: Breathtaking muscular size and always the lowest body fat percentile of any man onstage. Yates was the King of Bodybuilders, yet unlike so many elite bodybuilders, Dorian was never an adulation junkie. He had an intense personality and working class sensibilities that masked his innovative intelligence.

Somewhere along the way Dorian found physical and psychological solace in the intense solitude of intense weight training. He began redirecting his incoherent rage from the street to the gym. He discovered he possessed an uncanny ability to effortlessly impose rigid self-discipline. He became an Iron Monk. He immersed himself in the fringe sport of competitive bodybuilding and discovered he was genetically and psychologically predisposed towards it. He melded and shaped his body with an ease that flabbergasted his gym peers.

Isaac Stern once said of Mozart, "*In a single nine month period at age fourteen he composed five violin sonatas; the maturity between the 1st and 5th represented thirty years of growth.*" Dorian Yates underwent a bodybuilding version of Mozart's musical metamorphosis. He rose from obscurity to world class in an amazingly short amount of time. In 1991 he took second place at the Mr. Olympia, bodybuilding's Superbowl. In 1992 Yates' reign of utter and complete dominance commenced. Dorian won the Olympia title six successive years starting in 1992.

From the start he stood defiantly apart from the bodybuilding establishment in every aspect of his life, training and approach. The epicenter of the bodybuilding universe was, is, and forever shall be, Southern California. While the Southern California scene provides a terrific environment for those who want to center their entire existence on bodybuilding, that which makes it attractive also generates sameness in terms of the final finished physical products. Most of the top SoCal bodybuilders used the same nutritional and training methods and for this reason the top pros tended to look pretty much the same. As a result of this physical echo chamber there emerged a definable group with no major physical differences. This coterie of physique champions clustered together and became infected with inside-the-box group think. There was one glaring exception: the super symmetrical Flex Wheeler. He was awesome and formidable.

Dorian Yates was the antithesis of West Coast bodybuilding. He lived in dreary, overcast Birmingham, England ensconced in a dank dungeon. He trained and ate in a radically different way; completely counter to California bodybuilding. As a result he built a body unlike anyone else.

The Quantum Leap Forward

When Dorian took second place to Lee Haney in 1991 he weighed 239 pounds. He made his bones by coming in large and in "ripped" condition. He likely carried a 4% body fat percentile. Yates' symmetry and shape, while good, was not great. What set him apart that night was excellent size and astounding muscular condition; the best in the competition. In 1992 Dorian captured his first Olympia title weighing 242 pounds. He was infinitesimally better than the previous year. He had the same great condition with a few added pounds of muscle and it was a nice win.

The California professionals were uniformly unimpressed and began making disparaging remarks about the new Mr. Olympia, stating that his reign would last a single year and he should be grateful that he had won a single Sandow Statue. The following year, the intellegensia concluded, the competition would be held stateside, in Atlanta, not in some gawd-foresaken dump like Helsinki, Finland where Dorian had won. Then the rightful reign of the West Coast men would commence.

Yates heard the smack talk back in Birmingham and used the disparaging remarks to generate a cold fury that fueled his training sessions. He went deep into the proverbial Iron Woodshed. When he emerged, he had transformed himself from a large, extremely well conditioned bodybuilder into a gargantuan, ripped-to-shreds mega-monster. He was huge, bigger than anyone when viewed from front, side or back. He was now the biggest *and* the most muscular bodybuilder in the world. The moment he strode onstage at the 1993 Mr. Olympia contest, all the other bodybuilders knew that the only battle was for 2nd and 3rd place.

Yates was striated and defined; every tiny muscle visible beneath what appeared to be translucent skin. He was now the biggest *and* the most fat-free bodybuilding in the world. Yates had added 20 pounds of pure muscle in twelve months, unheard of at these stratospheric levels where men are already at 99% of their genetic capacity. Dorian blew up to just under 300 pounds in the off-season while not allowing his body fat to rise above 10%, even at his heaviest bodyweight. He carved that massive mound of muscle into a 260 pound piece of human marble.

At the professional level, bodybuilders are already at the peak of their awesome genetic potential and improvement is measured in tiny steps. A bodybuilder might be able to lean out a bit, or perhaps over the course of a good year add 3 to 5 pounds of muscle. This would represent a significant bodyweight increase if muscular clarity and crispness were maintained. For an Olympia winner to add twenty pounds of lean mass while actually improving muscular delineation was unprecedented.

The shock waves first hit when the December 1993 issue of *Flex* Magazine appeared featuring photos of Yates weighing 271 pounds. He displayed definition nearly matching what he had exhibited in Helsinki weighing 239. He whittled down to 257 pounds for the Atlanta Olympia and pounded the competition into dust. The Diesel ran over the competition with such yawning ease that no further smack talk was heard from the West Coast elite. Another reign was underway. Lee Haney managed a record eight straight wins and Dorian Yates picked right up where Lee left off, racking up six straight Olympia wins.

Blood & Guts: Film Noir Extraordinaire

Film noir literally means "black film" in French and features themes that are uniformly negative. The feel is always dark and shadowy and purposefully filmed in black and white. Most noir stories feature main characters who find themselves embroiled in hopeless situations, fighting against forces that threaten them.

In 1999 Dorian Yates made the greatest bodybuilding training film of all time, appropriately named *Blood & Guts*. It was unintentional film noir at its best. Dorian and his savage training partner, the incendiary Leroy, video taped their *exact* workouts, exercise by exercise, set by set, rep by rep, for an entire week of training. Not a word of commentary or explanation from Dorian. No charts, no graphs, no product whoring, no nothing other than the indomitable Dorian powering through four workouts. The stark black and white photography is crisp and grim. The setting is Yates' infamous Temple Street Gym, a claustrophobic downstairs dungeon with damp walls, cracked plaster, ill lighting, musty old exercise machines and tons of free weights.

Silent, stoic, stolid, grim and intense, Yates plowed through these brutal workouts. His workouts more resemble an Ed Coan power training session at Quads Gym in Chicago than a Southern California pump & preen session using pee-wee poundage. This is grim stuff; Yates pushes 425 for 6 reps in the incline press before Leroy steps in and provides an additional agonizing forced rep. Watch as Dorian does arms curls. Watch as Leroy provides barely enough impetus to keep the final reps moving. In another snippet, Dorian readies himself prior to pulling 400+ in the barbell row. He chides himself, saying out loud "*It's a big weight—for a little woman!*" With that he strides forward and pulverizes the poundage. Leroy, a former army drill sergeant, screams at the top of his lungs in indecipherable military profanity using a street-seasoned cockney accent that would scare the shit out of Tony Soprano.

> ***"Let's get Nasty! C'mon Mr. Yates, the one who's in all the BLOODY MAG-A-ZINES! Pull and squeeze. DIG DEEP! LET'S GO!—MIGHTY PULL! AGAIN!! ALL YOU—NOW ANOTHER—PULL! ONE MORE! MIGHTY PULL! AGAIN!!!"***

Spittle flies from Leroy's mouth as Yates inhales the exhortations and uses pent-up psychological fury to finish rep after rep. It is chilling, terrifying, painful and inspiring to watch...see Dorian finish the 12th rep with 1265 pounds in the leg press, then cry out in pain as Leroy blows off Dorian's "*Sissy talk!*" He exhorts Dorian to do yet another. Watch as Yates throws caution to the wind. He let's out a war whoop, unlocks his quivering legs and in fact does do yet another rep, barely locking out even with Leroy's help.

My friend, muscle writer supreme, Julian Schmidt, major domo at Flex Magazine, told me that during the filming the camera crew told Dorian that they had inadvertently messed up filming a top set of a particular exercise. They asked that he stage a re-shoot; he told them without hesitation, "Well I suppose you'll just have to return next week when I do that exercise again because I don't stage *anything!*" And so they did. Dorian weighed 295 pounds in the film and was so gargantuan that he appeared inhuman. His technical execution was beyond reproach.

Blood & Guts is pure genius: why talk to death that which can be far better understood by watching? Why spend 20 minutes talking about how to do a proper 70 degree barbell row when everything can be made clear by watching the perfection master perform the 70 degree row? Why *talk* about workout pace, show it. Show full range-of-motion, show technical subtlety, show good spotting, show the meaning of true workout intensity, show the meaning of the teeth-grinding effort required to trigger muscle hypertrophy.

Everything can be communicated so much better by showing: demonstrate how the real deal looks when done by the very best in the world as they actually ply their trade. You could watch Blood & Guts with the sound turned off and come away knowing every important lesson there is to know about building gigantic muscles. You come to understand that in order to build muscle you must work hard enough to trigger muscle hypertrophy. Going through the motions builds nothing of any consequence.

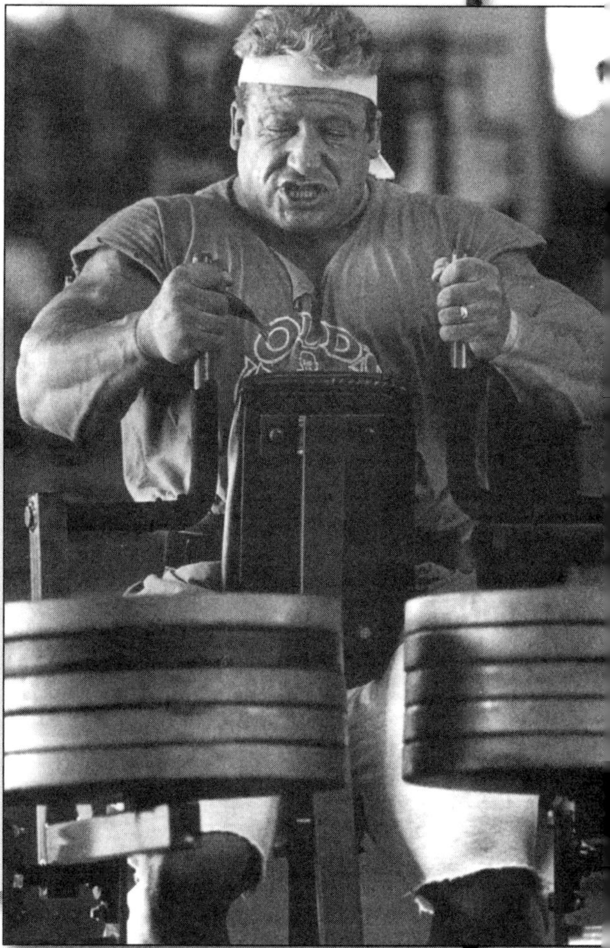

Dorian Yates built a physique unlike anything anyone had ever seen using techniques and tactics unlike anything anyone had ever used. The man was as strong as he looked. Yates hoisted incredible poundage adhering to the ultimate proviso: technical execution of each lift must be pure perfection. A bodybuilder seeking the most effective way to stimulate the maximum amount of muscle fiber needs to use a full and complete range-of-motion. Regardless if the exercise is a shrug or an overhead press, lateral raise or row. Yates' goal is to isolate the muscle being targeted.

He also ate like a man and never went below 3,500 calories. His food selections were sane and sensible. He was a smart and innovative bodybuilding theoretician whose unique approach to bodybuilding was incredibly effective. I loved his persona and attitude; he was a no nonsense individual who personified complete dedication.

My Day with Dorian

In 1996 I was the lead correspondent at the Chicago Olympia for *Muscle & Fitness* Magazine. I sat in the front row and would write the competition coverage and additionally interview the winner the next day to write a body part training article. I watched with glee as Dorian crushed the competition yet again. I wrote the feature lead on the competition in about 20 minutes and was really excited about the next day. I would be with a guy I really admired and was doing the body part feature article on what I considered his greatest physical attribute, his back. This was gonna be great.

Dorian's famous elbow warmers the photographer's nightmare: The Diesel always insisted that he wear these funky, torn and frayed elastic elbow sleeves in photo shoots. It was his way of saying, "I wear these when I train and you are taking training shots. The elbow warmers add realism into your posed and glossy photos." Many a photographer overstepped their bounds and asked that he take them off. Photographers were fearful and rightfully so, of incurring Dorian's wrath. Many were pressured mercilessly by management to "get the champ to use more poundage on the exercise shots." Sometimes if he was in the mood, he would.

I saw one rabbit-like artiste photographer confront the Diesel and his fearsome posse prior to a photo shoot. "Dorian, the boss asks if you can **please take off those things!** And use more poundage! The other contract bodybuilders are loading up 800 in the squats and 1600 on leg press photos...we **need you** to commit to the process." Need I explain the severity of the shit-storm that ensued? It was horrific. On that particular day, a back training session the day after the Olympia, he said, "One plate per side—that's it!" End of conversation! Plus he wore **those things**—the elbow warmers stayed.

After being put up in a penthouse suite; after seeing the prejudging and the Olympia finals from the front row; after having walked backstage into an atmosphere so strained and tense you could cut it with a knife; I would get to meet with the champ Sunday morning. I would be with Dorian for a lengthy photo shoot; interview him, write up a back training article and catch a plane home later that day. I made a lot of dough that weekend for the privilege of grilling one of my idols on what I wanted to know about most: how in the hell did you build a back like that? Dorian's back training photo shoot began at 10 am and went on for

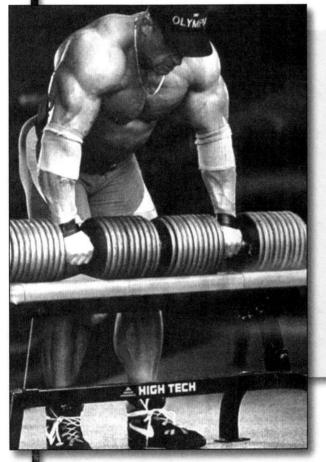

for hours. It was obviously draining but important: the two articles would be multi-page magazine feature pieces.

I was fortunate enough to see him in tiptop shape that morning, up close and personal, he actually looked better than he did the previous night. After winning the Olympia the previous night, he could not party. If he had eaten or drank anything he would lose his perfect condition and ruin the back-to-back photo sessions scheduled for the next morning. As soon as he was finished with the back body part photo shoot Dorian had to roll right into another body part photo shoot with a different photographer. I actually felt sorry for him.

I arrived early and he invited me to sit with him as the camera crew set up. He munched on a dry bagel and looked drawn and very tired. It had to be torturous to win the Olympia and not even be able to drink a beer or have a good meal afterwards. We would talk between exercise shots about his training. Leroy and Steve Weinberger were there to assist. Yates was very short and obstinate towards the photographers, but exceedingly nice to me. They were trying to get him to lift gargantuan poundage to make the photos look more dramatic and he was having none of it. A lone 45 pound plate on each side of the barbell or machine was all he would allow. The photographers were being pressured by headquarters to use massive weights and were tearing their hair out in frustration. Dorian also insisted on wearing the elbow warmers that he always wore for every single workout.

He told me he weighed 261 and standing 5'10" with an incredible tan, his skin appeared transparent. Every time he lifted his arm to take a bite of bagel, muscle and sinew shot across his forearm, upper arm and deltoids in waves. When he chewed, all the muscles of his face were visible and rolled in syncopation with every bite. His lower back and glutes were so stripped of fat that with every step cross striations appeared. He was at once, the most muscular and most defined human I had ever seen, before or since. He liked the two articles I had written about him in the past year. One article discussed the similarities between his training and that of Ed Coan. The other article talked about how he was whipping West Coast ass. He found the Coan article "fascinating stuff." He later gave my book on Ed Coan a great endorsement. My article on Dorian's back attack "wrote itself." I finished it on the plane ride home.

His body on that day was pure perfection. To see this great champion up close and personal after a steamroller win was fabulous. Yates was known for his single-minded dedication and would famously duck out of social events early saying, "I hate to part good company, but tomorrow is leg day and I need to go home and rest."

During his reign Dorian was the antithesis of a glad-handing ego maniac craving attention. Quite the contrary: he was a man of few words and at competitive events was ominous and unapproachable. One year I was at the Olympia and as I sat eating lunch with

Julian Schmidt, The Diesel and his posse strode through the restaurant. They stopped for no one; they were on the move. The eatery, crammed with elite bodybuilders, came to a complete halt for "The Man" and his Praetorians. No back slapping or greetings were offered or given. He avoided eye contact with everyone. He happened to glance in our direction and saw the two of us. He stopped and his crew pulled up. "Jul-eye-an...Martee." He said. He gave the two of us the slightest of nods and the faintest of smiles then wheeled around and his muscle armada continued onward. One boneheaded bodybuilding pro card holder yelled over at us, "DAMN! I have been saying hello to that *big bitch* for five years and he's never so much as smiled or acknowledged I existed! Who in the hell are you guys!"

It was a scene as I imagined it might have been in feudal Japan when a Shogun Samurai chieftain passed through a village. He had far more detractors and enemies than friends within the cloistered world of bodybuilding. Many bodybuilders are narcissists, adulation junkies that crave attention and applause. Not the iconoclastic Yates. For Dorian Yates the process was the reward. Competition was the requisite report card. In a sea of sameness, he stood out like a unicorn amongst a herd of sheep.

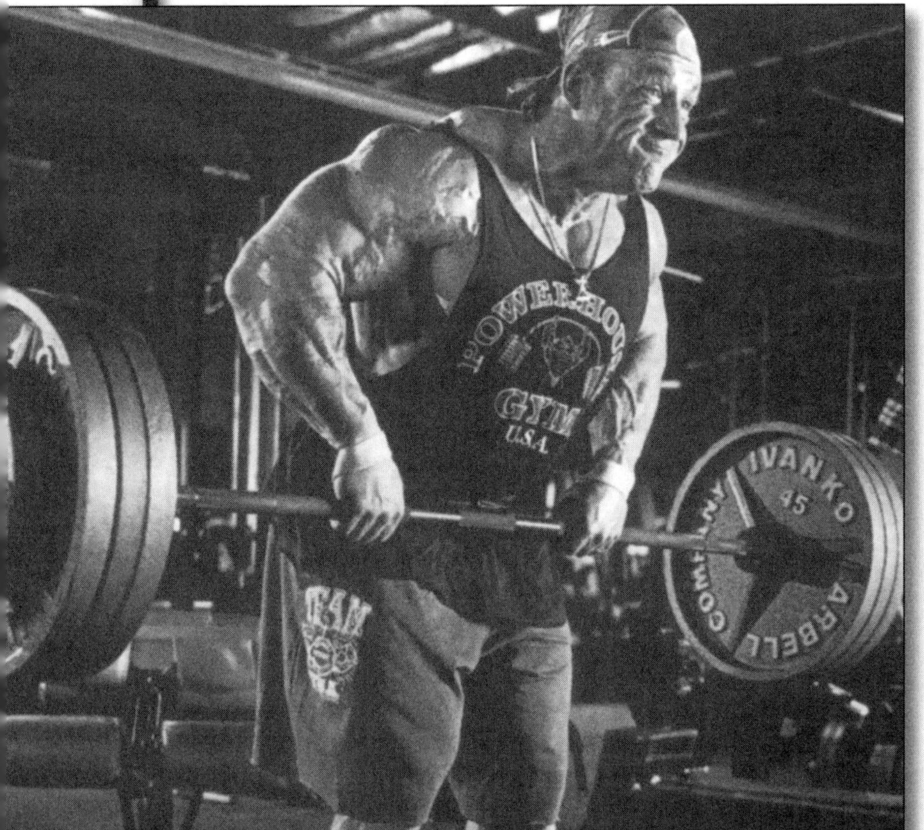

Bodybuilding, Blood & Guts Style

Dorian Yates trained four days a week. He would hit each body part once a week hard and heavy and allow that body part to rest for a full week. He worked up to one all-out set, usually in the 6 to 8 rep range before having Leroy step in and administer additional forced reps.

Day	Bodypart	Exercises	Sets/Reps
1	Deltoids	Smith machine press	1 x 15 - 120, 1 x 12 - 240, 1 x 8-10 - 440
		Seated lateral raise	1 x 12 - 50s, 1 x 8-10 - 70s
		On-arm laterals	1 x 20 - 35s, 1 x 8-10 - 70s
	Traps	Dumbbell shrugs	1 x 12 - 140s, 1 x 10-12 - 185s
	Triceps	Triceps pushdowns	1 x 15 - 80, 1 x 12 - 130, 1 x 8-10 - 180
		Lying Extensions	1 x 12 - 100
		One-arm pushdown	1 x 8-10 - 70
	Abs	Crunches	3 x 20-25
		Reverse crunch	3 x 12-15
2	Back	Hammer pulldowns	1 x 15 - 135, 1 x 12 - 220, 1 x 8-10 - 285
		Nautilus pullovers	1 x 15 - 220, 1 x 12 - 320, 1 x 8-10 - 340
		Barbell row	1 x 12 - 285, 1 x 8-10 - 375
		One-arm rows	1 x 8-10 - 245 each arm
		Cable rows	1 x 8-10 entire weight stack
	Rear delts	Rear delt machine	1 x 8-10 - 55s, 1 x 10-12 - 40s
	Lower back	Hyperextensions	1 x 10-12 - 40
		Deadlifts	1 x 8 - 320, 1 x 8 – 405
3	OFF	OFF	OFF
4	Chest	Incline barbell press	1 x 10 - 220, 1 x 8 - 310, 1 x 8 - 425
		Hammer bench press	1 x 10 - 220, 1 x 6-8 - 350
			1 x 10 - 50s, 1 x 8 - 110s
		Incline DB Flyes	1 x 10 - 50s, 1 x 6-8 - 70s
	Biceps	Incline DB curls	1 x 10 – 100
		EZ barbell curls	1 x 6-8 - 140
		Nautilus curls	1 x 6-8 - 100
	Abs	Crunches	3 x 20-25
		Reverse crunch	3 x 12-15
5	OFF	OFF	OFF
		Chin ups	2 x 8-10
		Pulldowns	2 x 8-10
		Bent over dumbbell laterals	2 x 8-10
	Calves	Seated calf raises	1 x 20
	Abs	Abs	3 x 20
6	Quadriceps	Leg extensions	1 x 15 - 130, 1 x 12 - 200, 1 x 10 - 270
		Leg press	1 x 12 - 770, 1 x 12 - 1045, 1 x 10-12 - 1265
		Hack squat	1 x 12 - 440, 1 x 8-10 - 660
	Hamstrings	Leg curls	1 x 8-10 - 130, 1 x 8-10 - 180
		Stiff leg deadlift	1 x 10 - 350
		Single leg curl	1 x 10 - 50
	Calves	Standing calf raise	1 x 12 - 900, 1 x 12 - 1300
		Seated calf raise	1 x 12 – 250
7	OFF	OFF	OFF

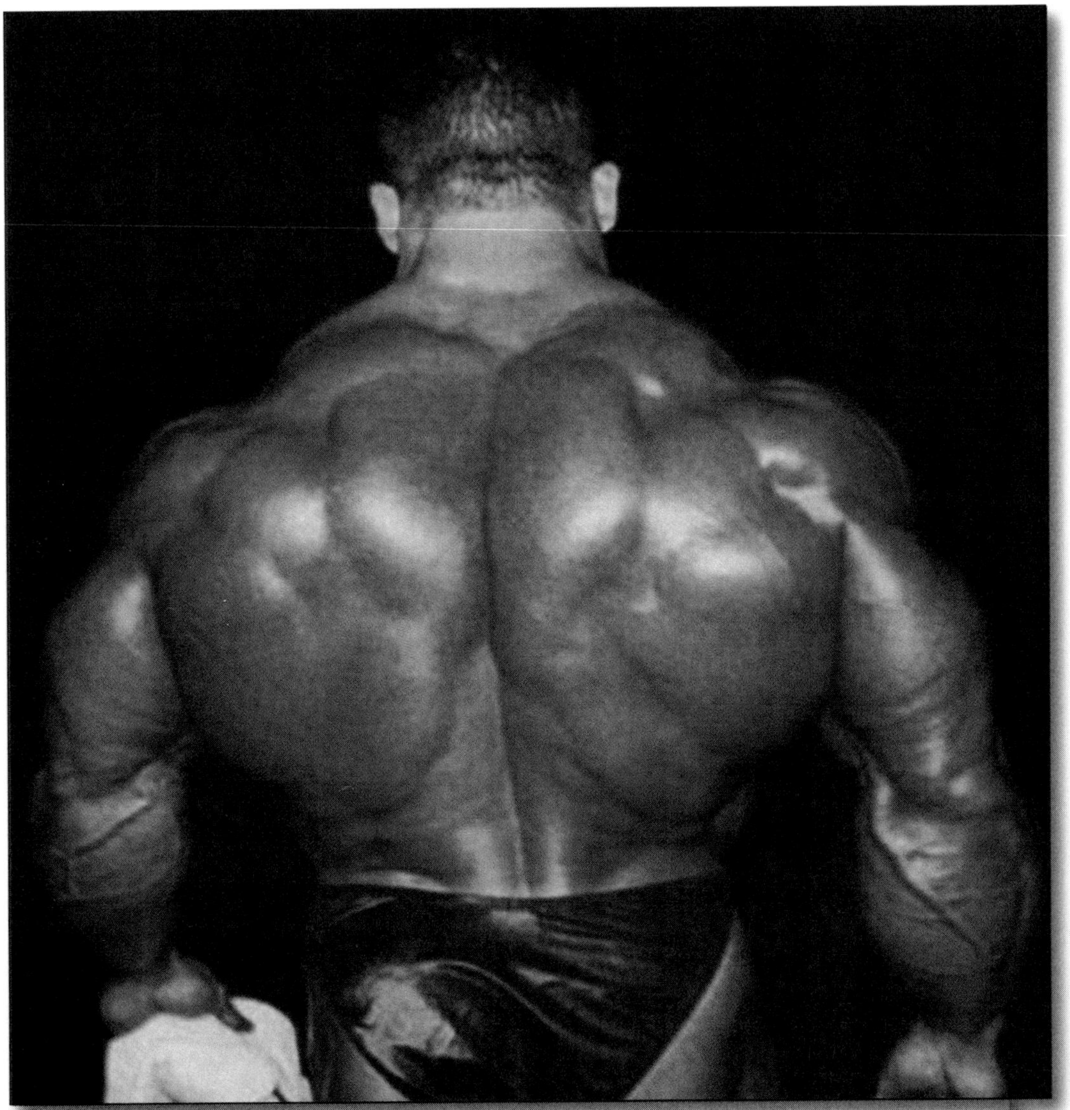

This is what I saw during "My Day with Dorian." This is the greatest back in the history of bodybuilding. This thickness and muscle mass, this sensational size wasn't built doing one-arm lat pulldowns with 100 pounds or some other pee-wee back exercise using puny poundage. This back was built doing 70 degree bent-over rows using a barbell and perfect technique pulling 450 pounds for reps. Yates was able to achieve a mind-muscle connection working a muscle that bordered on paranormal. I've seen lots of great traps and erectors on powerlifters and Olympic lifters over these many decades, but Dorian Yates had the best back; the thickest back, the most defined back I've ever seen; particularly his gargantuan central back region. This is comic book stuff. He reeked of strength and power because he was strong and powerful. His relaxed physique to me was more impressive then when he posed or flexed. His legs were nearly as incredible as his back. Note the gargantuan right forearm.

KIRK KARWOSKI

Prototypical Purposeful Primitive

Kirk Karwoski captured seven straight National Championships, six straight IPF World Powerlifting titles and got bored with it all. One evening at Maryland Athletic Club at about the time of year he would normally need to start serious preparation for the upcoming National Championships, training partner Bob Myers, and I reflexively tried to convince Kirk to mount yet another assault. We wanted him to win a eighth National and seventh World title. He informed us that he was bored to tears with the entire process and would not mount another campaign. It was final: he was "all done." The title was his for the taking. He had built up such a huge cushion over the rest of the world-level lifters that the "flee" phenomenon was occurring.

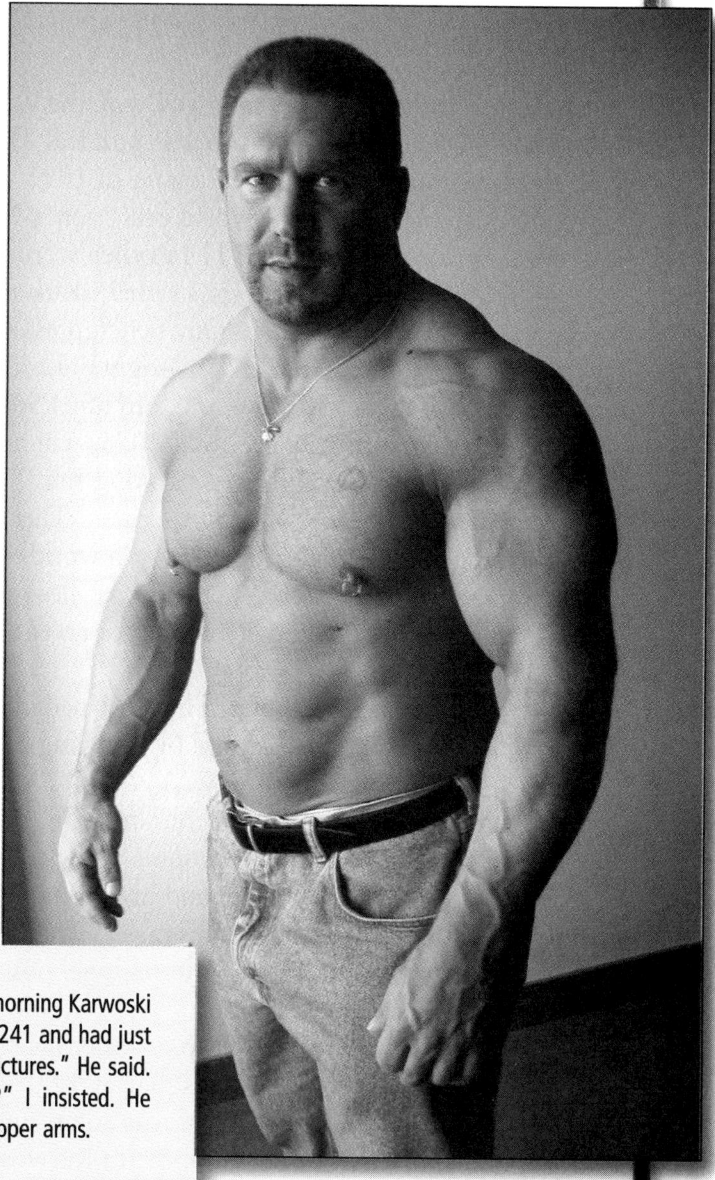

I took this photo in the hotel room the morning Karwoski lifted raw and squatted 826. He weighs 241 and had just rolled out of bed. "Let me take some pictures." He said. "Damn, can't I get some coffee first?" I insisted. He displays 16 inch forearms and 20 inch upper arms.

The flee phenomenon is when a particular lifter becomes so dominant within a weight division that the other contenders within that division "flee" to the next weight class either up or down to avoid the dominator. At that time, the only other IPF lifters in the world that inflicted the flee phenomenon were Ed Coan, Dan Austin and Gene Bell. Kirk was causing 275 pound lifters to add a few pounds and become heavyweights or drop down to the 242 pound class.

I suggested that Kirk might spice up the process by lifting at the World Championships wearing no supportive equipment. "What if you won the World Championships wearing no squat suit, no knee wraps, no bench shirt, and just a belt? Hell, you could still squat 850, bench 500 and pull 775 for 2125!" He steadfastly refused.

I had another idea. "What if you won the World Championships *without training for it?*" Kirk looked puzzled, Bob too was puzzled. The three of us stood in the main weight room at Maryland Athletic Club in winter of 1997. I related my "No Training" angle. "Has anyone in the history of the world ever won a National or World title in any sport *without training for it?* I think NOT! In other words, without any training at all you could still squat 825 wearing gear—am I right?" Kirk thought a minute and nodded. Encouraged I continued. "You could certainly bench press 475 using a shirt? Hell, you could roll out of bed in the morning and do that—right?" Kirk nodded. I delivered my closer: "And you can certainly deadlift 750 anywhere, anytime! So why not skip training! Take off *completely*! Show up at the Nationals, total 2075, win and get selected for the World Championship team! Now that would be a freaking first!" I was fired up and I loved the pure gonzo weirdness of the idea. I wasn't done. "Then…still not training…show up at the World Championships, total 2100 and win a world title! All without ever setting foot in the gym!" Bob and I hi-fived each other: *Genius*! Become the first National and World Powerlifting Champion to win without training for an entire year!

Kirk had had enough of our hair-brained ideas. Big Bob looked like Bluto trying to cheer up Flounder in *Animal House* by breaking a beer bottle over his head. Karowski got hot. "No, No, NO FREAKING WAY! NO!" I'M ALL DONE! Look: I've had it! I can't stand the idea of training—or not training—I'm sick of powerlifting and want out. Why am I going to go through all the trouble and aggravation? So I can do this?" Kirk took his left hand, licked his index finger and made an imaginary line on an imaginary chalk board. He wanted no more notches on his pistol handle. He left and that was the end of his complete domination of national and international powerlifting in the 275 pound class.

As this is being written, ten years after his retirement that night in MAC, Kirk *still* holds the IPF World Record in the squat at 1,003 pounds. His 2,306 World Record total was only recently exceeded and that was completely attributable to the allowing of bench shirts that inflate bench presses by 40%. In Karwoski's day, his bench shirt added 40 pounds to his bench press—not 40%. Had he worn the shirts allowable today, his 595 pound bench press would have turned into 700 and his total would jump for 2300 to 2450.

I worked with Kirk from the time he was 18 years old and over the subsequent decade helped guide him from being a really good lifter to a hall of fame power immortal. My role was that of a strategist and coach. When I started helping him, he was a tremendous squatter, albeit wild and inconsistent. He was not dropping his squats deep enough. Over time we developed a squat style that fit his unique proportions. I took him to bench press master Ken Fantano for help on his lagging bench press. Pre-Ken, Kirk was a 440 pound bench presser and had been stuck there for almost two years. Ken showed Kirk the Fantano technique and Kirk took to it immediately. He eventually bench pressed 600 using the patented, low touch-point, integrated leg drive style.

He worked the hell out of his deadlift and despite having the smallest hands I've ever seen on a big time lifter, he eventually pulled 800 for a dead-stop double and 825x1 without straps. He never duplicated these pulls in competition: his humongous squats affected his deadlifts to such an extent that he was unable to register more than 771. (He pulled 777 at 242 after a relatively light 826 squat.) His 950 to 1000 pound squats wreaked havoc on his pull power and 771 was all he could manage after walking out and squatting 940+ three times, as he would do in a competitive powerlift competition.

Kirk Karwoski succeeded because he had a fierce single-minded focus and a maniacal determination to be the best. He had a demonic work ethic and was a smart trainer. For ten years he centered his entire existence on powerlifting. His laser-beam focus paid huge dividends. Kirk totally revamped his physique.

At one point early in his career he was so disproportional and bottom-heavy he was called T-Rex. With huge thighs, huge calves and huge glutes, he had a smallish, underdeveloped torso and short arms. He looked as if God had accidentally grafted a 190 pound bodybuilder's torso onto a 350 pound football offensive tackle's lower body. Kirk looked like one of those mythical creatures, a half man/half horse Satyr. It was obvious why he was a great squatter and equally obvious why his bench press was okay and why his deadlift lagged so far behind.

He was his own worst critic and had a gift for seeing things as they truly were. It took five years to bring his torso into proportional balance with his massive lower body. Most men continually play to their strengths and avoid addressing weaknesses. Not Kirk, he ultimately achieved muscular balance because he steadfastly attacked his weak points. His approach towards training stayed basically the same throughout his career.

I broke my leg in 1983 and turned my full attention to coaching. I had been working with

Mark Chaillet, Ed Coan and Doug Furnas when Kirk approached me. He was a kid that I had first met at Marshall Peck's basement gym in rural Forestville, Maryland. At the time Kirk was a very junior guy among a crew of hard-ass men....Joe Povinale, Joe Ferry, Jeff B., Frank H, Pat Brooks from Baltimore, Pete Lumia...we'd gather and train all three lifts on a single day in long extended power sessions. Kirk was there, and already had a reputation for being a good squatter and not much else. Had someone told that crew back then that this kid would become one of the greatest powerlifters of all time, he would have been laughed out of the room.

Kirk could squat, though not as much as the guys at Marshalls. Jeff B for example could double 550 in the bench press without a bench shirt weighing 265. Lots of us had deadlifted 700-plus. We continually goaded and challenged Kirk. Marshall bet him he couldn't squat 500x10 without gear and within a month he did it. Even back then he rose to challenges. After we all gravitated to Chaillet's Gym, Kirk dropped out for a while to play college football and while he liked playing ball and the college coeds, he couldn't get his head wrapped around the books.

He got a great job as a Union Pressman and settled in. He bought a small condo and worked his union job. He'd get off at 4 every day and stayed in this groove for the next decade. Kirk wanted to lift in the Big Leagues, the USPF/IPF. I told him his squat depth wasn't near low enough. He held all kinds of records in the fledgling ADFPA, but in the USPF squats had to be unquestionably below parallel. Plus the level of competition in the 242 pound class was stratospheric: Thor Kritsky had played football at Virginia Tech with Bruce Smith; Dave Jacoby was the dominant 242er in the World; Willie Bell was a stud with an 800-plus deadlift; and Joe Ladiner was positively frightening...the 242 pound class was a meat grinder.

Still, he was the hottest young prospect on the scene. So we went to our first USPF nationals. He promptly bombed out: three straight squats, nine reds lights, and bam! He was gone! The next year the same thing: another bomb out! The following year we yet tried again. He was insistent about starting with 804 in the squat, a Junior World Record. I tried to talk him into starting lower, but he would hear none of it. His first attempt squat was turned down 2 to 1. Still, he had gotten one white light. His second attempt was turned down 2 to 1. He flipped out and threatened mayhem. He told me point blank that if he missed his third squat and suffered the embarrassment of bombing out in his third straight National Championships he would quit powerlifting forever. He was super serious and I believed him.

As we stood at the chalk box prior to the do-or-die attempt, he chalked his hands. I chalked his back to keep the bar from slipping and happened to notice Ed Coan and Doug Furnas sitting in the front row. All of a sudden they started laughing about something totally unrelated, I quickly jabbed Kirk, hard in the ribs, and said, "LOOK! Look at Furnas and Coan—they're LAUGHING AT YOU!" He looked over at his idols and instantly morphed into a demon. He finished chalking his hands and continued to glare at the dynamic duo of Doug and Ed. As they finished laughing at their private joke, they coincidentally happened to look at Kirk and I at the chalk box, their smiles still lingered on their faces, their shared joke must have been a funny one. The look on Kirk's face went from nervous, disjointed and apprehensive to a look of pure evil. Hatred cubed. "I'LL TEACH THOSE SON-OF-A-BITCHES NOT TO LAUGH AT ME!!!" He yelled. With that he stormed to the platform in front of a packed house and attacked the 804 like a maniac.

It would be nice to say he slaughtered the poundage and made it look easy...but I can't...it was absolutely agonizing. Kirk did something he had never done before; he took the barbell all the way down to parallel, his usual turnaround point...then he took the poundage down another 3-4 inches—way below parallel—before he began an ascent that was so slow, so horrific, so excruciating, so intense and torturous that the jaded, seen-it-all Mike Lambert, powerlifting's major domo and guru, later called this particular attempt, "*The single most difficult lift I have ever witnessed in my entire life.*"

Finished, Karwoski collapsed coming off the platform. The judge's lights came on...one white...one red... ("Oh SHIT! I heard him moan) then...a second white light! Pandemonium ensued! The auditorium went nuts! He had set a Junior World Record, stayed in the competition, placed third at the end of the day and went on to become one of the greatest powerlifters in history. We came within one red light of having him quit the sport altogether. Later on Ed came up and asked, "What the hell was going on with The Kid on that last attempt? He looked insane!" I shook my head and said, "I owe it all to you and Doug." Ed looked baffled. "Call it elemental child psychology." I said. The boy became a man that day.

Karwoski's Four Day/Week Power Training Program

Kirk was a methodical, determined, patient and intelligent trainer who took a long-term approach and never went crazy in training. Towards the end of his illustrious career, he never missed a rep over an entire 12 week cycle in any lift. Can you imagine? A man sits down with a pencil and paper four months prior to a National or World Championship, writes out the projected poundage, reps and sets for every single session for every workout for the next twelve straight weeks then *never misses a single predetermined rep*!

His prognostications were so realistic, his self-assessment abilities so accurate, he was so devoid of training ego and wishful thinking, that in each and every one of his four weekly workouts for each successive week, week in week out, he never missed anything. And it wasn't like he was handling pee-wee poundage and yawning his way through the workouts. Prior to his World Record squat of 1,003 his last five successive training weeks produced the following top squat sets: 900x5, 940x3, 960x2 980x2, 1000x2.

Interestingly, he used virtually the identical training template as Ed Coan, at least insofar as the workout structure. He was not near as comprehensive in his attention to the assistance exercises as Ed was, still Kirk's similarity to Coan's training template was no accident. I conversed weekly with Ed for years and purposefully infused Kirk's training template with Coan's ideas and strategies.

Karwoski 4 Day Training Split

Day	Bodypart	Exercises	Sets/Reps
Monday	Legs	Squat	7-10 x 2-8
		Leg curl	2-3 x 5
		Leg extensions	2-3 x 5
Tuesday	Chest	Close grip bench – touch & go	7-10 x 2-8
	Arms	Dumbbell curls	2-3 x 5
		Triceps pushdowns	2-3 x 5
Wednesday	OFF	OFF	OFF
Thursday	Back	Deadlift	7-10 x 2-8
		Grip shrugs	3 x 5
		T-bar row	3 x 5-8
		Pulldowns	2-3 x 5
		Dumbbell shrugs	2-3 x 5
Saturday	Chest	Bench press – competition grip	7-10 x 2-8
		Wide grip bench w/ pause	3 x 5
		Incline press	3 x 5
		Front raises	2-3 x 5
		Side raises	2-3 x 5

Kirk would take 12 weeks to prepare: week 1-2 he would work up to one top set of 8; weeks 3-8 work up to a 5 rep top set; weeks 9-12 a 3,3,2 and 2.

Ed, Doug and Kirk all felt that the 5 rep set, be it squat, bench press or deadlift, was the key to power and strength success. Each of these men sought to become as strong as possible in the key lifts in their 5 rep sets. Initially, each would use as little equipment and gear as possible, then as they moved deeper into the power cycle, they would add supportive gear in conjunction with dropping the repetitions. Each man felt that the key was becoming strong as possible in 5 rep sets without gear. When it was time to power train, they would be perfectly positioned to exceed previous bests. This love of 5 rep sets resonated with what I learned from Iron Scribe John McCallum, and later in my power apprenticeship with Hugh Cassidy. Hugh, Doug, Ed and Kirk all loved the 5 rep set. Ed, Doug and Kirk had squat "bests" of 900 x 5.

Karwoski Reemerges

I've seen a lot of great strength feats in my day: I stood twenty feet from Lee Moran when he squatted 1000 at a Pacifico competition in Dayton. Lee had a disastrous previous attempt when he came within an inch of being blasted in the kneecaps by five hundred pounds. A collar had not been tightened in the rush to get the weight ready for the World Record attempt and as Lee stepped back and set up, his side-to-side movement caused the loose collar to break away and the weights slid off one side of the barbell before anyone could do jack about it. The heavy left side, suddenly without equal counterweight, whipped downward around Lee's neck, a stumpy 22 inch fulcrum. The net effect was pure chaos and I had the perfect vantage point.

After a 25, 45 and a gold hundred pound plate fell to the ground, the imbalanced barbell, way heavier on one side, spun around Lee's neck and slung gold plates slingshot style over Lee's head. In rapid succession 100 pound plates were catapulted in the general direction of the audience. You have never seen people scatter so fast. By the time the 1st hundred pound plate landed there wasn't a human being within thirty feet. The 330 pound Hell's Angel leapt backward with the agility of Mikhail Baryshnikov executing a leaping twirl during the Nutcracker. He had to or he would have been slammed in the knees with the still secured 500 pounds.

The 45 pound bar whizzed around his neck and grazed a spotter's head. After the pandemonium died down MC Tony Carpino said to the packed auditorium, "WHAT THE F*&K JUST HAPPENED!" Lee composed himself and came back and made the lift on his subsequent attempt. I worked with Doug Furnas on successive occasions when he became the 1st man to total 2400 twice. At the first competition we basked in Maui and at the second we froze in Minnesota. I worked with the incomparable Coan for a decade and assisted him in whatever way he deemed appropriate. We worked together at National and World competitions.

You 'assist' you don't 'coach' men like Coan, Furnas, Chaillet, Karwoski, Jacoby, Lamar or Mike Hall. I assisted Ed when he posted the highest total ever (at the time) regardless of bodyweight. Ed was the greatest lifter I have ever seen, with the possible exception of Paul Anderson. I have assisted all-time great lifters like Lamar Gant, Dan Wohleber, Dan Austin, Joe Ladiner, Mike Hall, Dave Jacoby, Phil Hile, John Black and Bob Bridges during national and international competition. The point is—I've been around. I'm grizzled and tough to impress and I thought my time was over insofar as bearing witness to truly amazing strength occurrences. I was wrong.

Through a weird combination of chance and circumstance I bore witness to yet another absolutely incredible, all-time strength feat. It was an amazing display of pure hellacious strength. On December 9th, 2004 I assisted Kirk Karwoski when he totaled 2066 in the three power lifts wearing nothing, but a lifting belt. It was a retro-throwback powerlift festival staring Captain Kirk Karwoski in his first public lifting appearance in eight years. Physically he had never looked better: he lifted in the 242 pound class and was shredded and ripped. Through a combination of muscle maturity and low body fat, his arms and legs rippled and roiled with every step. Like a lifting Ulysses, Kirk had been away from powerlifting for nearly a decade and everything changed in the interim. At this competition, the AAU World Championship held in Laughlin, Nevada, Kirk went backwards in time. Rather than 'gear up' he decided to 'gear down.' He made eight out of nine lifts and started things off with a squat exhibition.

In staggering succession he made squats of 749, 804 and finally an explosive 826 pound effort. He wore a loose tee shirt and a wrestling singlet. Kirk experienced a severe thigh pull on his final squat with 826. On the previous 804 he barely averted a total wipeout. He lost concentration and tension on the descent for a split-second and his lapse caused him to be pushed downward way past his normal turnaround point. He caught himself and through sheer willpower and guts pushed 804 to completion. His post-lift analysis was that he had 'set up' with his feet slightly narrow. This gut-buster lift took a lot out of him and the selection of 826 pounds on his 3rd was conservative. Had the 804 gone the way it should, 840 was to have been the 3rd attempt. The 826 actually went a whole lot better than 804.

As Chuck Deluxe would say using another of his endless football analogies "Kirk 'jus needed to get the snot knocked out of him to clear his head." Karwoski took the 826 down quickly and exploded it upward from 3 inches below parallel to ¾'s erect. As he pushed through the sticking point, the vastus internus on his right thigh tore. He actually heard a noise. He recalled that, "I heard it {the thigh muscle} go 'pop,' but I was through the hard part and I was *not* going to lose this weight after getting 2/3rd erect." This lift was a thing of beauty; pure athletic poetry in motion, 8-and-a-quarter squatted deep and explosive by a guy weighing 239 in a lifting belt and nothing else. This was as fine a lift as I'd ever witnessed by anyone anywhere.

In the bench press Kirk made an explosive 446 opener and a fine 463 second before experiencing his only miss of the entire competition: a 479 3rd attempt bench press. He had trained hurt. "I had been nursing a torn rotator cuff for the last ten weeks. It was a work-related injury, nothing to do with training, and before injuring it I had bench pressed 500 with a pause without a shirt." Kirk said. "Even injured I had hoped for a double body weight 480 pound bench press." This was not to be.

The deadlift would be touch and go on account of the thigh injury. He decided to dramatically curtail the number of deadlift warm-ups. Julie Scanlon, Kirk's Lady, and myself, were his only handlers. We applied ice to the injury, but it would be anyone's guess if he would be able to deadlift effectively. He felt confident of being able to pull 705 regardless how bad the leg hurt. The competition was dragging on and on and on, and fatigue was becoming a real factor. His opening 705 deadlift "felt ok." His second attempt with 749 felt better than 705. The thigh injury was not a factor, but fatigue might be his undoing. Kirk had taken his first squat at 10 am and pulled his final successful deadlift, 776 pounds, at 7pm, a full nine hours later.

I remember way back when Kirk was campaigning as a kid 242 pound lifter, going against hall of fame guys like Dave Jacoby, Willie Bell and Thor Kritsky. Kirk was a young man trying to break into the ranks of the true champions and we were in shock-and-awe over the poundage these men were lifting. Clean, legal lifts wearing single ply squat suits, standard length knee wraps and single-ply bench shirts. That was twelve years ago. Kirk was now matching those awesome lifts made by those awesome men without wearing any supportive gear! At age 38 Karwoski's lifting was truly transcendental.

While still a young lifter, Kirk had been campaigning as a 240 pound lifter. He let his bodyweight increase to a full 275 pounds and really came into his own. When super-heavyweight champion Mike Hall unexpectedly dropped out of the National Championships at the last minute in 1990, Kirk and I thought our chances would be better in the super heavyweight division instead of lifting against Calvin Smith, the National Champ at 275. Karwoski captured his first National Championship as a super-heavyweight. At the 1990 IPF World Championships, Smith and Karwoski switched classes and Kirk lifted against The Fearsome Finn, three-time World Champion, Kyosti Vilmi. Karwoski electrified the crowd in his true coming out party.

US head coach Sean Scully called Karwoski's battle with Vilmi, "One of the most exciting lifting performances I've ever witnessed." Vilmi pulled his final deadlift to beat Kirk by a scant 5 pounds. I kicked myself in the ass for not having made the trip. As his longtime coach I felt my presence would have certainly been good for 5 pounds. I vowed to make the trip the following year. In Orebro, Sweden the very next year, I was present as a US team coach when Karwoski easily captured the first of six straight IPF world titles, including one at 242. The other five were as a 275 pound lifter. Kirk won seven straight national titles, including one at 242 and one as a super heavyweight. I was his coach at every national championship, including his final when he squatted 1003 and totaled 2303. Both were world records.

After winning his sixth straight world title, circumstance and boredom caused him to retire from powerlifting. He went into business with his parents. He had worked a union job for nine years. He leapt into the private sector and the 60 hour workweeks that go with it. In the subsequent years he contented himself by training and coaching. I saw him at a party and thought he looked really good at his reduced body weight. I suggested that he consider posting a 'raw' total. The idea of lifting raw intrigued him, but he did not want to compete. "I have zero interest in competing against others or winning titles or trophies. I would like an opportunity to lift in front of strict judging without wearing power gear of any type." Karwoski came through in the clutch per usual. Let us hope that we haven't seen the last of Karwoski's exploits. Regardless, 2,066 weighing 239 pounds without any gear is one hell of an accomplishment.

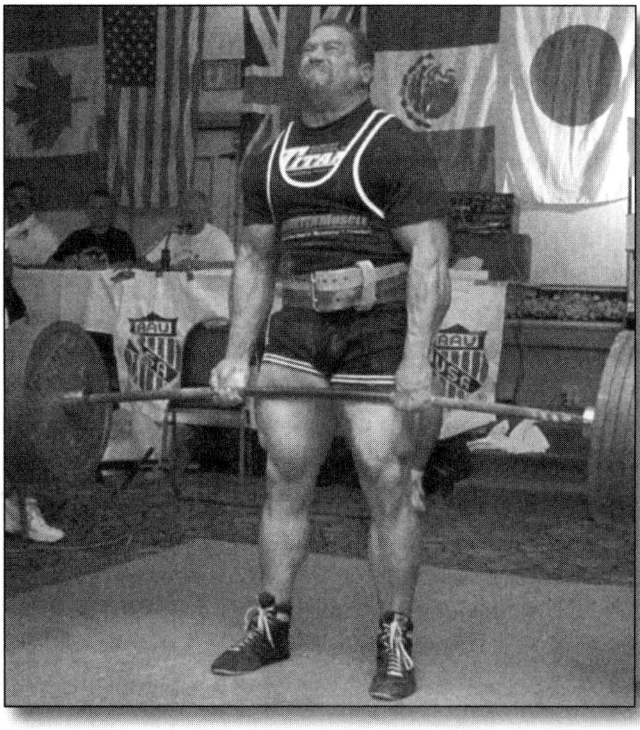

777 pounds was the most Kirk had ever deadlifted in competition. Over the years he physically transformed from disproportional to super proportional by working on his weak points. Too many athletes continually play to their strengths and this eventually results in physical and psychological imbalances that become impossible to overcome.

I had the great pleasure of working with this man from his athletic infancy through his ultimate maturation. I passed along to him the collective insights I had gleaned from my many mentors. He absorbed the collective knowledge and added his own unique training twists.

Iron Methods

"We are what we do repeatedly."
—Aristotle

The Purposefully Primitive Resistance Training Amalgamation

Amalgamate is defined as "merging into a single body." The Purposefully Primitive training amalgamation is not a merging of all methods into a single body, rather our amalgamation is the steady rotation of Master methods. Instead of throwing all the Iron Methods of all the Iron Masters into the equivalent of a philosophic blender to create a single diluted hybrid, our amalgamation is of a different flavor. We respect each approach and each method as if it were an amazing ethnic dish served at a gourmet restaurant.

We amalgamate by alternating methods or by *slight* modification. Each Method of each Master offers a splendid tactical template for use at different times during your resistance training career. One Purposefully Primitive tenet is that all systems eventually cease delivering results. When stagnation eventually and inevitably occurs we need to be ready with another equally effective resistance training regimen that contrasts dramatically to the approach being used.

When constructing a resistance training regimen, so much depends on the amount of training time you have available. Too often the individual feels that only having a few days a week to train is not enough to trigger progress. That is factually inaccurate. If you train hard enough, two or three days per week will work. In fact several of the Iron Masters purposefully limit training to two days a week.

I have devised five distinctive training templates, each based on available time. The templates range from 2 days per week to 6 days per week. In my studied opinion all five templates should be used at some point, regardless your level of proficiency. Each template uses a Master's Method as its architectural base structure. I have retained the essential essence gleaned from the Masters and made a few modifications. For example, Chaillet and

Cassidy each used a two day per week training template. Feel free to use the Master's exact template as specified in the Iron Master's section. I have constructed a studied amalgamation. Use the exact method or use my modest modification.

The wonderful thing about resistance training is that poundage can be adjusted; a beginner can perform the exact routine used by Dorian Yates or Bob Bednarski, albeit with 1/10 the poundage. Regardless the workout choice, follow the rules: start light and build technique as this will keep you safe. 90% of weight training injuries are attributable to two causes; too much poundage or straying outside the technical boundaries of the lift. Use realistic poundage for the rep range that you select.

Sync up the resistance training method with the goal. Are you seeking to add muscle? Use an intensity-biased method. Are you seeking to reduce body fat? Use a volume-biased approach. Place the goal into a periodized training template. Start off light and easy as this allows acclimatization to the workload while perfecting techniques and creating critical momentum. The biggest mistake rookies make is to start the periodization cycle off too heavy. Start the process off *below* capacity and end *above* capacity. A periodized approach requires you commit for 6-12 weeks. The sole goal of progressive resistance training is to build and strengthen muscle. Reverse engineer a training program that fits the realities of your life. Answer three key questions and you can construct a customized training regimen.

1. What are your realistic goals? Add muscle? Reduce body fat?
2. How many days do you have to dedicate to training?
3. What length periodization timeframe can you commit to?

Once you have decided on a goal and determined the number of training days you have available, select an appropriate training template. Determine a timeframe and break the long term goal down into weekly benchmarks. Systematically achieve the weekly goals and arrive at the predetermined final destination. For example; if you want to add muscle and have three days per week to train, you might decide to use my amalgamated 3-day training template. You might decide to commit for 10 weeks. Perhaps your goal is to add 10 pounds of muscle in ten weeks. Each week you push your bodyweight up one pound; each week you grow slightly bigger and stronger. The mass building periodized template starts off with higher reps and lighter weight. Each successive week, poundage is increased. The "lean-out" procedure is the mirror-image reverse. The 10-week mass building periodization plan stair-steps ever upward until you arrive at a series of predetermined final goals. Each week you improve poundage used and this steady increase in strength gains converts into steady increases in muscle mass.

To recap: determine if you want to add muscle or lean out. Pick one. Determine how many days you have to train. Select a weight training template that syncs up with your available days. Devise a 6 to 12 week periodization plan. Start with the desired end goal and work backwards to the start date, establishing small weekly benchmarks for each lift and for bodyweight. Lifting performance needs to be nudged upward weekly, in some manner or fashion. We synchronize nutrition and cardiovascular exercise with resistance training to accelerate progress. Regardless the selected direction (add muscle, lose fat) rest assured that if you abide by the precepts and principles, if you generate the requisite training intensity, the body has *no choice*, but to accede to your self-imposed biologic imperatives.

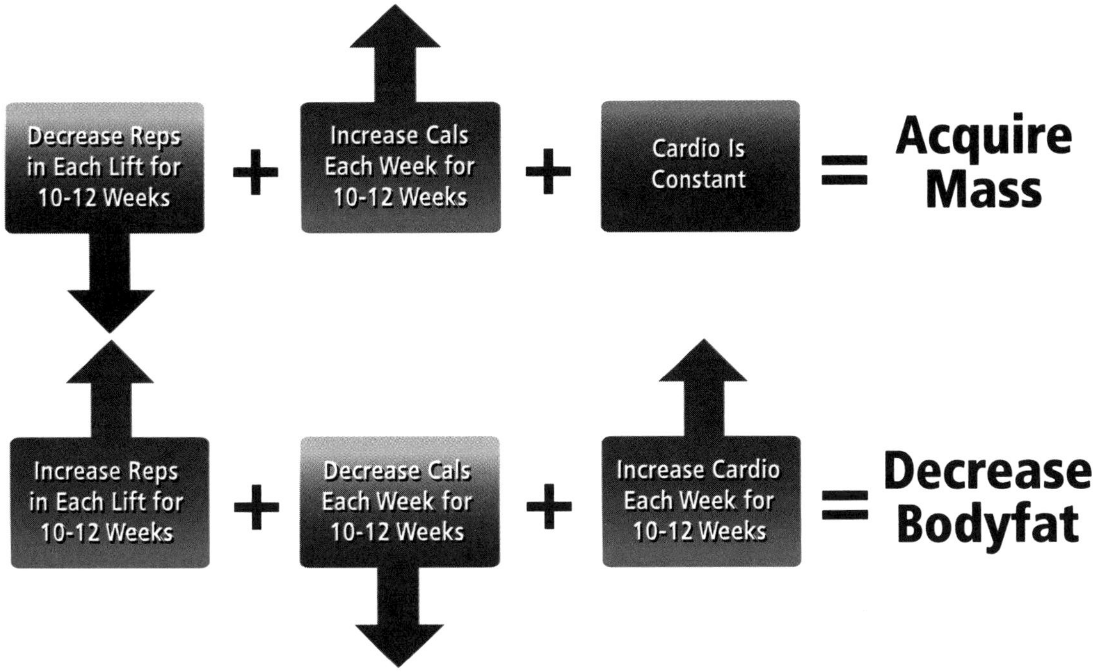

Recapitulation of Modes and Methods

Now that you have been introduced to the ten Iron Masters and their individualistic training systems, a recap could be beneficial: do any of the various approaches appeal to you? People have likes and dislikes and often being exposed to a new way in which to train infuses the individual's efforts with wild enthusiasm.

Progressive resistance training taught at local health clubs and YMCAs is uniformly boring, standardized and ineffectual. Round pegs (clients) are routinely jammed into square holes using cookie-cutter resistance programs that just don't work. The typical health club or YMCA offers pabulum resistance training programs that are a complete waste of time. Know-nothing "trainers" instruct wide-eyed clients how to perform meaningless exercises that produce zero results. There is no point in having trainees perform sub-maximal sets, particularly using inferior exercise machines. The intensity generated is insufficient to trip the hypertrophy trigger. The reason we lift weights is to grow muscle and become stronger—Period! There is no other physiological reason or rationale.

To compound the inanity of using sub-maximal training routines, personal trainers never change the blasé exercise menu. They don't know any other way to train. This is analogous to being forced to eat a diet of one bland meal comprised of the same insipid food every day. We offer a gourmet resistance training menu representing different disciplines, regions and cultures. There are three types of advanced weight training: bodybuilding, powerlifting and Olympic lifting. Let us open our eyes and hearts to the broad world of resistance possibilities. Regardless the system selected, you need to train with requisite intensity. To trigger hypertrophy, gut-busting physical effort is required. Accept and embrace the inconvenient necessity of progressive resistance.

Lifter	Training	Description
Paul Anderson 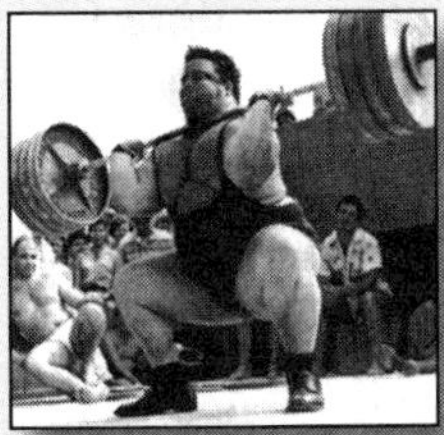	Olympic lifter & Powerlifter	The only man to bestride two categories, Anderson's training was broad and varied. He practiced the three overhead lifts, the three powerlifts and was an advocate of partial rep training. He would break rep strokes into thirds, and build strength within the partial rep range. This would convert into an improved regular rep. Paul enjoyed enduro training sessions and would take hours to complete a routine, often with thirty minutes rest between sets. **Recommended for advanced men seeking variety.**
Bill Pearl 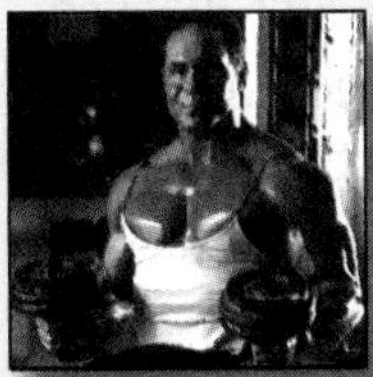	Bodybuilder	Bill was the master of classical "volume" bodybuilding training. He trained each muscle two or three times weekly and hit each muscle from a variety of angles. He would use three or four exercises for each muscle. Bill's session might take two hours to complete. He never went to failure. Bill sought the cumulative effect of lots of exercises and sets. His rapid pace elicited a strong cardio effect. **Recommended for use in lean-out phases.**
Bob Bednarski 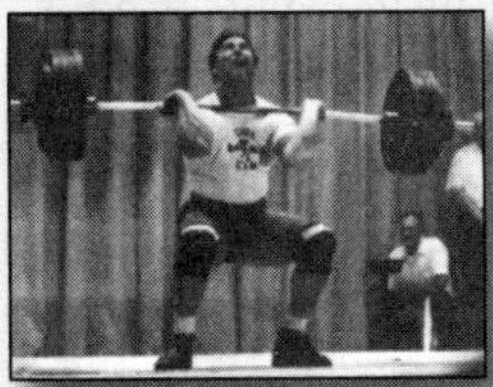	Olympic lifter	Bob used a variety of training methods and the routine we selected focuses on a single lift (or two per) in each session. This exclusivity allowed him to concentrate fully and completely on a particular lift and hold nothing back. Over a 5-6 day period he would hit all muscles using overhead lifts and squats. This "rolling split" is extremely effective. **Recommended for dramatic change of pace.**
Hugh Cassidy 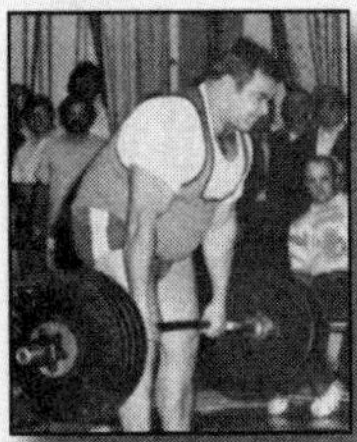	Powerlifter	Cassidy was an early power pioneer and believed in working the three powerlifts to near exclusion twice a week. He also believed that "back-off sets," should be done after working up to a big double, triple or five rep set. Back-off sets were the "hallmark" of his power routine. Cassidy would reduce poundage and perform three sets of either 8 reps, 5 reps or 3 reps with static poundage, usually 50 pounds below the top set. These "hallmark" sets forced growth. **Recommended for limited time-maximum power.**

Lifter	Training	Description
Mark Chaillet 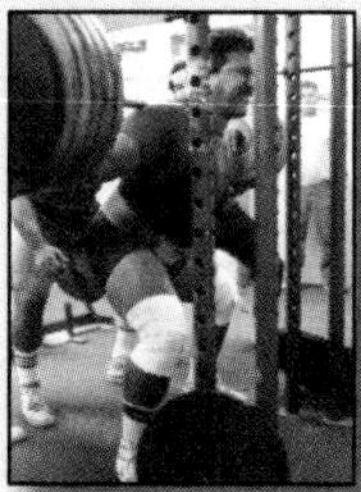	Powerlifter	Mark was the powerlifting minimalist who worked up to a single rep in three lifts once a week. Chaillet staged mini-power competitions every Monday and Thursday. On Monday he would work up to an all out single repetition in the squat and bench press and on Thursday he would work up to a single repetition in the deadlift. He would begin this process approximately 12 weeks before a competition. He did little, if any, assistance work. **Recommended for those pushed for time or for advanced men burnt out from overtraining.**
Doug Furnas 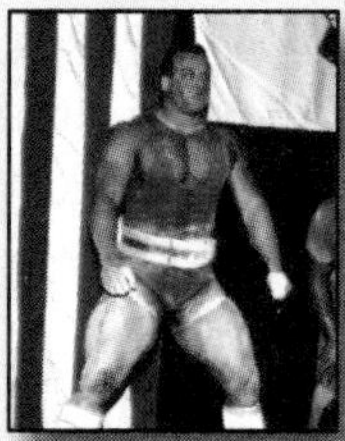	Powerlifter	Doug was subjected to a lot of high volume power training when he trained under Dennis Wright. He later dropped "light days" and established the "once a week per major lift" format. Furnas developed incredibly efficient lifting techniques. He found the right stance widths for his structure in the squat and deadlift and the optimal grip width for his bench press. He was extremely conservative by nature, and rarely missed a lift in training. **Recommended for competitive athletes.**
Ed Coan 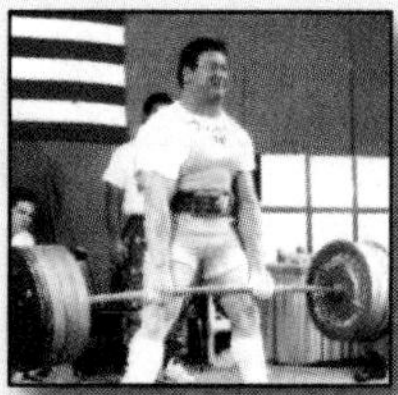	Powerlifter	The greatest powerlifter in the history of the sport used a five day per week training split. Ed religiously used a wide variety of assistance exercises. Coan's approach is highly applicable for normal individuals. His five day training approach allows for time to attack every muscle on the body fully and completely. This approach is genius! Ideal for those who have the time to train five times weekly. **Recommended for competitive athletes.**
Ken Fantano 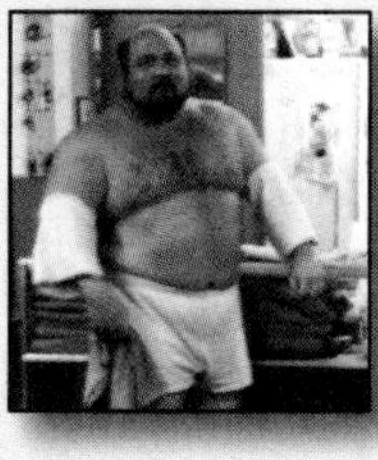	Powerlifter	Fantano developed one of the strongest raw bench presses in history using basic training tactics and a revolutionary bench press technique. His training was done in two or three weekly sessions and is a perfect template for those pressed for time. He made tremendous gains training twice a week. **Recommended for those seeking maximum return on a minimum time investment.**

Lifter	Training	Description
Dorian Yates 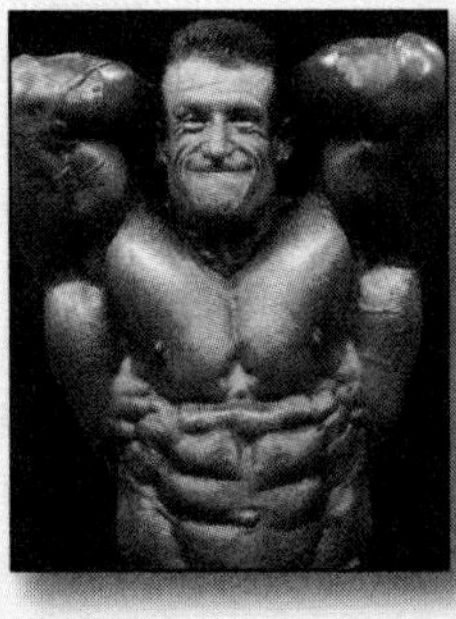	Bodybuilder	At the polar opposite of Bill Pearl lies Dorian Yates. The Diesel felt that intensity trumped volume and sought to blast a muscle thoroughly, once a week. He completely decimated the muscle, working up to one all out top set, including several forced reps, using two or three exercises per muscle. His approach was intensity based. He once famously quipped, "If you shoot a person through the heart with a bullet—he's dead. No need to pump more bullets into the body." Hit a muscle hard! Tax muscles past capacity; decimate the target. **Recommended for maximum muscle size.**
Kirk Karwoski 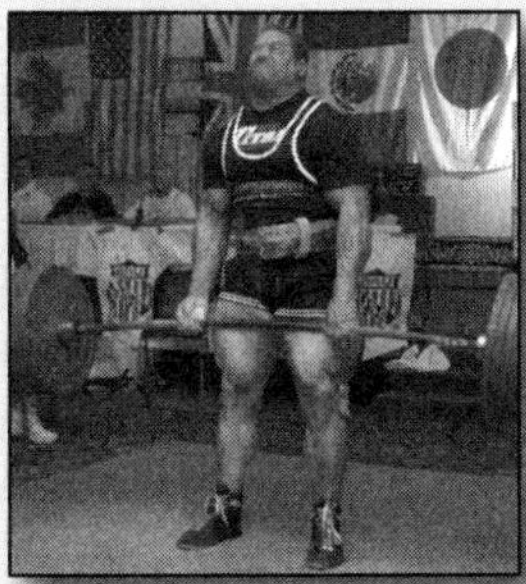	Powerlifter	Karwoski's training split was similar to that of Yates. Four weekly sessions in which each muscle was attacked thoroughly once a week. The key to making this type of routine work is generating sufficient intensity in the individual sessions. Each subsequent week slightly more poundage is used and small weekly increments result in huge cumulative gains over the course of an 8-12 week extended periodization cycle. Karwoski, Coan and Furnas could complete an entire 12 week cycle and never once miss a single rep on any lift. **Recommended for power and size.**

What the Iron Masters Have in Common

1. ***The elite use free weights to near exclusion***

   From Anderson to Yates, all the Iron Masters make barbells and dumbbells their weapon of choice because they are superior tools. The very rawness of hoisting barbells and dumbbells is what makes them so effective for muscle and strength building. Smooth and efficient is not nearly as good as crude and difficult when the name of the game is triggering hypertrophy. Free weights trump mimicking machines every single time and in every single instance.

2. ***Sessions are centered on core compound multi-joint exercises***

   The Iron Elite start off every training session with one of the core compound multi-joint exercises. These exercises force groups of muscles to work together in synchronous fashion to complete the assigned muscular task. The synchronized interaction between contiguous muscles actually amplifies muscular results by allowing muscle overload. Large, sweeping exercises allow individual muscles to exceed individual capacity: their neighbors pitch in to help. Perform isolation exercises *after* the lead multi-joint exercise. Performing an isolation movement prior to performing the compound multi-joint exercise sabotages strength available for the multi-joint movement. Avoid pre-fatigue.

3. ***Sessions are intense***

   Master resistance trainers know that in order for muscle growth to occur, and muscle strength to increase, the targeted muscle must be stressed in some manner or fashion. Unless some element of stress is present, the adaptive response will not be triggered. Muscle fiber does not thicken and strengthen in response to sub-maximal effort. However, stress sufficient enough to trigger the adaptive response can take many forms: multiple "top sets," one top set, high reps, low reps…ad infinitum.

4. ***Sessions are short***

   If the resistance trainer is working hard enough to trip the adaptive response, muscles are traumatized and fatigued. While more experienced elite resistance trainers are able to go longer and harder than people new to weight training, even the elite recognize that after an hour or so of intense training, a point of diminishing returns sets in and further training is not only fruitless, but counterproductive. Pearl is the exception: he uses extended training that could be called a version of 3rd Way cardio training. By purposefully extending workouts he amps-up the cumulative stress effect.

5. *Shocked and traumatized muscles need to be rested before training them again*
   When a muscle is trained properly, using effective resistance procedures, the muscles are traumatized, decimated, torn down. To subject that muscle to intense stress before it has recovered from the initial pounding is counterproductive and disruptive to the recuperation/adaptation/growth cycle. Rest is critical. Avoid genuine overtraining.

6. *Technical proficiency is sought in all exercises*
   There are beneficial and detrimental techniques connected with every progressive resistance exercise. Different motor-pathways elicit different muscular results. Rep speed, length of stroke and attention to technical execution need to be factored in and mulled over prior to and during each and every set. Exercise techniques need to be refined and honed over time. Eventually signature techniques unique to the body structure of the trainee are developed.

How to Build Muscle

Let us be clear on what a sensible progressive resistance program will and will not do: a sensible weight training program builds and strengthens the 600-plus muscles of the human body. Weight training alone will *not* make you leaner, nor will it melt off stored body fat. The caloric cost of weight training is insignificant when compared to sustained cardiovascular exercise. A torrid weight training session lasting 45 minutes *might* burn off 200 to 300 calories, depending upon the size of the trainee. Resistance training, with its rest periods and uneven exertions, is not a particularly effective calorie oxidizer. Even cardiovascular exercise is too often overestimated as a calorie burner. Tooling along at a heart-pounding, 15 calorie per minute pace, even after 30 minutes the trainee has only burned 450 calories; the exact caloric content of a medium size order of McDonald's French fries.

The profound purpose of proper resistance training is two-fold: trigger muscle growth and increase strength levels. Nothing else should be sought or expected.

A nice metabolic bump does occur after an intense weight training session. Intensely trained muscles will generate a thermogenic effect that lasts for hours after the cessation of the session. The body's thermostat is effectively turned up; additional calories are required to feed the metabolically activated muscles. In this post-workout state, the body burns calories at an accelerated rate as energy demands are ratcheted upward. The famished body demands fuel: so feed it after training. If preconditions are right, the body will burn fat as fuel.

The purpose of resistance training is to trigger hypertrophy, build muscle and increase muscular strength. When a person new to resistance training begins using a sensible weight training program, when they follow the correct procedures, triggering hypertrophy is relatively easy. Lyle McDonald stated in *The Ketogenic Diet* that every new pound of muscle requires 30 to 40 additional calories per day to survive. Ten pounds of new muscle will burn off 400 additional calories per day, the caloric equivalent of a 40 minute cardio session. From Scientific American Magazine,

> ***"Skeletal muscle is the most abundant tissue on the human body and also one of the most adaptable. Vigorous training with weights can double or triple a muscle's size...a muscle can become more massive only when its individual fibers become thicker."***

By subjecting muscle fiber to external stress, systematically and repeatedly, the fibers thicken in order to cope with the imposed stress. The end result, over time, is that the stressed muscle becomes thicker, larger—and stronger. Experience has shown that certain resistance training procedures are incredibly effective at causing muscle fiber to thicken and strengthen. The Iron Master section illuminates the methodology of the World's greatest resistance trainers. Each attacked their respective situation using widely divergent strategies and procedures; yet when we step back and search for commonalities, we find many among our Iron Masters; the reason being that each respective method is rooted in science and biology.

Here is another Purposefully Primitive tenet: *Certain exercises done in certain ways using certain tools and exerting certain intensities invariably produce certain results.* There are key core exercises that have been proven to be superbly effective at building and strengthening muscles. You can find these key core exercises (or subtle variations) in all the training templates of all the Iron Masters. This is profound and a signal that you too should include these exercises in your resistance training template. Certain exercises done in certain ways can be used by regular individuals to elicit extraordinary results. The Masters have identified these effective exercises and training tactics.

Getting Started

The Nine Critical Free Weight Exercises

Building muscle and strength has been made overly complex by a fitness industry dedicated to selling exercise equipment. Truth be known, there are nine basic free weight exercises that can and will deliver all the results a serious individual can expect from a progressive resistance routine. There are a half dozen or so additional auxiliary free weight exercises that are legitimate variations on the nine core exercises.

You need only a barbell, dumbbells, a sturdy exercise bench that inclines and a primitive set of squat racks. A safety power rack is needed by intermediate and advanced trainees that train alone. Effective muscle and strength building is a raw, brutal undertaking and anyone who tells you different either doesn't know what they are talking about or are trying to sell you a product.

The Iron Masters know that the diligent use of a basic free weight program, done consistently, will deliver more results than any other muscle building/strength-infusing system known to man. Further, there are certain key exercises that rise to the top of all advanced trainers' regimens: key lifts, or close variations, repeatedly appear and these lifts should form the structural backbone of every effective resistance program.

In our Purposefully Primitive approach, the nine key exercises are sub-divided into three tiers: on the top tier are the three most important free weight exercises: the squat, bench press and deadlift. The 2nd tier is occupied by the overhead press, curl and triceps press. The 3rd tier contains the Romanian deadlift, single leg calf raise and abdominal exercise. These nine exercise and their related variations will provide an infinite number of training possibilities and a lifetime of study.

1st Tier	**Squat**	**Bench Press**	**Deadlift**
	Quadriceps	Pectorals	Erectors
	Glutes	Front deltoids	Glutes
	Hamstrings	Triceps	Rhomboids
	Erectors	Latisimus	Teres
			Latisimus
			Trapezius
2nd Tier	**Overhead Press**	**Curl**	**Triceps Press**
	Front/side deltoids	Biceps	Front Triceps
	Triceps	Brachialis	Side Triceps
	Upper pectorals	Forearms	Rear Triceps
3rd Tier	**Romanian Deadlift**	**Calf Raises**	**Abdominals**
	Hamstrings	Calves	Upper Abdominals
	Glutes	Soleus	Lower Abdominals
	Erectors		

Primary Exercises

Squat

Free Weight Squat

I have new trainees work up to 50 free weight squats without poundage before I allow them to transition to plate squats. After all, if you can't do a proper weightless squat, how will you be able to do a correct one holding a heavy plate, much less a barbell perched precariously on your back? Assume a shoulder width stance, inhale, break the knees, push the butt *rearward*; knees out as you descend and ascend. Maintain a bolt upright torso. Knees are not allowed to travel forward out over toes. Descend with tension and precision, squat *deep* then arise explosively.

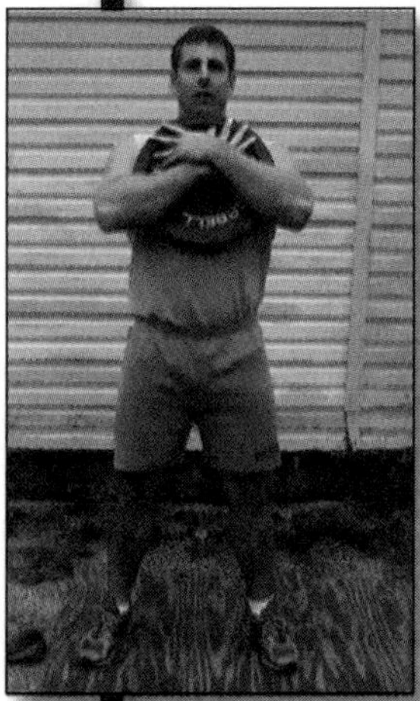

Plate Squat

The plate squat is an interim step. The trainee clutches a plate to their chest as they squat. (Photo 1) Observe all the free weight squat rules: sit *back*—not down! (Photo 2) Spread the knees and keep knees pinioned out throughout. The knees are not allowed to travel forward out over the toes. Keep the knees over the ankles. Inhale mightily on the way down; exhale while arising.

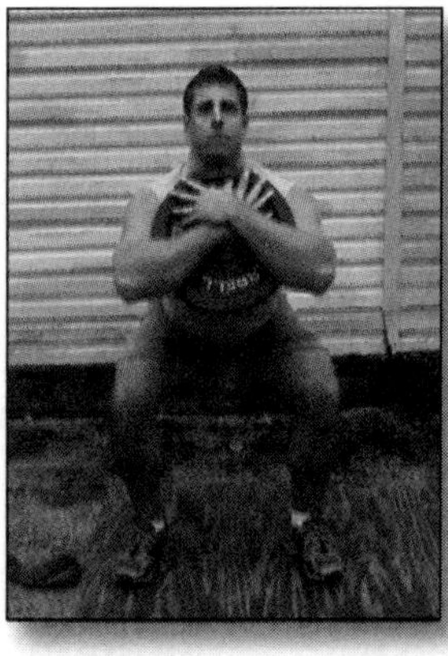

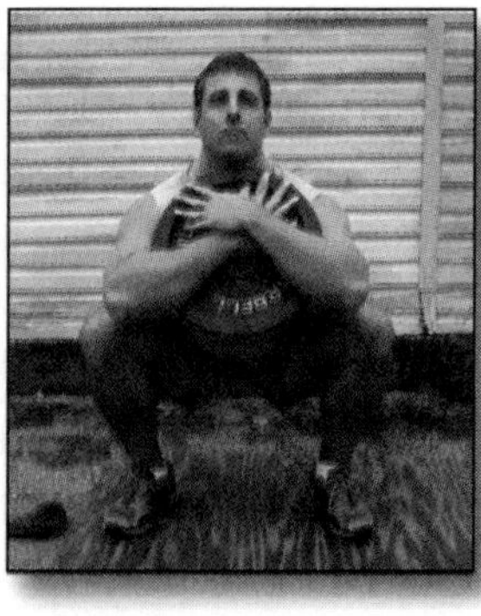

Barbell Squat

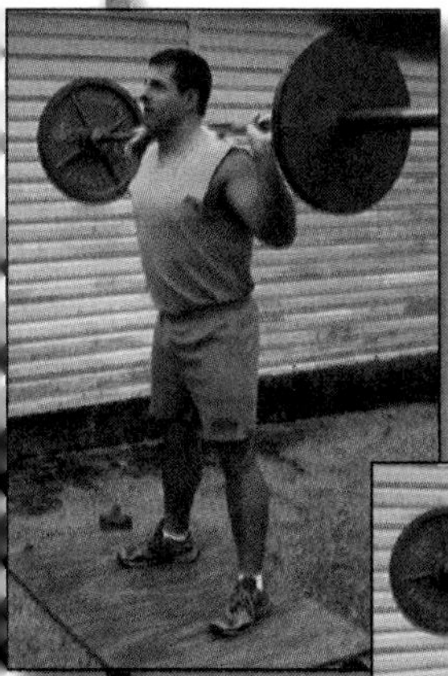

After mastering free weight and plate squats, graduate to the barbell. Never allow the hips to rise up to get a squat moving upward: the butt must stay *under the torso* as you push upward. Stay upright, head back. Do not let the torso bend forward as you rise up. This technical flaw, leaning forward as you arise, turns the great thigh exercise into a potentially injurious exercise.

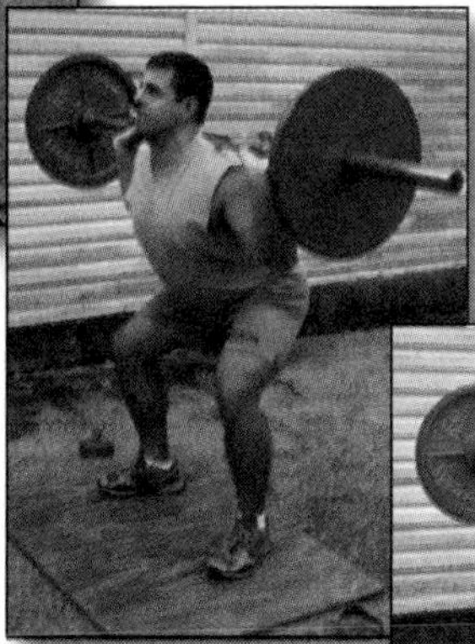

Stance width makes a huge difference in the muscular effect. A wide stance with an upright torso isolates the quads. A legal depth narrow stance squat requires great hip flexibility and cause thighs, glutes and hamstrings to share the workload.

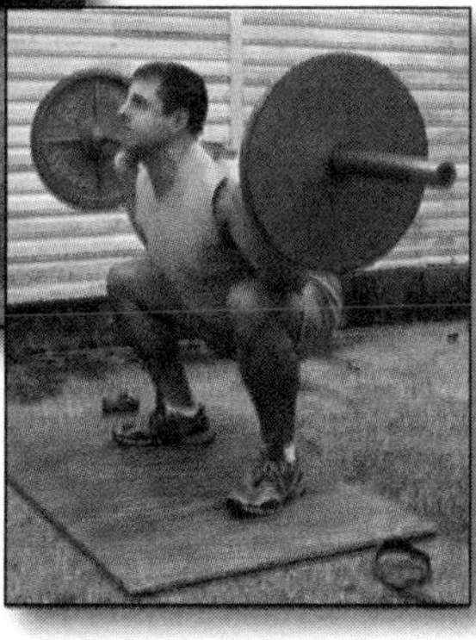

Shallow squats are worthless squats. For maximum effectiveness try pause squats. Pause squats are terrific for ingraining proper technique: use less poundage, squat down, stay upright, pause at the bottom position for 1-5 seconds. Push up on the heels, not the toes. Pauses work great on any stance width.

Bench Press

Incline Free Weight Pushup

Some beginners cannot do a single bench press with the lightest dumbbells. Find a sturdy support 3-4 feet off the ground. Stand three feet away, extend the arms and keep the body straight. Lower to the support. (Photo 2) Push back up while keeping the body rigid. The lower down the push-surface the more difficult the upward push. Three sets of however many reps you can do, three times a week. Lower the surface when you can perform 3 sets of 12 reps. On alternate days shift grip width between wide and narrow.

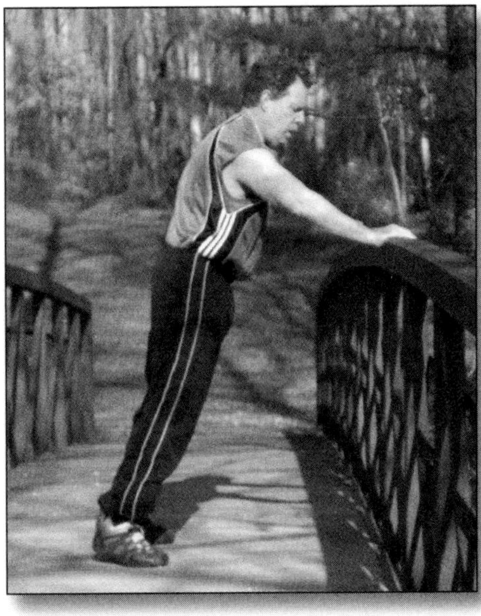

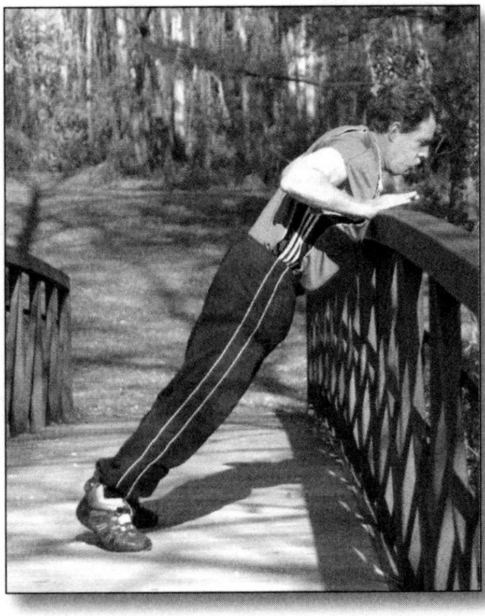

Dumbbell Bench Press

(not shown) Dumbbell bench pressing forces each arm to carry its fair share. Sit upright on an exercise bench, pull two dumbbells, thumb up, close to the torso, lay back and rotate the arms outward. Allow the bells to settle and stretch downward. Push them up while exhaling. Lock the elbows completely. Inhale on the descent and allow the bells to stretch the shoulder girdle downward at the bottom. Lower with control, push explosively, pause every rep Fantano style. The path of the dumbbells arcs slightly rearward, ending over top of the eyes.

Barbell Bench Press

Lower the bar to just below the pectoral muscles. The wider the grip the more pectoral used. (Photos 1 thru 3) A medium width grip causes the muscular stress to be distributed among pecs, front delts and triceps. The narrow grip (Photos 4 thru 6) stresses front delts and most particularly, the triceps. *Pause* poundage on the chest, regardless the chest exercise, before firing the weight to lockout. Pausing bench press reps forces far more muscle fiber to fire than bouncing a barbell off the chest to create momentum; momentum means muscle fiber gets a free ride. Take the momentum out of the bench press; pause barbell bench presses using all the different width grips. Synchronize a gigantic inhalation with the lowering of the bar. Pause and on a full breath use compensatory acceleration to explode the barbell upward.

Wide Grip Bench Press

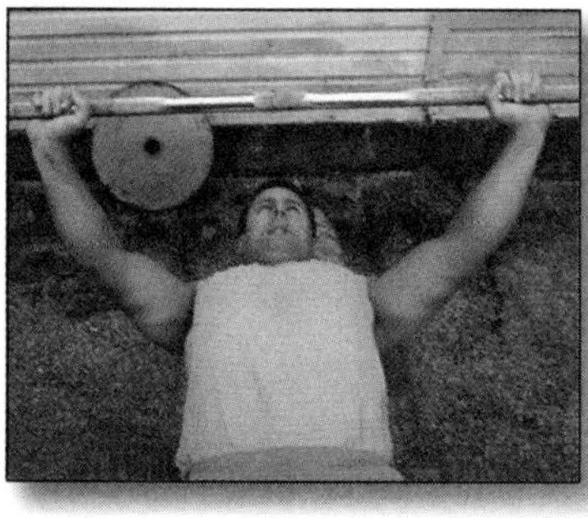
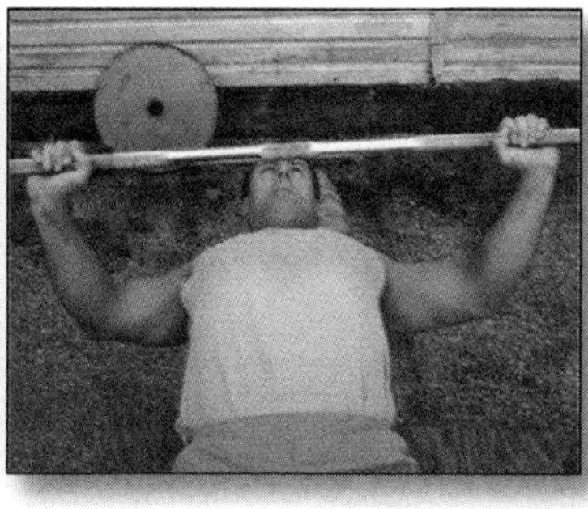
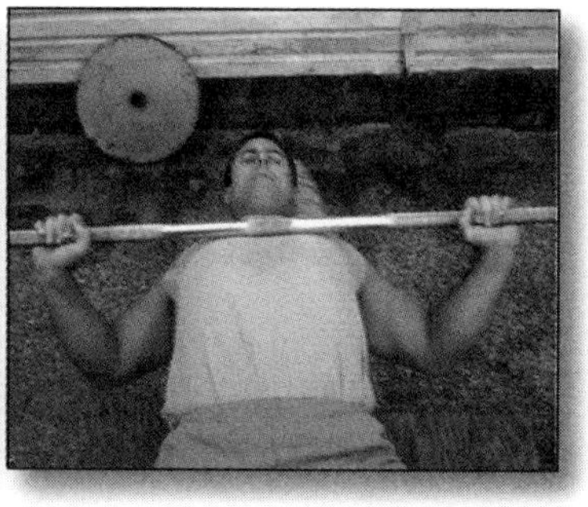

Narrow Grip Bench Press

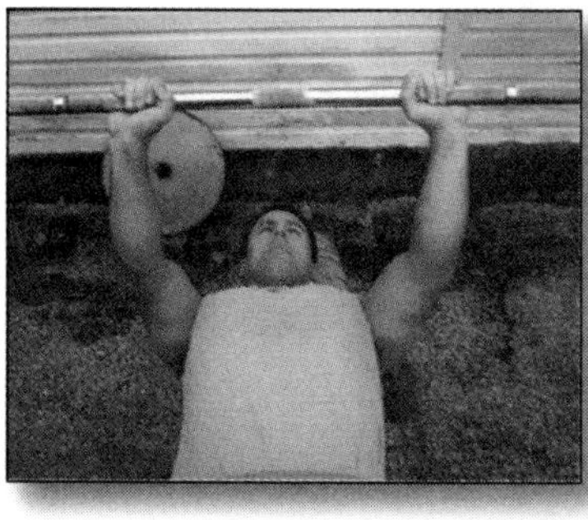
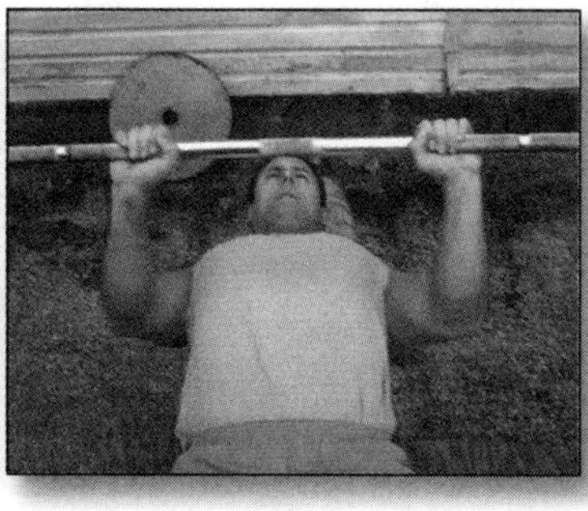
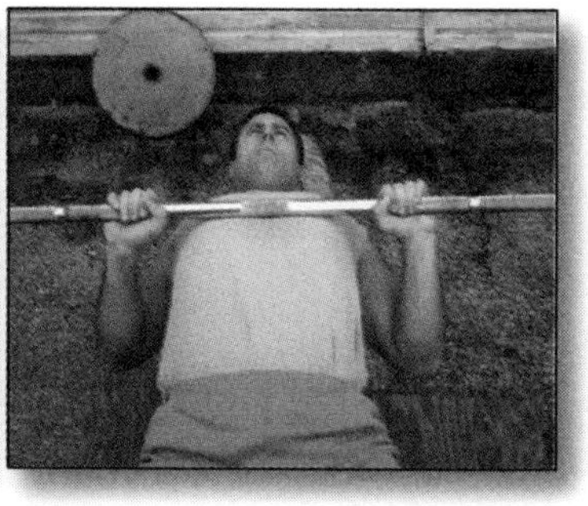

Deadlift

Sumo Deadlift

The easiest deadlift to learn is the sumo deadlift. Think of the Sumo deadlift as a reverse squat. Use the same stance that you use in your wide stance squats. Never *bend over* to pick up a deadlift, squat down to grasp to bar.

Note Chuck's takeoff position: he freezes in this position, generates muscle tension and breaks the bar from the floor by pushing downward with the legs. He maintains his upright torso throughout, no matter what! This is the key technical point to the Sumo. Those with good flexibility can start with an empty bar or pair of light dumbbells. A kettlebell can make an ideal sumo deadlift implement. Keep the knees over the ankles when pushing upward and when lowering the barbell. Keep the hips *under* the shoulders at all times! Lower with tension, precision and control. No bouncing off the floor between reps. At the top of each rep exhale. Inhale mightily on the descent. Done properly, the thighs are stressed, not the lower back.

If the back hurts after a session you are bending over, not squatting down. Bad technique!

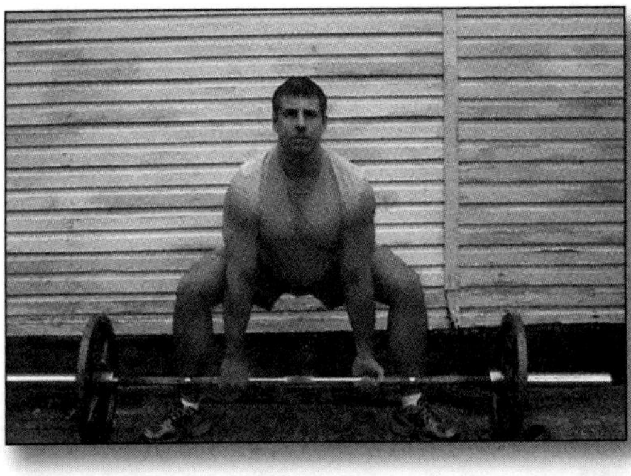

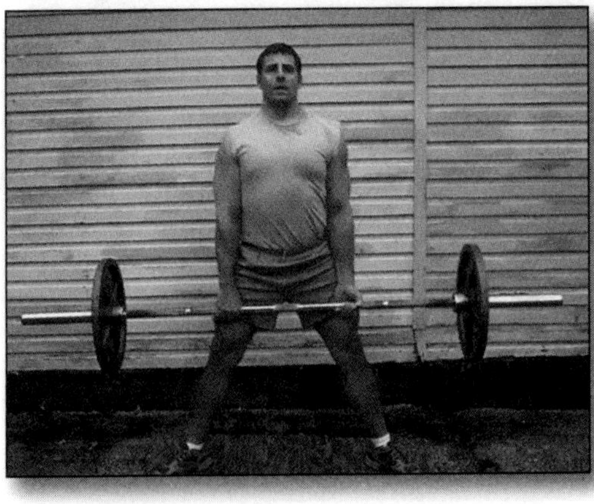

Conventional Deadlift

Stand over top of a loaded barbell. Look down; you should be able to see your toes under the bar. Set feet 8 to 15 inches between heels. Every muscle on the back is tensed. The spine is kept rigid as you *squat back and down.*

Squat down until you can grasp the barbell with a shoulder width grip. The eyes look up. Using leg power alone, break the weight from the floor. The bar travels up the vertical shins, staying in continual contact with the shins and thighs before achieving lock-out. The pull commences when the shoulders are directly over the bar in the lowest position. Pull upward in a straight line to completion. Lower the bar without losing any muscular tension. *Quietly* touch the weights on the floor before instantly reversing direction to begin the next rep.

Tension ensures precision and control. The spine and the muscles of the back stay arched, tight and upright at all times. Never, ever allow the butt to rise up as you start a rep. The butt is kept *under* the torso. Keep the shoulders over the bar throughout the pull.

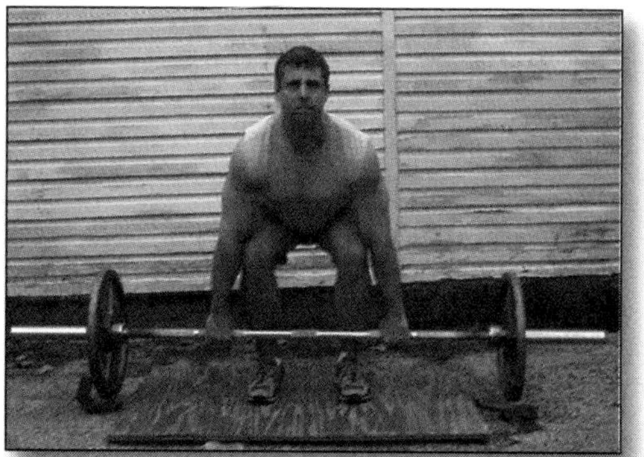

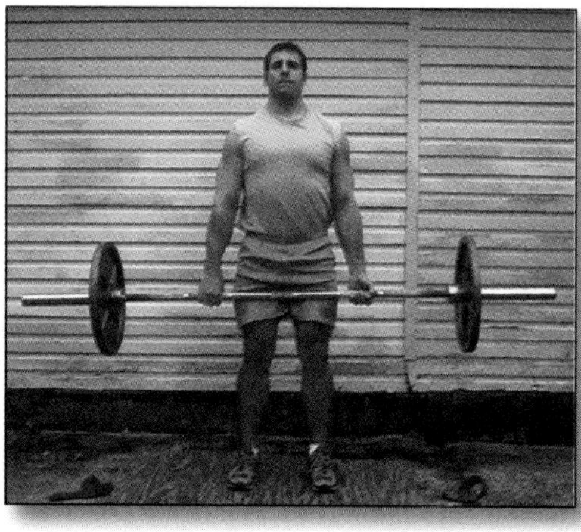

Secondary Exercises

Overhead Press

There are three distinct overhead press variations. Each one can be done standing or seated: the barbell press, the dumbbell press and the press behind the neck (PBN). In the standing overhead barbell and dumbbell press, power clean a weight to the shoulders, lean back ever so slightly, lock the legs and freeze the back. Now push upward as close to the face as possible. Use a shoulder width grip. In the PBN, set the loaded bar in the squat rack, shoulder it and step back. Use a wide grip, same as the wide grip bench press. Press the weight overhead. Be careful to not bonk the back of your skull. Lower to the hairline or ear lobes before pushing upward. Use standing and seated versions for variety. Always lock the elbows fully and completely. Hold the top position for a full second. Lower slowly and with great control. Push explosively!

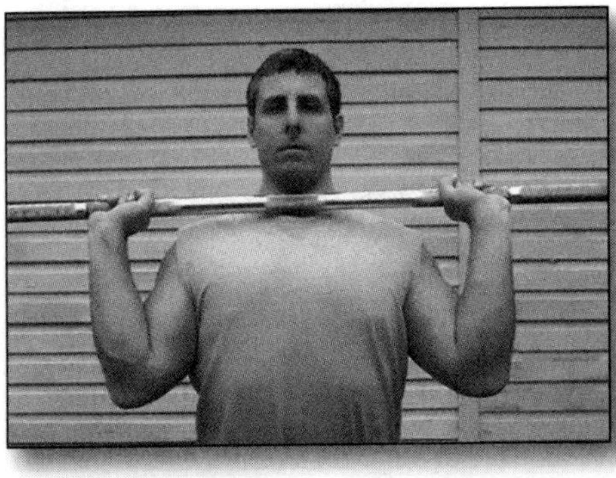

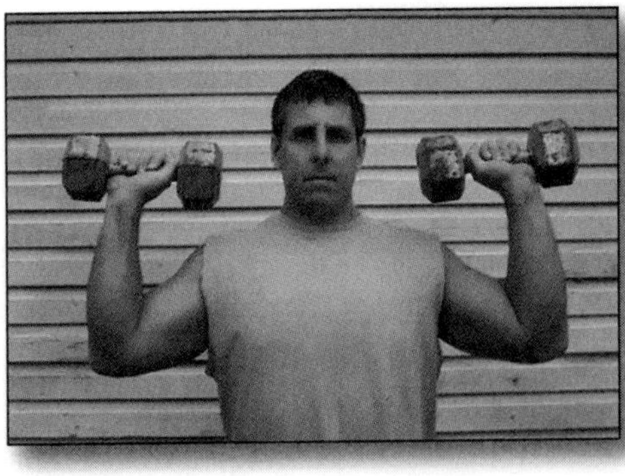

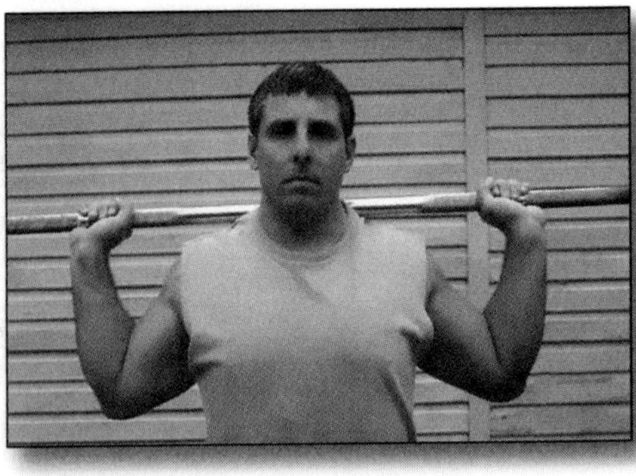

Biceps Curl

Keep the elbows back regardless of what curl variation you select. Don't turn curls, a terrific biceps exercise, into half-ass deltoid front raises. Most trainees allow the elbows to move forward as they curl. This makes the curl easier; the biceps calls on its neighbor, the deltoid, to help lift the poundage. Isolate the biceps by keeping the elbows back. Alternately, uses pads or braces that immobilize the upper arm: preacher bench, spider curl bench, any of the various curl machines.

Utilize different arc paths using barbell and dumbbell curls. Try curls done close to the body, curls angled out from the body. The trainee will be able to isolate the inner or outer biceps head by honing isolative curl techniques. This is *not* a compound multi-joint exercise! Feel the biceps contracting as you are performing the curl; avoid using the front deltoids to lift the weight. Curls have a nearly limitless number of variations. The name of the game is making the mind/muscle connection with the target muscle. "Feel" the biceps work as the rep is happening. Muscle contraction is only achieved with fierce concentration.

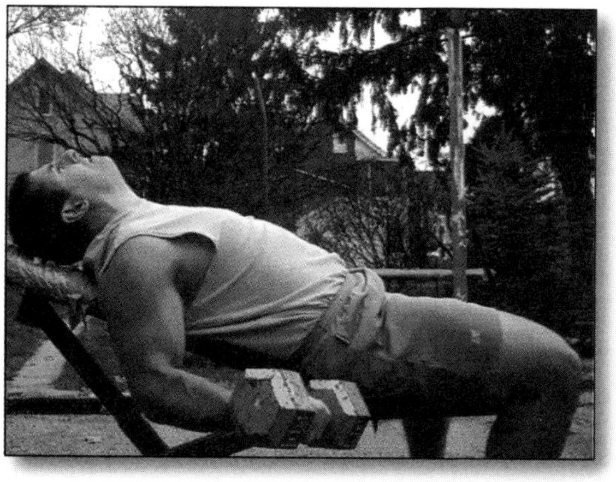

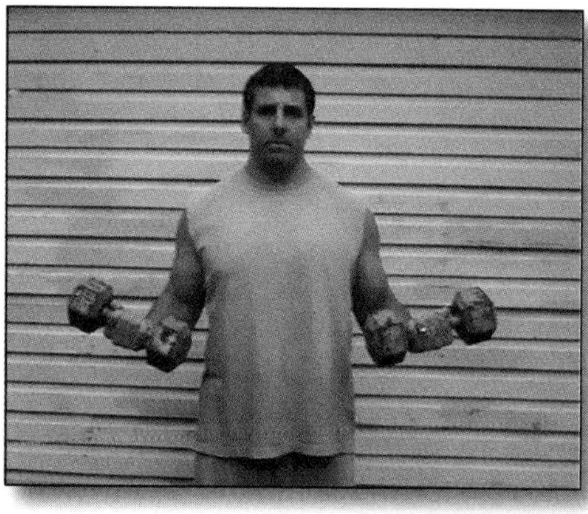

Triceps Extension

Triceps extensions are an isolation exercise and can be done standing, seated or lying. They can be done with one or two dumbbells, or a single barbell. Using a very narrow 4-6 inch overhand grip, palms facing up, push a *light* barbell, dumbbell or pair of dumbbells overhead. Stabilize the upper arms. Once the upper arms are immobilized and frozen, lower the poundage until the triceps is stretched. (See photo)

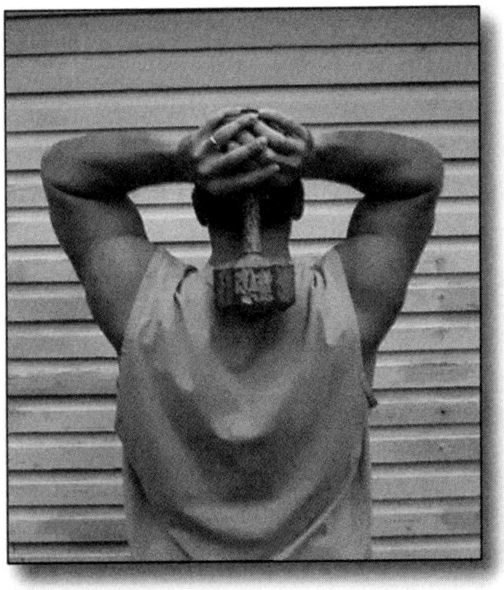

Allow the poundage to stretch downward, behind the head. When the lowered weight has bottomed out, push upward, and do not allow the lower arms to shift or sway or try and find some better push position. Freeze the lower arms and use triceps power alone to push the poundage from the stretched position to complete lock out. You will feel the triceps contract intensely as the upward push is occurring. Smoothly lower and raise the lower arm. The smooth upward push culminates in a full and complete elbow lock. Tense the triceps hard in the completed position before lowering. Looking at the lift from afar, only the *forearms* move.

TERTIARY EXERCISES

Romanian Deadlift

The Romanian deadlift is traditionally done while holding a barbell and is a spinal erector exercise. Our version is done holding a single barbell plate and is a hamstring isolation exercise without peer. This is the most intense and effective of all hamstring exercises and is difficult to describe. Done with improper technique, this exercise disintegrates into a worthless, sub-maximal erector exercise.

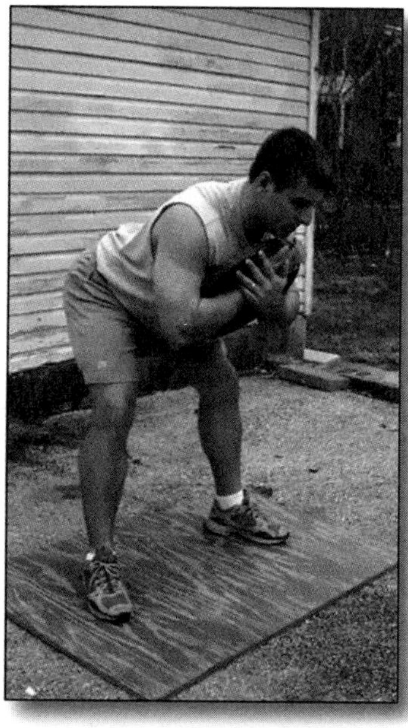

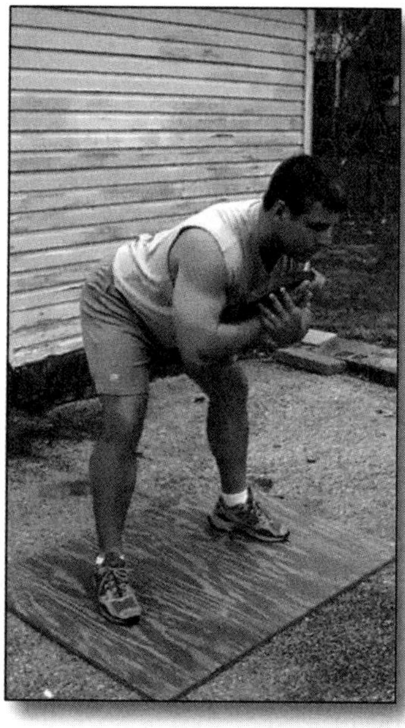

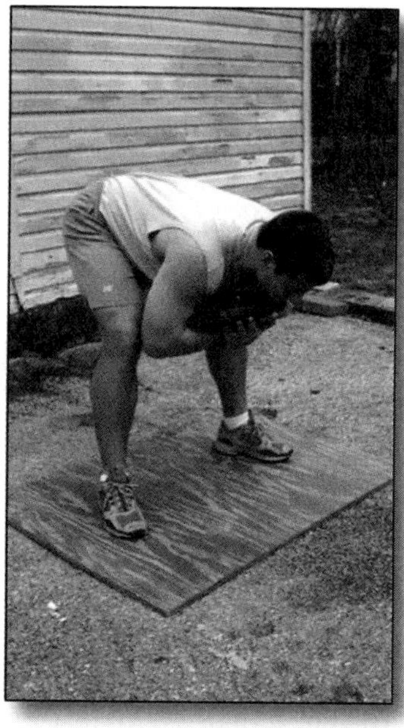

Assume a Sumo deadlift stance and stand erect holding a plate. (Not shown) Break forward at the hip joint while maintaining a tight arched back. Lean forward, (photo 1&2) descending slowly. Allow the poundage to pull the torso downward. The hip joint is the fulcrum. At the lowest point, exhale all remaining air. This allows the poundage to pull the torso downward another 3-6 inches. Rise up slowly, *very slowly*. Use the HAMSTRING POWER ALONE to come erect. Feel the hamstring struggle to ratchet the torso into final lockout position. Slow-motion is the key to the effectiveness of this exercise. You will feel a stretch in the hamstrings lowering to the bottom position. You feel an intense hamstring contraction while arising.

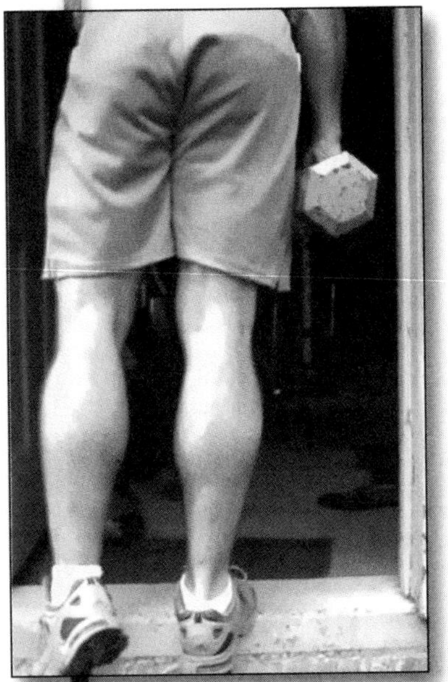

Calf Raise

Seated or standing, there are a couple tricks of the trade worth sharing. First, periodically alter toe positions: heels flared out and toes pointed inward, rise up onto the outer portion of the foot. Toes pointed straight ahead rise up onto the middle of the foot. Heels close and toes are turned out, rise up onto the inside ball of the foot. Always commence each rep from a totally stretched position. At the top of each rep hold the completed position, high on the toes, for several seconds.

High reps work best for both calves and forearms. Sets of fifteen to fifty reps are used to attack the dense tissue of the calf. Our selected ultra-basic calf raise is the single-leg calf raise done on a step holding a dumbbell.

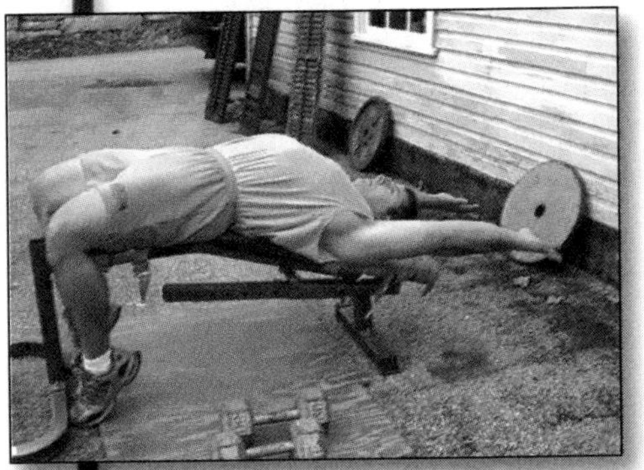

Decline Sit-up

There are a million abdominal exercises and lots of people have favorites. Essentially you have upper abs, lower abs and external oblique, side muscles. We like the decline sit-up and per usual have some trade tricks: note Chuck's toes are barely held in place by a thin rail. This way he is unable to push upward with thigh flexion and take stress off the frontal abs. The exaggerated ROM with the head-below-shoulders start position makes the first 1/3rd of this exercise the most difficult. We hold our arms overhead to make the difficult more difficult. Initially do these with arms crossed on the chest. These can also be done holding a barbell plate.

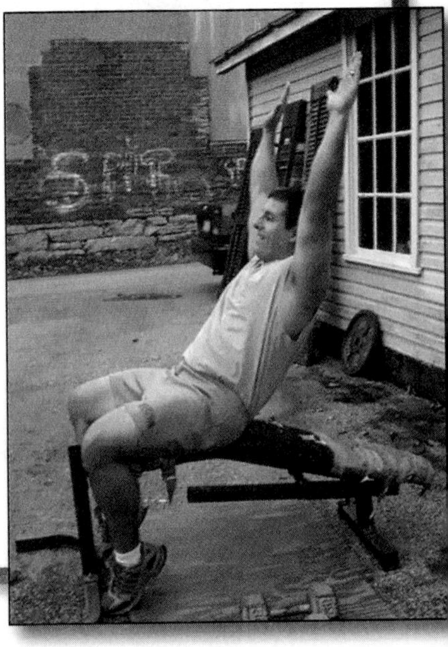

Sit back all the way, until the back of the head touches the bench pad, that's you signal to come erect—but slowly—roll up one vertebra at a time. This is another continuous tension isolation exercise. Start each rep from a dramatically twisted position and blast the external oblique muscle. Lower slowly to the other side, twisted that direction. Touch the shoulder and while maintaining the twist, power erect. The slo-mo decline sit-up is excruciatingly effective.

AUXILIARY EXERCISES

Legs

Front Squat

This is a fabulous exercise; next to back squats, the second best leg exercise known to man. Load a barbell on the squat rack, step under the poundage using front squat hand position. (Photo 1) Break the bar from the squat rack, step backwards and set the feet in a back squat stance. Now take a huge breath and squat down. Upon breaking the knees, push the butt rearward while maintaining an upright torso. (Photos 2&3) The stance is wide enough to allow you to squat deep. Squat flat-footed and maintain balance. The thigh stimulation is incredible, even using light poundage. The movement is very similar to the front squat holding a plate.

The trick is to squat deep while maintaining flat-footed balance. Inhale as you descend and exhale as you come erect. When your set is done, simply return the bar to the squat rack. Wrist ache will pass, the wrists loosen up eventually.

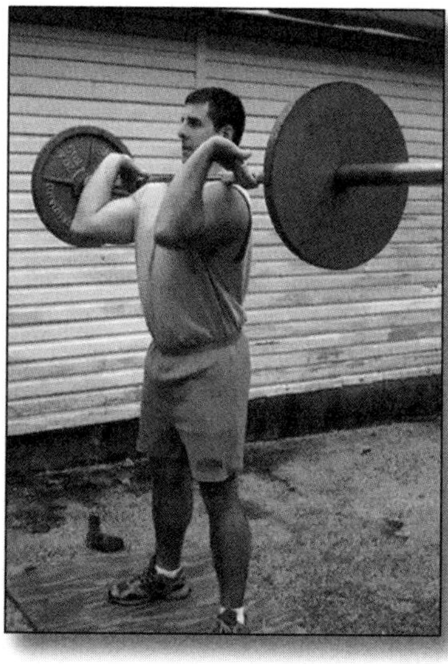

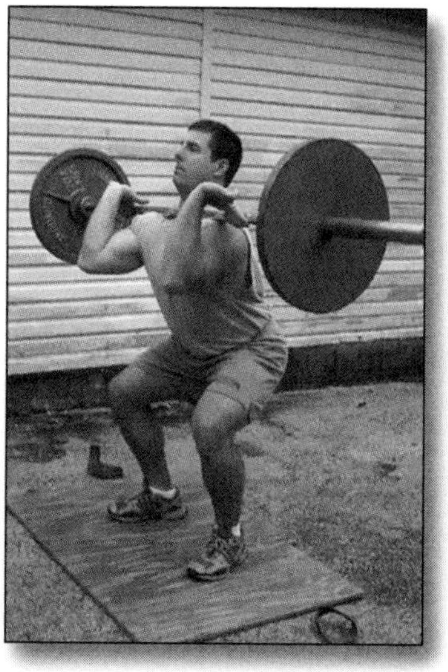

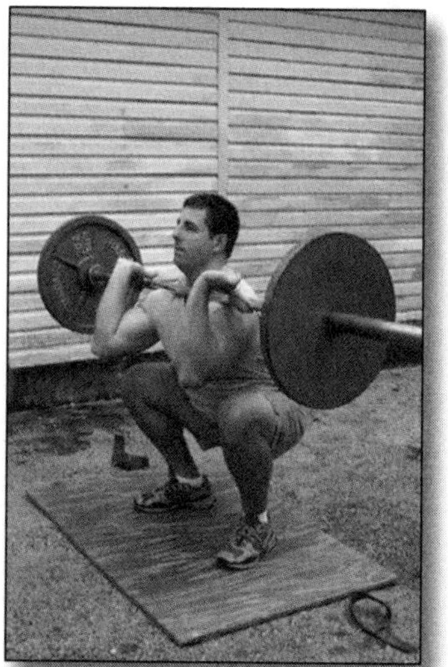

Lying Leg Curl

This is a good hamstring stimulator made better by using a few Old School technical tricks. Our variation is the excruciating "slow start leg curl with full pull-though." Sounds like a dish at a gourmet restaurant. Leverage is extremely good for the first 4-6 inches of a leg curl rep. The trainee can generate an explosion at the start of a leg curl and *fling* the poundage upward to completion. By using a violent start you can create and ride the momentum to completion. We purposefully use a slow start that eliminates momentum. Suddenly the payload seems four times heavier—which is exactly what we want. Another tip: push the hips into the bench pad as you pull on the weight. The natural inclination is to let the hips rise up during the pull. This makes the leg curl easier—which is exactly what we don't want. We want harder! Slash poundage, use the slow start; push the hips downward into the bench.

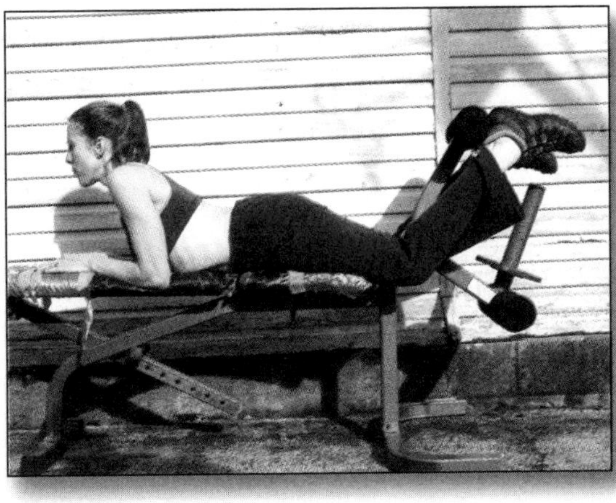

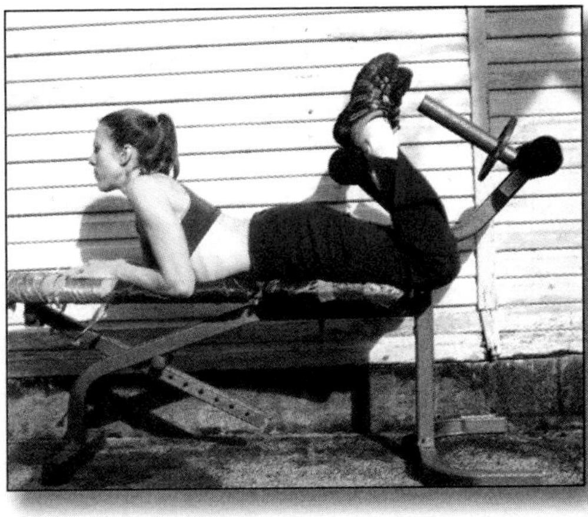

Chest

Incline Press

We could rename the incline dumbbell press, The Irish Pat Casey Press or the Italiano Fantano press. Both men could push 200 pound dumbbells for a half dozen paused reps.

We expropriate Ken's incline technique: make sure the lower back adheres to the 45 degree bench pad at all times. Please do not turn inclines into flat benches by bridging upward when the rep gets rough, thereby turning an incline into a flat bench. Pause the weight on the chest on every rep and hold an ultra-flexed lockout for 1-2 seconds before lowering for the next rep. Ken demanded the bells be touched together at the conclusion of each rep. (Photo 3)

Push on an upward motor pathway using a barely discernable rearward arc. At the start of the push, the elbows are under the payload. Explode the poundage upward, using compensatory acceleration, i.e., push as fast as possible through ever inch of the concentric phase. Push up, slightly back and inward. Bump the bells at the top. Feel the upper pecs contract when pushing to completion.

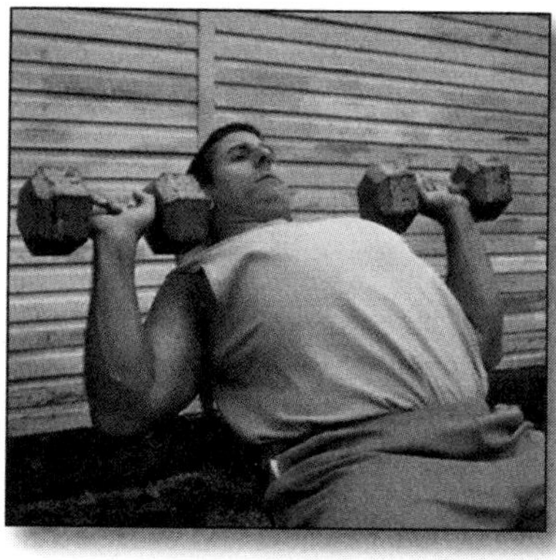

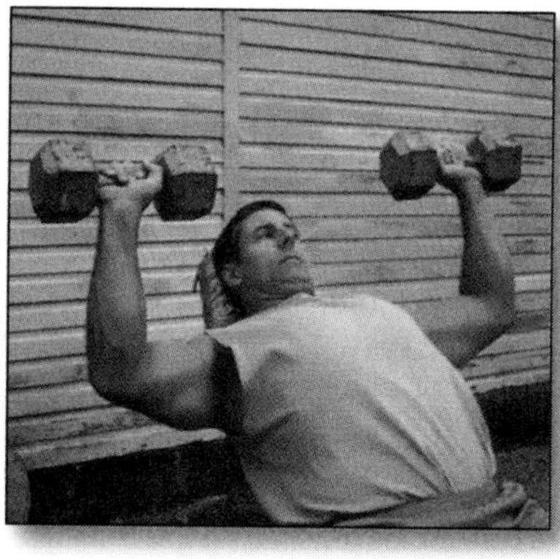

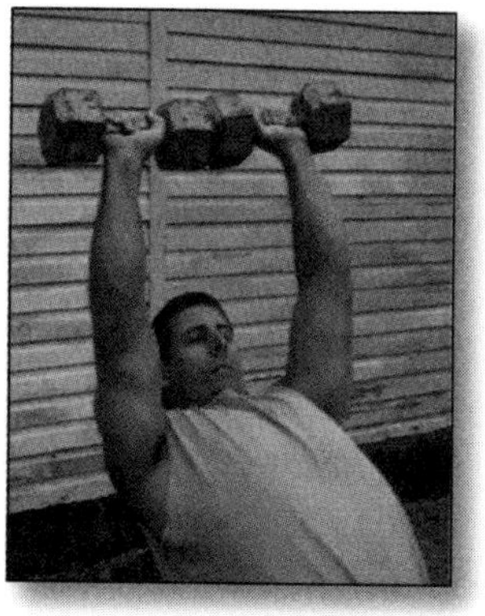

Dips

Many dip variations: one can be done between two benches. (photo 1) The between-bench dip is the easiest because you are dipping with less than your full bodyweight. Dip deep, slump forward, relax and stretch in the bottom. Then power upwards to complete elbow lock-out. Hold lock-out for two full seconds, flex the triceps to the point of cramping. A partner can set a plate on your lap to increase resistance. Standard dips use fixed bars. For triceps, dips can be lowered until the upper arms are parallel to the floor. Free weight dips done deep work pecs while weighted dips are the Mac Daddy. Master bench dips before progressing to "regular" and finally, weighted dips.

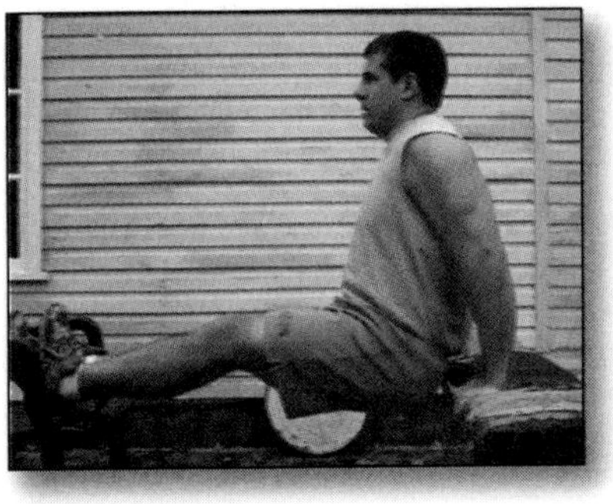

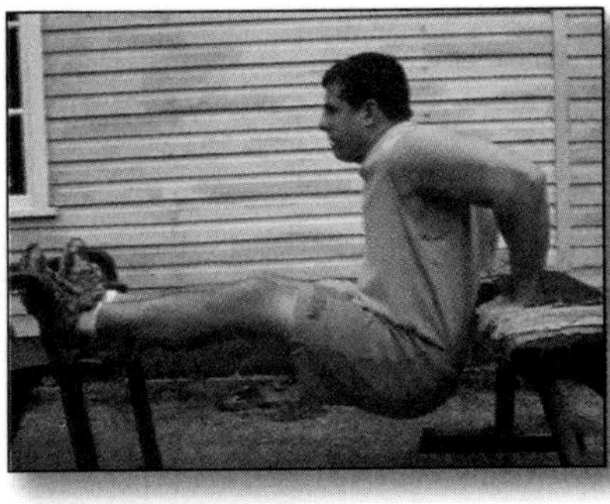

Dumbbell Flyes

Don't let dumbbell flyes morph into some weird combination of flye and dumbbell bench press. A proper flye is done with pristine technique and (relatively) light weight. Poundage needs to be light thus allowing the arms and especially the hands to be held *wide* as possible while the weight is raised and lowered.

Arnold called himself "A master of flyes" and described the correctly performed flye, "You should feel as if you were hugging a giant tree." Raise the arms upward *slowly* keeping the hands flung wide. Lift the bells using pec *power* alone. Continual tension flyes allows complete pec isolation. The bottom stretch is critical: allow the bells to pull the arms downward: lift with pecs alone!

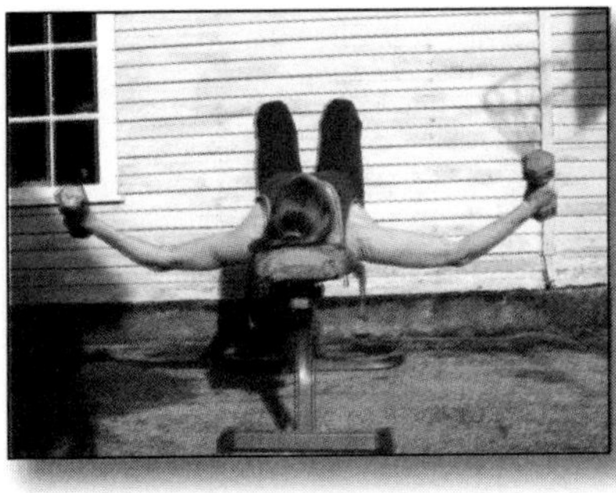

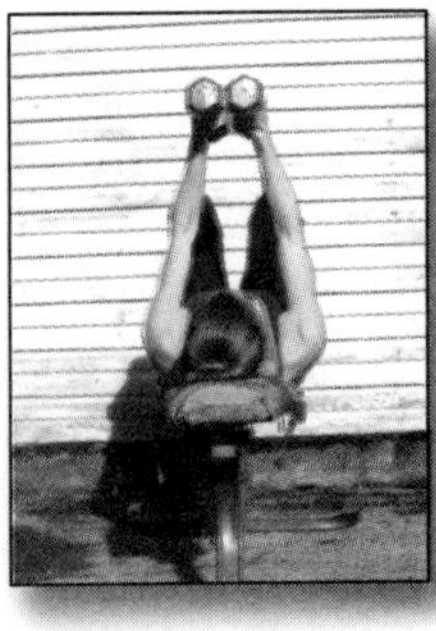

Back

Power Clean

Technically tricky, this is an outstanding overall back developer. The power clean is the second best of all back exercises, next to the deadlift. The PC blasts traps, spinal erectors, teres, lats and rhomboids.

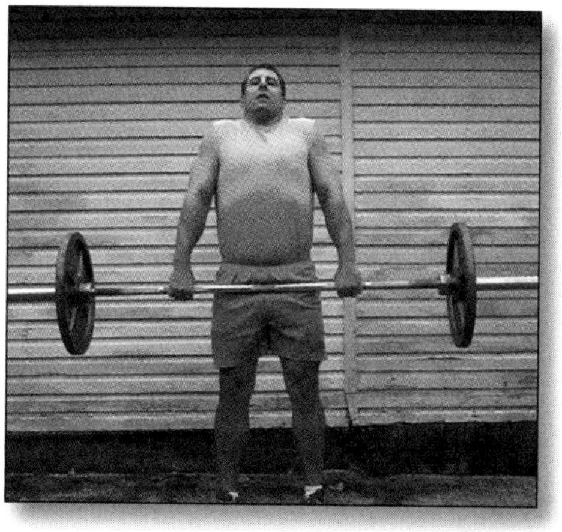

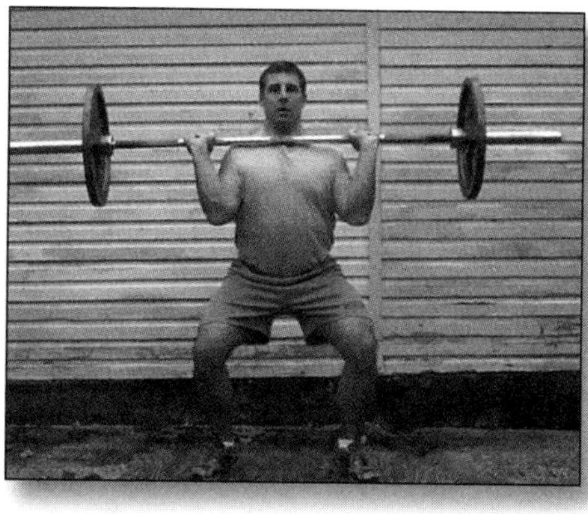

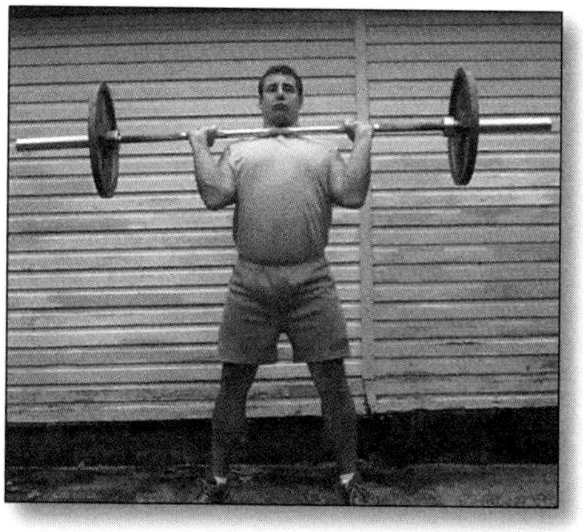

Use a shoulder width stance and shoulder width grip. Squat down in a conventional deadlift start position. Now pull a light barbell upward in one fluid motion. (Photo 1) The barbell is pulled *straight up*. Use a weight that you can pull to shoulder height for 10 reps *easily*. At the pulls peak, snap the wrists under, catching the barbell on the shoulders. (Photo 2) Stand erect cradling the bar. (Photo 3) This is one rep. Flip the bar off the shoulders and replace it on the floor. Begin the second rep immediately using a tight, flexed, flat, arched back. The bar travels upward in a straight line, always and forever the shortest distance between two points. The optimal starting pull position, be it power clean, high pull or deadlift, commences with shins as near vertical as possible. The barbell is never jerked at the start; apply power slowly at the takeoff and accelerate as the bar moves upward. Go up on the toes to add height. Elite lifters jump down and under and splay the feet outward, catching the barbell in a splendid iron ballet worthy of emulation. Lower the bar to the platform using great restraint and control.

A poor lifter bounces and crashes his reps off the floor while the elite lifter's plates touch in near silence. This is a technique lift so please work on precision, speed and position using modest poundage.

Barbell Rowing

This is a terrific lat builder, but alas, performed improperly (no lat isolation) rows are worthless. In Photo 1, Chuck's barbell is actually being held an inch off the ground; he has "frozen" his torso position. He will pull the bar to the chest maintaining this position throughout the set. Rows can be "arm pulled" instead of "back pulled." From the dead hang, pull the bar upward and touch the stomach. The torso stays parallel to the floor throughout. Do not dip and heave from the hip joint to get the bar moving—that makes the lift easier and we want to make the lift harder. With a torso frozen and immobile, *pull* the bar to the chest using the back instead of the arms.

Another key technical point: pull back and up with the *elbows*, not the biceps. This causes the target muscles, the upper and lower latissimus dorsi to activate. Try to hold the bar on the chest for a split second before lowering: this creates further contractions. Heaving upward from the waist to start each rep turns a great lat exercise into a so-so erector exercise. Grip widths can be altered to create different muscular effects: try a wide 32 inch grip and lighter poundage. Alter under-grip width.

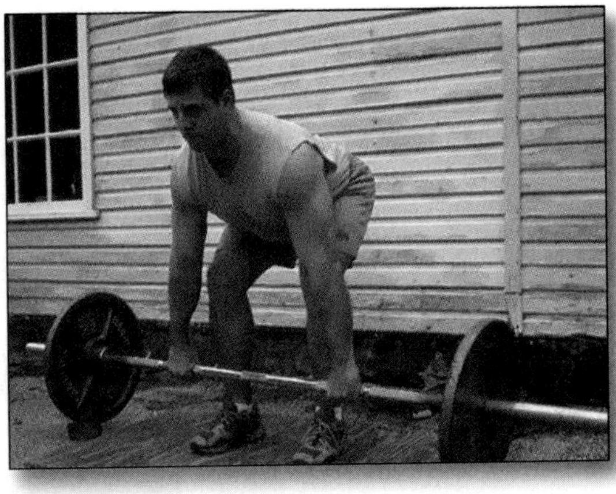

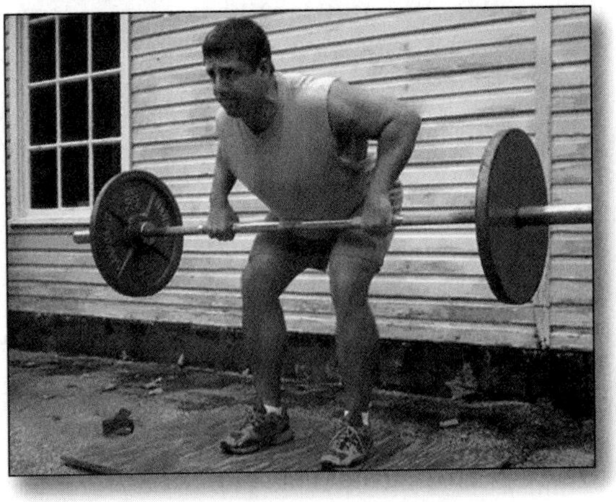

Two Day A Week Training

Weight training twice a week is the bare minimum. Even in the primordial world of the Purposeful Primitive, twice a week is the *least* amount of training required for a serious effort.

Our amalgamated template for twice-a-week training is super simplistic: perform the three 1st Tier core lifts or their close variations twice a week. A beginner would perform three sets of each. Advanced trainees might want to add "back-off sets." This routine is the barest of the bare and must be executed with sufficient intensity. This routine can be *extremely* productive. It is a result-producing legitimate strength approach that is the absolute best entry-level program for a beginner.

It can be amped-up for advanced trainees by adding the Hugh Cassidy "Hallmark Back-off Sets." Then barebones basic becomes brutal. To incorporate back-off sets, work up to the top set then slash the poundage by 25% and perform three static sets. If you are a serious trainer experiencing burnout, twice-a-week training is a great way to rejuvenate. Often, advanced men train so often their training loses its effectiveness. Twice a week squat/bench/deadlift *only* training is a great way to cut back yet stay serious. Cassidy's expanded version turns barebones into an Iron Inferno. Minimalist routines are wonderfully remedial for chronic burnout.

For a beginner, performing the three lifts exclusively twice a week is ideal. Total homage is paid to learning, *really learning* proper technique in the three most important exercises in all of resistance training: squat, bench press, deadlift.

This is iron immersion: you repeatedly practice at tugging and pushing on ever increasing poundage and become exceedingly proficient at the squat, bench press and deadlift. What a fabulous base, what a terrific progressive resistance foundation on which to construct all future efforts. This routine is ideal for someone with limited time and each session can be completed in 30 minutes (or less) by a beginner. The truly strong might need an hour. If you have a crazy work schedule or hectic life situation, this is for you.

Mark Chaillet squatted and bench pressed on Monday and deadlifted on Thursday, working up to a single rep in each lift. That was it! He used this approach to deadlift 880 and squat 1,000. Beginners should perform three sets of 10 repetitions in the squat, bench press and deadlift twice weekly. A good rule of thumb is on the first set, use 50% of the final poundage. If you intend to work up to 100 pounds for 10 repetitions on the third and final squat set, the poundage menu would break out as follows...set #1, 50 pounds for 10 repetitions; Set #2, 75 pounds for 10 repetitions; Set #3, 100 pounds for 10 repetitions. Use the 50% 75% 100% poundage approach for all three lifts.

Two Day Split: Simplistic, Time Efficient, Deadly Effective!

Day I	Squat, Bench Press, Sumo Deadlift
Day II	Squat, Bench Press, Conventional Deadlift

Advanced men can add back-off sets: if you were to bench 405x5 on the top set, the back-off sets would be 345x8 (85% of 405) for the three static sets. Advanced trainees need more sets. A 650 deadlifter might go 135/255/345/455/545 before 585x5 on the top set of the day. Peck and I used four 4-week cycles: 8 rep top set, then 5, then 3 with back-off sets of 10, 8 and 5 for 3 sets.

Three Day A Week Training

The three day a week Purposefully Primitive amalgamated training template is the last of the routines wherein the entire body is blasted, head to toe, in the same session. I used this template successfully for the first five years of my own lifting career. This approach is classic: I got it from the Mac McCallum and Bill Starr in ancient *Strength & Health* Magazines.

A three day a week routine always works well for athletes involved with competitive sports as it allows plenty of time for other athletic activities. The stronger you get, the longer it will take to get through this "Big Man" Routine. You will *need* a couple days to recover. Then you hit it again. In the three day a week training regimen, add Tier II exercises: standing overhead press, barbell curl and triceps press/extension, to the existing menu of Tier I Exercises. Periodize the squats, bench presses, deadlifts and overhead pressing. No need to cycle arms. This approach works phenomenally well for intermediate lifters, athletes involved in other sports, and serious fitness devotees. If you don't feel blasted, you're not exerting enough. You need to sustain the effort from the beginning until the end of the workout.

Anybody can kick ass on the 1st exercise of a routine, but whose ass is being kicked on the third set of the 5th exercise? This routine is a lot of work; beginners should complete it in 45 minutes or less. Advanced men—who are stronger and who need more time to get up to that all-out top set—might need 60-75 minutes. This is at the outer limits of muscular endurance. Always do arms last! We begin using core exercise variations.

Three Day Split: Work the Whole Body Thrice Weekly

Day I	Squat, Medium Grip Bench Press, Sumo Deadlift, Barbell Standing Press, Barbell Curl, Lying Triceps Extension
Day II	Pause Squat, DB Bench Press, Romanian Deadlift, DB Seated Press, Incline DB Curls, Dips
Day III	Front Squat, Wide Grip Bench Press, Conventional Deadlift, Press-behind-neck, Barbell Curl, Standing Triceps extensions

Beginners: 3 sets of 8 reps progressive: 1st set, 50%, 2nd set, 75%, 3rd set 100%
Advanced Trainees: Note that we incorporate our exercise variations and options. Instead of regular squats three times a week, perform squats, pause squats and front squats. Dumbbell bench presses make for a terrific bench variation. Switch from sumo deadlifts to Romanian to conventional deadlifts. Use seated dumbbell press, incline curls and overhead dumbbell triceps presses. Dips are a fabulous triceps exercise.

A word about periodizing for advanced trainees: in a classical 12 week periodization cycle, the cycle is broken down into three 4 week cycles. Week 1-4 try working up to an all-out set of 8, in week 5-8 work up to all-out set of 5 reps and in week 9-12 hit triples. If you are reverse periodizing, looking to lean out, try starting off with 6 rep sets, jump to 8s and end with 12s. Again, this is a tough routine and young aggressive testosterone-laden men will make excellent gains. It is important to smart bomb with a protein/carb shake after training to replenish the traumatized body. By using basic exercises and their close variations this template hits muscles from slightly different angles and eliminates boredom.

Four Day A Week Training

If you engage in serious progressive resistance training long enough you become stronger. Biological fact: if you train the way we tell you, you will make size and strength gains.

Basically, when your strength reaches a certain point, *whole body routines* take too long. The exercises at the end of the elongated whole body routine invariably suffer. What good is it to handle 150x6 in an exercise at the ass-end of a whole body session when you can handle 150x10 when fresh? Session stamina and pure fatigue comes into play more and more as you become stronger.

Recovery is another issue that becomes more intrusive as you become stronger: it takes a muscle a lot longer to recover from 455x5 than it does to recover from 155x5. It takes a hell of a lot longer to recover from 655x5 than it does to recover from 155x5.

If a man can get to the gym for 60 minutes four times a week, incredible gains can be realized.

I have created an amalgamated version of a four day Yates/Karwoski template. Feel free to use either man's *exact* routine as outlined in the Master's Method section. Periodize the lifts. In our four day routine muscles are blasted to smithereens once a week:

Four Day Split: Ground Zero Split Routine

Day I	**Leg Day:** Squat Front Squat Romanian DL or Leg Curl Standing Calf Raise	Start with squats, continue with front squats, follow up with assistance exercises.
Day II	**Chest & Triceps:** Competition Grip Bench Wide Grip Bench Narrow Grip Bench DB Flyes Dips Lying Triceps Extension	Three bench grip widths, followed by a few sets of very light DB flyes. Dips make a terrific segue into triceps. If dips are problematic substitute bench dips. End with lying or overhead tri extensions.
OFF	OFF	Rest for a day in the middle of the split.
Day III	**Back & Biceps:** Deadlift 70-Degree Row Power Clean Preacher Bench Curls Spider Curls	Deadlifts followed by regular rows or 70-degree rows. Power cleans are light and precise. Feel free to substitute Progressive Pulls. Pick two types of curls, perform 8-12 reps.
Day IV	**Shoulders & Abs:** Overhead Standing Press Press-Behind-Neck (PBN) Lateral Raises Abs	Press, behind-the-neck press, laterals. Some men add light chest, more triceps or another 'lagging' part. Hit abs hard.
OFF	OFF	Take two days off to be prepared to start the routine over again.

Beginners: This is not a beginner routine!

Five Day A Week Training

I like to use an amalgamated variation of Bob Bednarski's rolling training split. You could also use the "straight/no chaser" Ed Coan program pulled directly from the Master Method section. The choice is yours. My Bednarski-inspired rolling progression concentrates on a single body part or lift per day for five straight days in a row. I love this approach; you focus totally and completely on a single body part or lift each day. Ed's routine is pure power perfection.

Five Day Split: Iron Immersion

Day I	**Quads:** Squats, pause squats or Front Squat	Pick one: squat, pause squats or front squat. Do up to 10 sets. Work up to a maximum 3-5 rep set then hit 2-3 static sets of 5 to 8 reps.
Day II	**Chest:** Bench Press Dumbbell Bench Incline Bench	Pick one: bench, dumbbell bench or inclines. Do up to 10 sets. Work up to a maximum 3-5 rep set then hit 2-3 static sets of 5 to 8 reps.
Day III	**Back:** Progressive Pulls	Progressive pulls could be used. (See Iron Essays for description). Other possibilities include: deadlifts alone, power cleans alone, deadlifts off a plate or high pulls. Perhaps chins or pulldowns alone for upwards of 10 sets.
Day IV	**Shoulders:** Front Barbell Press Dumbbell Press Press Behind the Neck	Pick one: Front Barbell Press, Dumbbell Press or Press Behind the Neck. Work up to a maximum 3-5 rep set then hit 2-3 static sets of 5 to 8 reps.
Day V	**Leftovers:** Biceps Curls/Triceps Ext Calf Raises/Leg Curl Abs	Super-set day: super-set curls and triceps. Calf raises can be super-setted with hamstrings. A good day for extended ab session.
OFF	OFF	Take two days off to be prepared to start the routine over again.

Beginners: This is <u>not</u> a beginner routine!

Advanced Trainees: Cycle the squat, bench, progressive pulls and overhead presses. Sessions should be concentrated. This routine works for both power/strength and for leaning out. It can also be used by those pressed for time. A beginner or intermediate trainee can blast the hell out of one exercise in 20 minutes—I mean blast to the point of complete exhaustion. I usually hit 7 to 10 sets on a single exercise. On day V hit the "minor" exercises. You must not rush and you must not let technique disintegrate. This approach is pure simplistic genius as long as you obey the rules. Do not skimp on range-of-motion. Use spotters for safety.

Six Day A Week Training

Some people *love* to weight train. They have the time, they have the situation, they have the energy and they have the inclination to train and train often. Some people are psychologically adapted to *do more*, but to *not do it as hard.*

At one polar opposite of the bodybuilding world stands Dorian Yates, the mover of mountains, the power and bulk monster. The Diesel has more in common, from a training approach and workout prospective, with the likes of Kirk Karwoski or Ed Coan (or Kaz) than he does with Bill Pearl or Arnold Schwarzenegger. Dorian trains like a powerlifter that uses forced reps on the last set of each exercise.

At the other extreme of the bodybuilding world stands Bill Pearl. Bill trains each muscle two or three times a week. Dorian trains a muscle once a week and uses much heavier weight. Bill uses a blistering workout pace and gets an intense cardio bump during his weight workout. Bill Pearl is a *volume* trainer. Dorian is an *intensity* trainer. Bill, like Arnold and Sergio and Franco and all the other volume training greats of the early 70s, routinely performed 16-20 sets for a *single* body part. Pearl works through his entire body over a three day period: Monday, Tuesday and Wednesday. He immediately begins the sequence anew taking three days to train the entire body *again* on Thursday, Friday and Saturday. He rests on Sunday. His routines use different exercises in the second three day blitz of the same week.

This approach does not lend itself to strength training; it is a volume approach that emphasizes more exercises, more angles and quicker pace.

Pearl emphasizes *feel* over poundage. To Bill, poundage is secondary to muscular contraction. He uses a barrage of exercises in order to exhaust the muscle completely. He wears the muscle down whereas Dorian knocks the muscle out. Because Bill doesn't use bar bending poundage, he is ready to hit that same muscle once again two or three days later. He never uses forced reps or other intensity-amping tactics, as that would cut into his energy reserve and not allow him to recover in time for the second weekly entire body session.

Dorian Yates expends so much energy and uses such incredible poundage, amplified further by forced reps and drop sets, that he needs a full seven days for his shattered muscles to recover. I find the six day a week, pure bodybuilding approach, works best for times when the goal is to lose as much body fat as possible. For use during a maximum lean-out phase, the volume approach cannot be beat: lots of exercises, lots of sets, high reps, fast pace.

Six Day Split: Volume Over Intensity!

Day I	Chest, Triceps, Upper Back
Day II	Quads, Hamstrings, Shoulders
Day III	Lower Back, Biceps, Forearms
Day IV	Repeat Monday Using Different Exercises
Day V	Repeat Tuesday Using Different Exercises
Day VI	Repeat Wednesday Using Different Exercises
Day VII	OFF

Beginners: This is not a beginner routine!
Advanced Trainees: This routine will take 60 to 80 minutes to complete and works best if used in conjunction with a 'lean out' phase.

The Purposefully Primitive Training Week

The snapshot on the next page is from my training log for the week of August 13, 2007. It lists what I did on each day. I was using the *Warrior Diet* eating regimen and was in the midst of a summer "lean out" phase. My Triad was biased towards aerobic activity and I was using a Bednarski-inspired "rolling split." I would concentrate on one body part per session. I used this approach five days running: legs, chest, back, shoulders and arms. I used two bi/tri exercises per session.

Monday 8-13	**Bodyweight AM: 206** **Bodyweight PM: 203**
7:00am	Cardio: mountain jog, 69 mins, 900 cals, 134 avg ARHR max*
9:30 am	Weight Training: bench press 3x5, wide grip 2x5, narrow 2x5, triceps
10:15 am	Post-workout shake
2:00 pm	Racquetball: three games with Chris, 40 mins, 455 cals
4:30 pm	Main Meal: flattened chicken, fiber vegetable mix
Tuesday 8-14	**Bodyweight AM: 204** **Bodyweight PM: 200**
8:00am	Cardio: mountain jog steep grades, 40 mins, 534 cals, 138 avg ARHR max*
9:30 am	Weights: deadlifts 1x8, 1x5, 1x5, 2x3, 1x5
10:00 am	Post-Workout Shake
4:30 pm	Main Meal: giant smoked shrimp, black rice, salad
Wednesday 8-15	**Bodyweight AM: 204.5** **Bodyweight PM: 202**
8:00am	Cardio: kettlebell/clubbell 3rd way session, 30 mins, 400 cals, 145 avg ARHR max*
9:30 am	Weights: front squats 1x15, 1x8, 1x6, 1x6, 1x3, 1x12
10:30 am	Racquetball: three games with Chris, 51 mins, 405 cals
11:00 am	Post-Workout Shake
4:30 pm	Main Meal: grilled rib-eye steak, fiber vegetable mix, beer
Thursday 8-16	**Bodyweight AM: 204** **Bodyweight PM: 201**
8:00am	Cardio: swimming laps with fins, 45 mins
9:30 am	Weights: overhead BB press, dumbbell press, light press behind neck
10:15 am	Post-Workout Shake
5:30 pm	Main Meal: cod, fiber vegetable mix with brown rice and goat cheese
Friday 8-17	**Bodyweight AM: 203** **Bodyweight PM: 201.5**
8:00am	Cardio: mountain jog, 60 mins, 720 cals, 130 avg ARHR max*
9:30 am	Weights: biceps/triceps super-sets 12 sets/8-10 reps
10:15	Post-Workout Shake
4:30 pm	Main Meal: restaurant – steak, lots of beer
Saturday 8-18	**Bodyweight AM: 203** **Bodyweight PM: 203**
8:00am	Cardio: off
9:30 am	Weights: squats 5x5 progressive
4:30 pm	Main Meal: dozen egg vegetable omelet with goat cheese
Sunday 8-19	**Bodyweight AM: 202** **Bodyweight PM: 199.5**
8:00am	Cardio: free day – kayaked/fished at mountain lake for hours, exhausting!
9:30 am	Weights: free workout – leg curls, calf raise, kettlebell work
10:15	Post-Workout Shake
6:30 pm	Main Meal: smoked BBQ meat, fiber carbs medley

** average age-related heart rate maximum*

PERIODIZATION AND PREPLANNING

Stair-Stepping Progress Upward Via Creeping Incrementalism

Periodization is a tactical template used by elite athletes to morph from out-of-shape into best shape ever.

After a competition athletes let themselves detune and soften up a bit. Attempting to hold 100% of peak condition year round is physiologically impossible and psychologically a ticket to the mental ward.

Understand that peak condition is a ebb and flow proposition, and the logical question becomes, how can we maneuver the body from out-of-shape, coming off a competition, into best-shape-ever, leading up to the next competition?

Periodization is not so much a *method* as it is a *template* into which a method is placed. Periodization is precision preplanning for peaking every aspect of physical condition in a methodical and systematic fashion. Once the goals are established for the next competition, small sequential steps are reverse-engineered into a periodization timeline.

Elite athletes typically take 12 weeks to prepare for a competition and incrementally increase training demands each succeeding week. The entire process is called a *macrocycle* and subdivided into monthly *mesocycles* and weekly *microcycles.* Each week slightly more is demanded of the body.

Let's construct a hypothetical example for clarification purposes: a shot-putter is peaking strength for the National Championships. He has cycled his resistance lifts and his body-weight to peak on the competition date. Here are his logged results: this is what actually happened in his training during the last four weeks leading up to the competition. In our example, all projected training and body weight goals were met.

4 Week Peaking Cycle

Week of	Lift	Sets	Reps	Poundage	Bodyweight
August 7	Power clean	3 top sets	5	245	260 lbs
	Squat	3 top sets	5	505	260 lbs
	Jerk off racks	3 top sets	5	275	260 lbs
	Incline bench press	3 top sets	5	300	260 lbs
August 14	Power clean	3 top sets	3	275	263 lbs
	Squat	3 top sets	3	535	263 lbs
	Jerk	3 top sets	3	290	263 lbs
	Incline	3 top sets	3	315	263 lbs
August 21	Power clean	2 top sets	2	290	266 lbs
	Squat	2 top sets	2	550	266 lbs
	Jerk	2 top sets	2	300	266 lbs
	Incline	2 top sets	2	330	266 lbs
August 28	Power clean	1 top set	1	300	269 lbs
	Squat	1 top set	1	585	269 lbs
	Jerk	1 top set	1	315	269 lbs
	Incline	1 top set	1	350	269 lbs
September 9	**US National Track & Field Championships**				**272 lbs**

So what's going on here? He is systematically creeping incrementally upward in four key lifts while simultaneously creeping his bodyweight upward. The plan was constructed ahead of time. Our shot-putter has rolled into the final month leading up the National Championships in excellent physical condition. He uses the final month leading up the competition to peak pure size and strength.

In previous shot-put competitions he has weighed 263 pounds with a best toss of 60 feet 9 inches. His previous best lifts weighing 263 were: power clean 275x1, 550x1 in the full squat, 295x1 in the jerk and 320x1 in the incline press. He has had a terrific 12 weeks leading up to the last month and has nearly duplicated his highest bodyweight, 263 and matched his best training lifts four weeks out. He had thrown 61 feet in practice.

He commences the final month feeling great and looks forward to pushing his bodyweight upward three pounds a week for four consecutive weeks. Each succeeding week he becomes larger and more powerful. At the competition he achieved a lifetime best throw of 62'9".

PERIODIZATION AND CREEPING INCREMENTALISM

All Purposefully Primitive resistance trainers use periodization, pre-planning, in order to morph from current physical condition into vastly improved physical condition. The use of a timeline allows us to convert small weekly gains into huge cumulative gains. Monthly mesocycles are broken into weekly microcycles.

Empirical experience has shown that four weeks to six weeks is about the right amount of time to work a particular progress vein. Less than four weeks and the individual could be accused of not giving the selected mode or method enough time to bear fruit. Staying with a non-productive mode for longer than 4-6 weeks is counter-productive and betrays an unhealthy allegiance to a system gone dry.

We construct a periodization cycle that further illustrates our method. Periodization principles are perfect for resistance training; cardiovascular training and nutrition can also be periodized. The Purposeful Primitive always has a plan. "Cast a Cycle", create a game plan, establish weekly goals in the interrelated elements. For example, weight training, cardio, bodyweight and nutrition can be cycled. The first order of business is to establish realistic goals. Reverse engineer the process, move backwards from the goal to the beginning and create weekly mini-goals. Hit the micro goals and the meso goal takes care of itself.

Let us construct another periodized game plan, this one for an average person of average capacities and capabilities. We will layer on a half dozen progress benchmarks and use an 8 week cycle. In this case we will assume the person would like to lose 10 pounds and add a few pounds of muscle during the process. Experience has shown that a stone beginner (less than six months training) can lose fat while simultaneously growing stronger. Those new to the progressive resistance experience will find that new muscle is easily built, even in the face of consistent weekly body weight loss.

The hypothetical individual is male: he stands 5'10", weighs 200 with 20% body fat and would like to shed 10 pounds in eight weeks: a realistic goal. Because his is a total beginner, with limited time to weight train, we select a Cassidy-inspired twice a week training regimen that concentrates on doing the three powerlifts to exclusion. The three lifts are performed in two 30 minute weekly sessions. We project and track five inter-related categories: bodyweight, bench, squat, deadlift and cardio.

Beginners should warm up with 50% of the day's top poundage on the 1st warm-up set. 75% on the second warm-up set. The third set is the 100% top set weight. Log sessions and track results. The cardio column lists the length of each cardio session and the frequency; how many aerobic sessions are performed each week. For the first four weeks the trainee is expected to lose two pounds of bodyweight per week. For the final four weeks, a 1 pound weight loss per week will suffice. Beginners find it quite easy to lose weight during the 1st month of a new training regimen. We take advantage of that phenomenon. The 8 week periodization cycle is designed to create physiological and psychological momentum.

8 Week Beginner Periodization Cycle

Week	Bodyweight	Squat	Bench	Deadlift	Cardio
1	200	70x8	60x8	100x8	20 min/3x
2	198	75x8	65x8	105x8	22 min/4x
3	196	80x8	70x8	110x8	25 min/4x
4	194	85x8	75x8	115x8	28 min/4x
End of first mesocycle—now we drop reps, increase poundage, increase cardio					
5	193	95x5	85x5	125x5	30 min/5x
6	192	100x5	90x5	130x5	32 min/5x
7	191	105x5	95x5	135x5	35 min/5x
8	190	110x5	100x5	140x5	40 min/5x

At the end of this hypothetical 8-week periodization period, the individual will be 10 pounds lighter, in markedly better shape, stronger with much better cardio conditioning. Muscle has been added. Squat poundage increases by a whopping 57%. Legs are much more muscular. Bench press poundage has improved by a staggering 67%! Chest, arms and shoulders are considerably stronger and more muscular. The deadlift is up by 40%. The muscles of the back and hips are significantly shapelier. The scale weight loss of 10 pounds is factually inaccurate. Our beginner has also added 5 pounds of muscle during the 8 week period.

There is no way the person could realize these across the board strength increases without concurrent muscle gain. This fellow actually lost 15 pounds of fat while adding 5 pounds of muscle. This muscle "add back" resulted in a 10 pound bathroom scale loss. Cardio exercise is critical for elevating the metabolism. By incrementally increasing both the duration and frequency of cardio, body fat loss is accelerated. Nutrition is critical for providing the requisite nutrients for speeding up recovery and muscle growth. The entire training effort could be undermined by improper nutrition. Not eating enough, or eating too much of the wrong kind of food, could easily derail the process. This example is an actual person, a student of mine, a person that realized this degree of progress in the timeframe outlined. This is not atypical for trainees new to our approach.

Logging Entries

Almost without exception elite athletes log training results and do so in real time, as the workout is actually occurring. Immediately after finishing a set, you'll see the elite pick up their little spiral notebooks and with hands still shaking from exertion, jot down what just happened.

Why do they go to the trouble?

The athletic elite review results every week to detect trends, mull over what has occurred and plot the next step. Based on the data, they make "in-flight" corrections and institute minute or substantive changes.

Often outsiders will mistake this continual, slavish adherence to written detail as unchecked ego, just another example of Narcissistic tendencies exhibited by people overly concerned with their bodies. In fact virtually every serious competitive athlete has a written game plan that structures workouts and plots training leading up to a competition. The log is the daily report card that identifies how reality is stacking up against projection. Progressive resistance training is particularly suited for logging since the results are numerical.

Again, the elite athletes set the game plan into a timeframe (typically 12 weeks) and project ahead of time where they want to be each successive week. If, by way of example, a shot-putter preparing for the Collegiate National Championships wants to peak his incline barbell press (past experience has shown him that when his incline press improves his shot-put distance improves) he might structure the projected 12 week periodization game plan as follows:

Week 1:	250x10 three sets
Week 2:	260x10 three sets
Week 3:	275x5 three sets
Week 4:	285x5 three sets
Week 5:	295x5 two sets
Week 6:	305x5 two sets
Week 7:	315x3 two sets
Week 8:	325x3 two sets
Week 9:	335x2 one set
Week 10:	345x2 one set
Week 11:	355x1 one set
Week 12:	365x1 one set

Typical logged entry for a single workout

August 24, 2007; BWT 259lb; Noon; Campus Gym
Incline Bench - 135x15, 185x5, 225x5, 275x1,
295x5, 295x5 - top sets ridiculously easy!

Dumbbell Flat Bench - 100 x10, 110x10, 120x10
all three sets also easy; chest extremely pumped!

Power Cleans - 135x8, 225x5, 265x5, 275x4
missed 5th rep, cut the pull/need more wrist snap

Barbell Row - 225x5, 275x5, 315x5, 365x6 new
PR 365x6 - used straps, felt easy, 6th rep was PR

Finished in 74 minutes: no rush between sets -
Smart-Bomb shake afterwards - 8 weeks to go!

During each workout, results should be logged. So much data is conveyed with so few words. Valuable empirical data needs to be collected. The log book covers what actually happened and offers instant impressions as to what occurred and why.

At the conclusion of each training week, the athlete should take 15 minutes to look back over the previous week's training. The savvy athlete determines how they are doing in relation to the projected training template: are they on schedule? Has the projected poundage matched the gym reality? Those serious about physical progress establish and maintain a detailed training log in order to keep track of where they *are* in relation to where they *should be*.

Logging is the opposite of a runaway ego – it's a reality check!

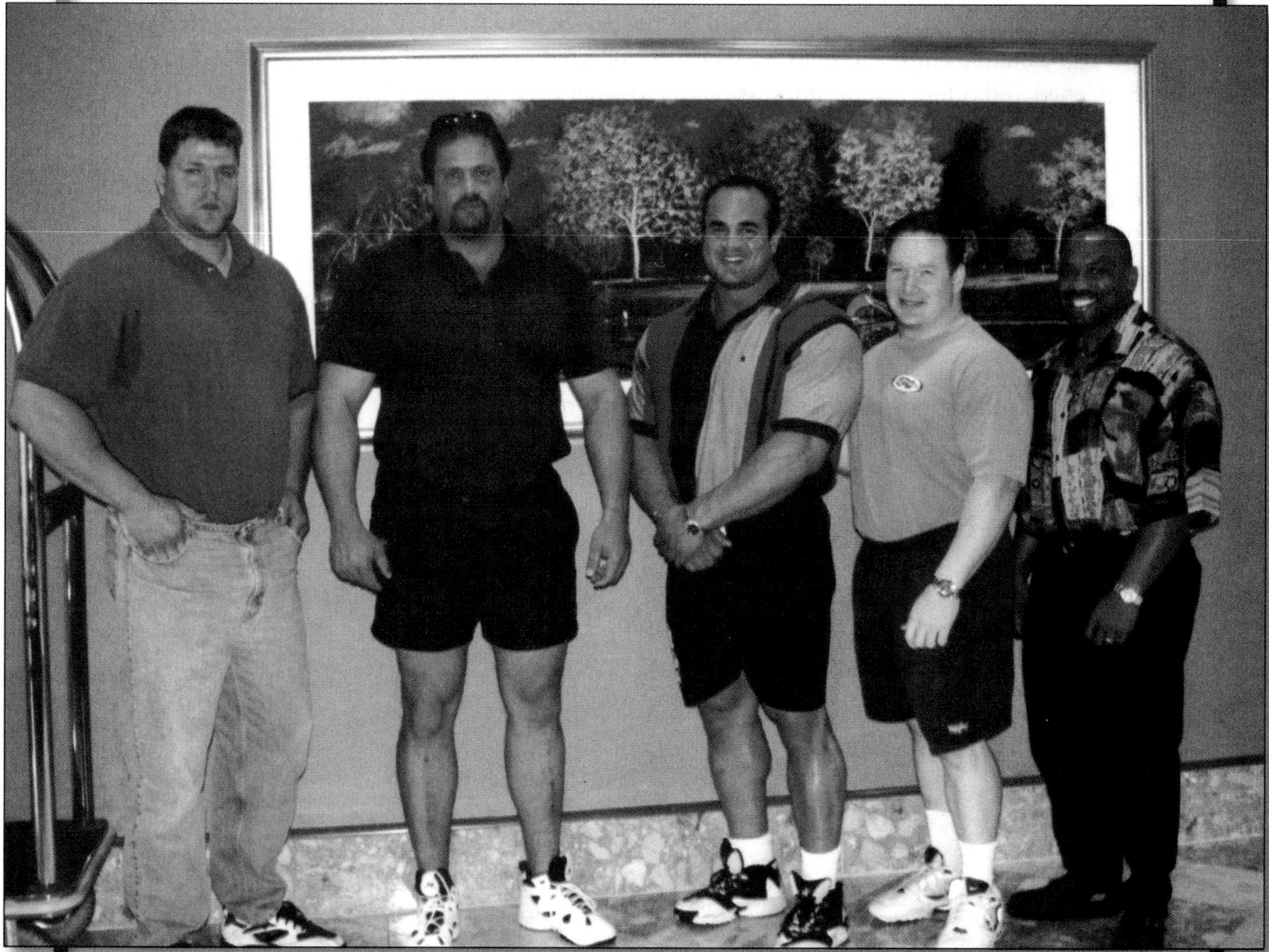

Left to right: Brad Gillingham, Bob Myers, Anthony D'Arrezo, Ed Coan, Gene Bell

"We don't pick 'em – we recognize them!" At the National Powerlifting Championships in the mid 90's I called Ed Coan and said, "Let's take that new guy Brad Gillingham to breakfast – he lifted incredibly well." Ed too was impressed with the gigantic newcomer from Minnesota. "His pop was Gale Gillingham. Played guard for the Packers during the Vince Lombardi era." Ed said. I then made a call to Brad and asked casual-like if he could meet me for breakfast. As far as he knew it was just he and I. When Ed, Gene Bell, Bobby "Nacho" Myers and Anthony D'Arezzo (RIP) our gigantic bodybuilder buddy all appeared, Brad seemed a bit shocked. I told him that every one of us wanted to meet with him and tell him personally how impressed we'd been with him and his lifting. I believe it was Brad's first National Championships; his clean crisp lifting technique, his competitive attitude, his brains and his incredible family support apparatus, made him destined him for lifting greatness we all felt. We toasted him at that breakfast: as I write this, Brad just retired from the sport. In the intervening years he captured the most prestigious of all power titles, the IPF World Championships, several times. He was a man built all wrong for squatting yet able to eventually squat 860. He had a 600 bench press and then pulled out his competitive shotgun to use on opponents: an 860 deadlift. He did it the hard way. Brad was an unstoppable force of Nature.

Iron Essays

A woman simply is, but a man must become. Masculinity is risky and elusive. It is achieved by revolt from woman, and is confirmed only by other men. Feminist fantasies about the ideal "sensitive" male have failed. Manhood coerced into sensitivity is no manhood at all…The quest for masculinity recapitulates the birth of civilization and the birth of high art…a work of art is a protest against nature…Modern bodybuilding is ritual, religion, sport, art and science, awash in Western chemistry and mathematics. Defying nature, it surpasses it.

—Camille Paglia

PRIMITIVE ROOTS

I commenced my own transformational odyssey in 1962 when at age 12 my Irish father bought me a 110 pound set of weights for Christmas. I wanted to transform myself from what I was—an average boy—into what I wanted to be—a muscular giant. I was a daydreamer, a comic book reader, a superhero worshipper and in my mind's eye I would visualize myself transformed into Herculean proportion.

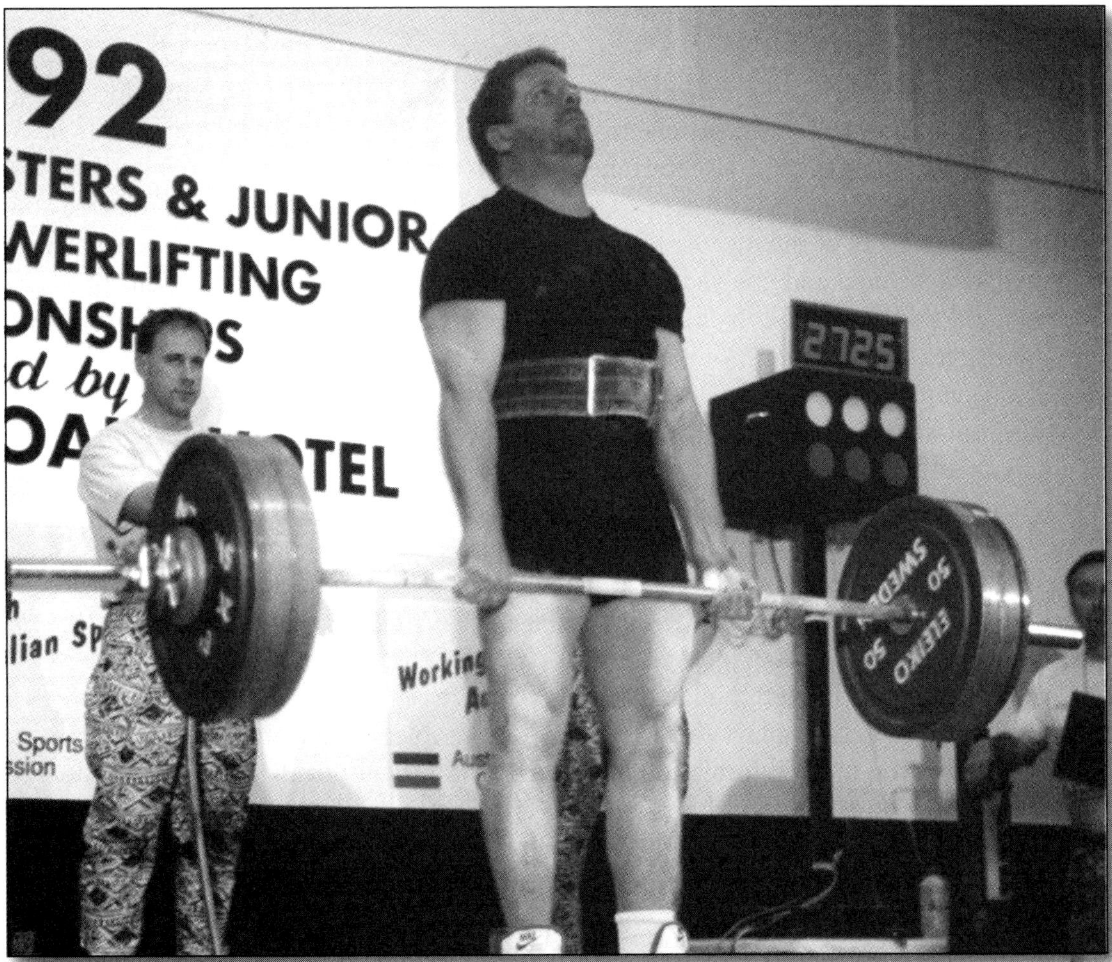

Here I am winning the IPF World Championships as a master lifter in Australia in 1992. This is my opening 272.5 kilo deadlift. I weighed 212. I had lost 13 pounds on the trip and lifted just enough to win. I was sick with a horrible sinus infection. My head clogged with thick green mucus. I ran a 100 degree fever and was told not to lift. I had squatted 704, benched 374 (without a shirt) and deadlifted 683 to secure a spot on the World Team. I was 42.

As a preteen I read Greek, Roman and Norse mythology and became a sport idolater. I wanted to become larger than life and instinctively sought out the tool that would enable me to achieve my imaginary physical goal: a barbell. My extremely supportive father enabled me to remake myself by purchasing the weights. He was a widower who worked long and hard and because of his work schedule I grew up with a lack of parental supervision.

Being a baby boomer, I had lots and lots of neighborhood mates and cohorts. Preteen males, we formed a roving tribe of "lost boys" and we actively and enthusiastically engaged in all types of organized athletic games. In those days parents sent children out to play; mothers particularly wanted the boys outside to preserve their sanity. Every single day we had enough male participants to form full football or baseball teams. The younger boys stood on the sidelines, anxiously awaiting their turn to be rotated into these massive sandlot games.

Once I obtained the tool of my transformation, my weight set, I set up a training area in my unfinished basement. Immediately my comrades and I began working out and my basement became training central, a subterranean wolf's lair for all our tribal activities. My Dad was a lonely, stoic type who had seen combat in WWII and won a silver star. Whereas the homemaker mothers of the nuclear families in my neighborhood wanted peace and serenity my dad welcomed and enjoyed the beehive buzz of young boys in the basement lifting weights and socializing. We even had guys come by who didn't train; they would arrive, meet and greet, then sit on one of the picnic benches that lined the concrete walls and watch the always intense, apparently entertaining, lifting action. We competed every single day amongst ourselves and always strove to improve. We pushed each other mercilessly to see who could lift the most.

We sought increases in strength, increases in muscle size and improved athletic performance. Progress became the benchmark, the report card as to whether or not our methods were working. I would walk to the newsstand once a month to buy *Strength & Health* muscle magazine for training information. We were in the informational Stone Age as far as bodybuilding and strength building techniques were concerned. In retrospect this was a blessing in disguise. Nowadays there is a very real problem with informational overload; there is literally too much information and it makes it difficult for the serious individual to sort through the possibilities and find truly effective methods. Back in those days there was very little confusion. The lack of sophistication and lack of choices (regarding exercise theory, modes, equipment and tactics) turned out to be an absolute advantage.

What information we had tended to be sound. The lack of choice kept us focused on the things that mattered: we lifted hard; we lifted heavy and we lifted often. We used basic barebones barbell exercises because we had no other equipment. We ate like young colts because we were young colts. The copious calories we continually ingested kept us anabolic and in a constant state of Positive Nitrogen Balance (PNB) though we had no earthly idea what anabolism or PNB were or why it was beneficial.

The huge amounts of food we ate caused us to recover quickly from the eternal pounding we subjected our bodies to. As a direct result we grew muscle and became inordinately strong. Fat kids, back in the day, were the exception; nowadays they are the rule. Our young metabolisms were akin to nuclear reactors: we could eat anything without consequence. We participated in innumerous athletic activities, both organized and informal. Our cardio was simply a natural outgrowth of our eternal participation in football, basketball, baseball and wrestling. We thought nothing about running for miles or biking for hours to get where we needed to go.

Our games were deadly serious and of the bone-bruising variety. We were athletic kids unwittingly melding intense cardio with intense weight training and 'supporting" all the intense physical activity by eating and eating and eating. In retrospect the area that modern knowledge could have benefited us the most was nutrition: we ate too much saturated fat and sugar. We were ignorant idiot savants; primitive kids who came up in primitive times and used primitive tools and primitive methods; we were spared the curse of too many options.

Raised without any feminine counterbalance in a harsh, stark masculine environment, I naturally evolved into an alpha male. I was never a follower. I was the leader and the schemer, the guy who got the games organized and the guy who other guys looked to for the next move. I never demanded it. My status was bestowed upon me by the others. Having no mother or any feminine influences, I unwittingly became a Spartan boy.

I was popular yet I never had any problem being alone or by myself. My wife says I was raised by wolves and in some ways that is dead on accurate. In my pre-driving years, if no one was around or nothing was happening, I might shoot 500 baskets or bounce a tennis ball off a street curb with great precision. I could make the tennis ball rebound fifty feet back and shoot twenty feet into the air. I would sprint and leap to catch the crazed rebound. I could entertain myself this way for hours.

Luck and circumstance conspired to catapult me into adult athletic competition at a very early age. I entered high school at age fourteen, the same year a new teacher arrived. This guy was a *bon vivant* Italian Wildman named Roy Patmalnee. He started a weightlifting club and my wild boy tribe showed up en masse and simply took over. As Sonny Barger once told Ken Kesey when asked how Hell's Angel's were selected, "We don't *select* 'em, we *recognize* 'em." My crew and I were recognized—immediately.

We were not suburban pussies; we were street toughs who fought with each other often and swore and smoked and pushed each other into the creek for no reason. We'd already made phenomenal physical progress. Roy looked like Robert De Niro and treated us like mates, not like children. He rubbed his hands gleefully and unleashed us on other schoolboys. He began trucking us around to intramural Olympic weightlifting competitions. As a team we went undefeated, eventually winning the Eastern Regional United States high school team title. Other teams would compete in cute uniforms and bring cheerleaders. We'd show up with our hair greased back with Brylcream, wearing black leather jackets and Chuck Taylor high top shoes. We made overt passes at the cheerleaders. We were aggressive and physical. We were primordial archetypes, "Here little man; hold my 1st place trophy while I French kiss your cheerleader sister."

Soon the "basement boys" were entering adult male Olympic lifting competitions. Suddenly we were comrades in arms with adult men and this accelerated the maturation process of already mature youngsters.

There was a ferocious Olympic lifter named Robert Lancaster who went to Howard University and later became a fighter pilot. He lifted at the time in the 181 pound class. Roy entered our team into the DCAAU Potomac Valley Regional Senior Men's Championships in order for us to get bitch-slapped in open men's competition. "This mauling will be good for you." I remember him telling us in a philosophic moment during the van ride to the meet.

I was given a life lesson that day, one that still serves me well. It was a demonstration of the relationship between muscle strength and muscle size. We were at the competition beforehand preparing to weigh in when AAU President Pete Miller excitedly said, "Marty! Hurry! You've got to see this!" As I followed, Pete explained, "Hey Marty, have you ever wondered why Robert Lancaster can lift so much more than you?"

Before I could answer we turned the corner into the men's locker room, "That's why!" Pete pointed at Bob stepping down off the scales in a pair of shorts looking positively Herculean, like Arnold Schwarzenegger on his best day. I turned to Pete and said, "DUH! Of course he can out lift me! With those massive muscles and that low body fat percentile, next to him I look like a point guard or a baseball second baseman. I got to get a lot more muscle and lose a lot of body fat if I'm going to look and lift like Lancaster." That was a profound formative moment for me.

The functional muscularity Lancaster displayed that day became my lifelong physical benchmark. Lancaster's physique had *function*: He could clean and jerk 410 when the world record was 413 and at 5'8" could slam-dunk a basketball.

Roy had been insistent that we undergo this trial by fire. We were scared shitless, ready to pee our pants. Lancaster was in my division and his degree of dominance created the "flee" phenomena as grizzled veterans in the know avoided his weight division. At the competition I pressed 215, snatched 195 and clean and jerked 260 weighing 171. Bob missed all three of his presses with something like 315 and was out of the competition. I ended up beating the remaining lesser lifters and won the Senior Men's title at age 14 to become the youngest winner in the history of the DCAAU. To my coach and my mates, it was as if I had miraculously beaten Cassius Clay or run 85 yards for the winning touchdown in the Super Bowl.

I became a boy sensation. Needless to say this lucky win fired me up and caused me to redouble my efforts. I went on to win my first National Teen title at age 17, pressing 260 and snatching 225. Both were AAU National Junior Olympic records at the time. I cleaned and jerked 315, but was disqualified for "press out." I dead-hang cleaned 295 for a triple weighing 193 at age 18. I was a holy terror and my status in the male community could not have been higher. When we got our driver's licenses, our whole world changed. We rode around in 400 horsepower muscle cars without seatbelts smoking Marlboros, drinking booze and throwing the empties out onto people's lawns. We trained hard, but now drank, smoked, fought and chased women who didn't run away too far or too fast. As Balzac noted in Cousin Bette, "All men are conscious of a woman's susceptibility to pugnacious masculinity." I personally can attest to the validity of that aphorism.

I had zero interest in high school studies. I was struck hard by wanderlust and romantic ideas about travel. As soon as high school was over, I hit the road. The lone wolf alpha male left home on good terms as soon as I turned 18. My dad remarried and I was happy for him. I hitchhiked back and forth across the country three times before I turned 20 and lived in a commune for many years. It was the sixties and I was a free spirit, a restless youngster who made male friends easily. I ended up in Portland, Oregon living in the twilight world of professional musicians and dope dealers.

I eventually ended up back in Maryland and got deeply involved with martial arts for five years. I studied under an internationally famous master of the Chinese "internal" martial arts, Robert Smith, a senior student to T'ai Chi God, Chen Man Ching. I became immersed in that world, but it was not my world and eventually I came full circle and got back into competitive lifting at age 29. Within 11 months of commencing powerlifting I squatted 600 raw weighing 198 pounds. I began writing articles on weight training and was published right away. I had always been a voracious reader and as a teen had been introduced to Hemingway, Conrad and Jack London. Getting published caused me to broaden my literary horizons. I had the good fortune to come across the Russian short story writers. They were the perfect mentors for a guy who wrote magazine articles. I needed to tell my training tales in 1500 to 2500 words and the plain-speak short stories of Turgenev, Tolstoy, and Chekhov (to lesser degree Dostoyevsky) gave me a template for my own Iron Tales.

Most people hear "Russian Literature" and mistakenly think it dense and obtuse, akin to wading through Emanuel Kant's *Critique of Pure Reason* or James Joyce's *Finnegan's Wake*. Not so. The Russian Masters were plain-speak writers who told their tales quickly, efficiently and with great economy and precision.

I stumbled across Turgenev's "A Sportsman's Notebook" early on and his compact density and passion for his subject matter made him my article writing mentor. Tolstoy's *Hadji Murid* and Dostoyevsky's *The Gambler* provided further literary benchmarks for my own tales. Later Anton Chekhov had a huge impact on me: his ability to underplay, his subtleness, his humanity, his humility, everything about the man moved me deeply. I read a quote of his I use to this day as a guideline. *"One should write so that the reader requires no explanation from the author. The actions, conversations and meditations of the characters need be sufficient."* I took that to heart. In the Iron World where I lived there were plenty of great characters and I needed to let them speak, unimpeded, without any of my feeble embellishments.

Another great writer, Truman Capote, gave me another applicable writing formula when he talked about writing *In Cold Blood.*"I am bringing fictional techniques to reportage."

I immersed myself totally within my chosen field. I was passionate and knowledgeable and continually excited about my little pie sliver of expertise: muscle, strength and how to acquire it.

I wrote of the men and events that populated this strange uber-masculine world. I was able to get paid to quiz my strength idols about how they morphed themselves! I was an insightful interviewer. I had a real point of view and I was, as Alfred Kazin once said of William Blake, *"Like so many self-educated men, he was fanatically learned. But he read like a fundamentalist—to be inspired or to refute."* That was me cubed. I had a voice and a viewpoint and considerable life experience at a young age. Some writers are incredible technicians, but have no worthwhile life experiences to draw upon; others are real adventurers with tales worth retelling, yet they can't communicate.

I never sought to write "over my head" and I never sought to write about anything that I was not intimately familiar with. I wrote of the world of weights and lifting and men who excel at it and my episodic training treatises were recognized and well received right from the start.

Hugh Cassidy was instrumental in helping me shape my craft. He focused my thoughts in my initial articles. He tore my prose apart as surely as he tore me apart in the gym. He was a tough taskmaster who taught me that the goal was clear communication and communicating trumped trying to impress.

In the intervening decade I continued a parallel course: furthering my own competitive aspirations while writing about what I learned from the world's best. I had ambitions and was driven to learn more and more and more. This made me an ideal interviewer. I knew my stuff and when I talked with athletes about their training they sensed immediately that I understood them. I created persuasive and compelling articles because I took the time to capture their idiosyncrasies, *patois* and mannerisms. I related with precision and care what it was about their training or nutrition that differentiated one great athlete from another.

I would suppose that it is no exaggeration to say that I have interviewed over 1,000 athletes about how and why they train the way they do, about how and why they eat the way they eat. I also had the privilege of coaching hall-of-fame strength athletes, often in the very competitions at which they turned in their all-time best performances. Certain men, it seems, are driven to improve upon the human body they are given. I was one of them.

What was it that drove myself and men like me? What was it that I was writing about? Was there an irreducible core question? Is that not the question: how best do we trigger *physical transformation*?

I made my bones by competing, by observing, by listening and by trying new things. I have come to a basic conclusion that in this day and age of unlimited choices and unlimited distractions, some very important and productive strategies have been obfuscated, discarded or ignored. I have come full circle in my attitudes and choices and now feel certain that those who earnestly seek to transform themselves physically can benefit from using my Retro Man Methodology, much of what I first stumbled on as a boy-child.

Those ancient methods turned out to be timeless. If you scrape away all the different rationale and reasons people engage in fitness-related activities, the bottom line is that they want to modify their physique, change their body from what it is into what they *want it to be*. Being dissatisfied with their physical status quo, they will rearrange their lives and devote time, money and effort towards triggering transformation. In almost every case they fail miserably.

People who successfully transform physically transform psychologically. I've seen this phenomenon occur repeatedly: self image undergoes an astounding metamorphosis when a successful physical metamorphosis is achieved. People who make radical physical changes reinvent themselves, not just physically but psychologically and emotionally as well.

For 45 years I've been in hot pursuit of those methods and modes that trigger physical transformation. I have come to the conclusion that the finest methods for triggering true transformations are based on modified versions of those ancient, purposefully primitive ultra-basic modes of training and eating I first stumbled upon four decades ago.

People nowadays chase their metaphorical tails in feverish pursuit of change, using fragmented and ineffectual methods. There are just too many choices and too many slick marketers with silky smooth raps that they relate with great conviction. They tell the gullible with pompous profundity that they have discovered a secret method. They disguise fallacious facts with absurd pseudo science and are seductive and persuasive.

People run in crazed circles all around the fitness Mulberry Bush, chasing one exotic mode, method, procedure or product after another. They all seek the mythical magic bullet of fitness: a method or mode that will enable them to effect a transformation *without* the disciplined deprivation, without the teeth-grinding physical effort, without the struggle. Life is struggle. I love what my Purposefully Primitive brother-in-arms, Ori Hofmekler says, *"Life in paradise should be rugged!"* We are primordially programmed for struggle yet we seek to avoid struggle at all cost. Struggle is the precursor to true transformation: without struggle there is no transformation.

45 years later and so many of those ancient adolescent epiphanies still ring true and still strike me as profound. Basic barbell and dumbbell exercises done with incredible intensity then backed up with lots of calories result in the construction of new muscle. If you are selective about the ample calories you eat, if you practice periodic cardiovascular exercise, stored body fat is mobilized and oxidized. If eating and training are perfectly attuned to one another, synergy takes hold and results are dramatically accelerated.

Significant change without significant struggle is a fitness myth perpetuated by people looking to sell you products. When I thought about writing this book, I posed myself a question: how simple could the transformational process be made without losing effectiveness? What would you need? How little could you get by with, in terms of tools, time, and effort? The answer was you would need a barbell and food from the grocery store. No need for personal trainers; no need for a gym membership; no need for a treadmill; no need for miracle devices or magic bullet products. You need a few tools, some regular food and a plan. I can provide the plan.

Build a Retro Home Gym

Old School Tools of the Trade

In this age of high-tech glitz and dazzle, the quest for physical transformation can confuse and confound the most astute and analytical individual. A serious fitness devotee seeks nothing less than complete physical renovation, but awash in a sea of conflicting methods and modes, who can sort the proverbial wheat from the chaff, the real-deal from the jive, the effective from the ineffectual?

Commercial gyms and omnipresent fitness infomercials continually churn confusion and purposeful obfuscation, promoting one exercise mode, machine or device after another, endless types and varieties, each presented as "the ultimate." Use of the device, we are told with the easy assurance of the unconsciously ignorant, makes transformation quick and effortless. If rapid and radical physique renovation were so damned easy the planet would be overrun with Arnold-clones and that just ain't so.

The cold truth is the process is damned difficult and the old cliché still rings true: success is 10% inspiration and 90% perspiration. Human nature is fickle and always seeks the path of least resistance. True physical renovation requires that we seek the path of *maximum* resistance, both figuratively and literally. Given a choice humans will always choose to sit or lie down when exercising and equipment manufacturers purposefully cater to this subconscious psychology.

Here is an irrefutable truth: any machine that mimics a free weight exercise can never equal the results from a free weight exercise. Why? Machines eliminate *the third dimension of tension*, control of side-to-side movement. This in and of itself makes machines that mimic 33% less effective than the corresponding free weight movement from a kinesiological standpoint. Machines are seductive, but not nearly as effective.

Good old barbells and dumbbells blow machines that mimic them into the weeds, every single time. It boils down to biomechanics and hard science. A machine locks the user into a super-specific, motor-pathway, a preordained groove that confines, constricts and eliminates any sway in the stroke path. A machine groove has two dimensions: up and down. Free weight training adds the critical third dimension: side-to-side control. In addition to up and down, the free-weight user fights to avoid wayward lateral movement. When a free weight is pushed, tugged or hoisted, it follows a path of its own making and the user has to prevent the weight from straying from the proscribed technical boundary.

From a muscle-building standpoint adding the third dimension is a marvelous thing and as a result free weight exercise always trumps the mimicking machine. The third dimension of tension activates muscle stabilizers that keep the poundage proceeding along the proscribed path. Triggering stabilizers results in additional muscle fiber stimulation which converts into additional muscular growth.

Can unglamorous Old School tools and tactics compete with splendiferous exercise machines that allow you to engage in fitness-lite always while sitting or lying? Are free weights a hopeless anachronism and are practitioners the modern incarnation of John Henry versus the steam engine drill? Not if results still count.

Does any of this inspire or kindle within you an urge to bail out of the subtle seduction of all-machine/all-the-time training to which so many are addicted? If you had a thousand dollars to construct a *serious* free-weight home gym, here is how I'd advise you spend that hard-earned disposable income. Here's a further tip: you could likely cut the $1,000 amount in half by purchasing equipment described *used*. Try used sporting goods stores that have sprung up everywhere. Look in the newspaper want ads under "exercise equipment." People are always looking to unload fitness equipment they no longer use.

Equipment	Cost
1. Olympic barbell: 310-pound set	$99
2. Fixed Dumbbells: 10 to 40 pounds @ $.40 cents per pound	$140
3. Bench: adjustable w/curl and leg curl/leg extension/curl attachments	$199
4. Power rack: w/overhead and floor pulley attachment	$499
5. Jump rope: leather professional	$14
6. Abdominal wheel: wheel with handle for core torso exercise	$11
Total	**$962**

Stone-Age Tools for Accessing the Third Dimension of Tension

1. Olympic Barbell

At some point if you use free weights you'll need to graduate from the pedestrian "exercise set" to an Olympic style barbell. The ball-bearing sleeves allow smooth, non-binding rotation of the load and the seven foot length is necessary for use in a power rack. Downside: the empty bar weighs 45 pounds so for exercises requiring less poundage you'll need to use dumbbells.

2. Dumbbells

We've selected six pairs of fixed poundage cast iron dumbbells, one pair each of 10, 15, 20, 25, 30, 35 and 40 pound dumbbells. You can save money by buying empty dumbbell handles and loading plates onto the handles for each set. Given a thousand dollars to work with and the ease and quickness of fixed poundage dumbbells, a $140 dollar investment, seems well worth the expense.

3. Bench

On an adjustable bench you can do flat benches, incline presses, seated curls and overhead presses. Pick a bench that allows you to add a plate-loaded leg extension/leg curl device and an incline curl pad. This piece of equipment is invaluable, enabling you to perform twenty plus free weight barbell/dumbbell and machine exercises.

4. Power Rack

The key critical piece of equipment, a power rack is a steel cage with four vertical posts set two feet apart. Seven feet in height, round holes are drilled every two inches. Two long bars are inserted in the holes allowing you to do every imaginable variation of squat and bench press safely. The 'pins' are set in such a fashion that if you miss a rep you simply ride the poundage down to the pre-set pins and walk away. Ours is equipped with supplemental pulleys allowing various types of pulldowns, triceps press-downs, seated cable rows and pulley curls. The front crossbar serves as our pull-up and chin bar and can be used for hanging leg raises. For serious free-weight training a power rack is not an option. It is invaluable and irreplaceable.

5. Jump Rope

We had a few dollars left and decided to purchase a leather jump rope for indoor cardio. Jumping rope is a lost art and when it comes to generating an elevated heart rate, the goal of all aerobic exercise, continual hopping is amazingly effective at raising the HR.

6. Ab Wheel

Our final purchase was the deceptive and devilish Ab Wheel. Available at any sporting good store for around $10; this simple device is deadly effective when it comes to building core strength. Kneel down and motor forward rolling on the little wheel until your nose touches the floor. Pull back to the starting position. This killer exercise strengthens the entire abdominal region while simultaneously stimulating the latissimus dorsi.

No this isn't the Ukraine…this is my home gym in the unheated garage out back of my country home in South Central Pennsylvania. Our coldest training session was conducted in 19 degree weather and our summer warmest was 102 degrees. The power rack pictured is the heart and soul of my gym. I have barbells, dumbbells, a few benches, and a single pulley device used for pushdowns and pulldowns (our one machine). Many a World Champion has trained here and the sessions are manic and intense. Some of the best deals in all of fitness can be had purchasing hardcore exercise equipment used. Check the local paper or the advertiser paper stuffed in your mailbox. People are always trying to unload exercise equipment. I purchased a second power rack for $150 out of the Sunday paper. Like classical literature at the used bookstore, hardcore exercise gear is a bargain because no one reads anymore and no one works out hard anymore.

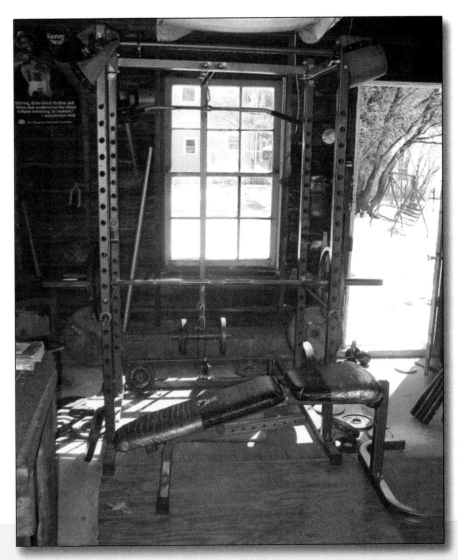

For a thousand dollars you can build a Retro Old School home gym and perform every imaginable progressive resistance exercise: buy it all used and save 50%. That is a lot of bang for the buck. The correct use of a power rack allows you to train alone and in complete safety—assuming you utilize the correct pin settings, adhere to proper exercise techniques and stay within reasonable poundage and repetition limits. The muscle-building attributes of three dimensional free weight training are unbeatable and irrefutable. An unbelievable variety of free weight exercises can be performed using our simplistic set up. The possible variations boggle the brain and are enough for a lifetime of study and application. The possessor of this Old School home gym will be limited only by imagination and motivation. Our rustic set up provides every conceivable tool for transformation, all right at your fingertips, nestled just a few steps away in the comfy confines of your garage or basement.

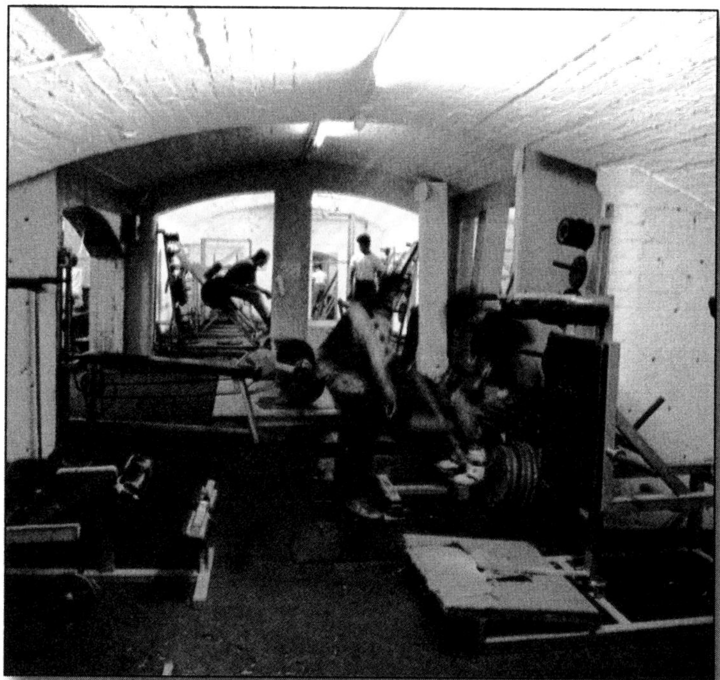

Here is the decaying dump in which the best body in the world was built. Dorian Yates won six straight Mr. Olympia titles. He did all his training in this dank gym he owned and operated in Birmingham, England. The Temple Street Gym was a tough place in a tough section of a tough city run by a genuinely tough guy. It was inhabited by tough, no-nonsense dudes who trained hard, heavy, and often. They offered profane encouragement to one another.

Compare this stark reality to the chrome and steel, machine-centric, Swiss ball spas where patrons moan and threaten lawsuits if someone forgets to wipe a few beads of sweat off the Pilates machine. Physical transformation is all about struggle and effort. People do not want to come to grips with that biological reality. One reason the fitness supplement industry always thrives is subconsciously they appeal to an inherent human character flaw: we want to believe a magical pill or potion can transform us.

YOU'VE GOT ABOUT AN HOUR

Don't Apply Chronologic Boundaries to an Organic Undertaking

People often ask, "How long should a resistance exercise session last?" Is there a tipping point, a point of diminishing returns where energy nosedives so dramatically that further exercise effort is futile, if not downright counterproductive? The answer is yes. Experience and science converge on this one.

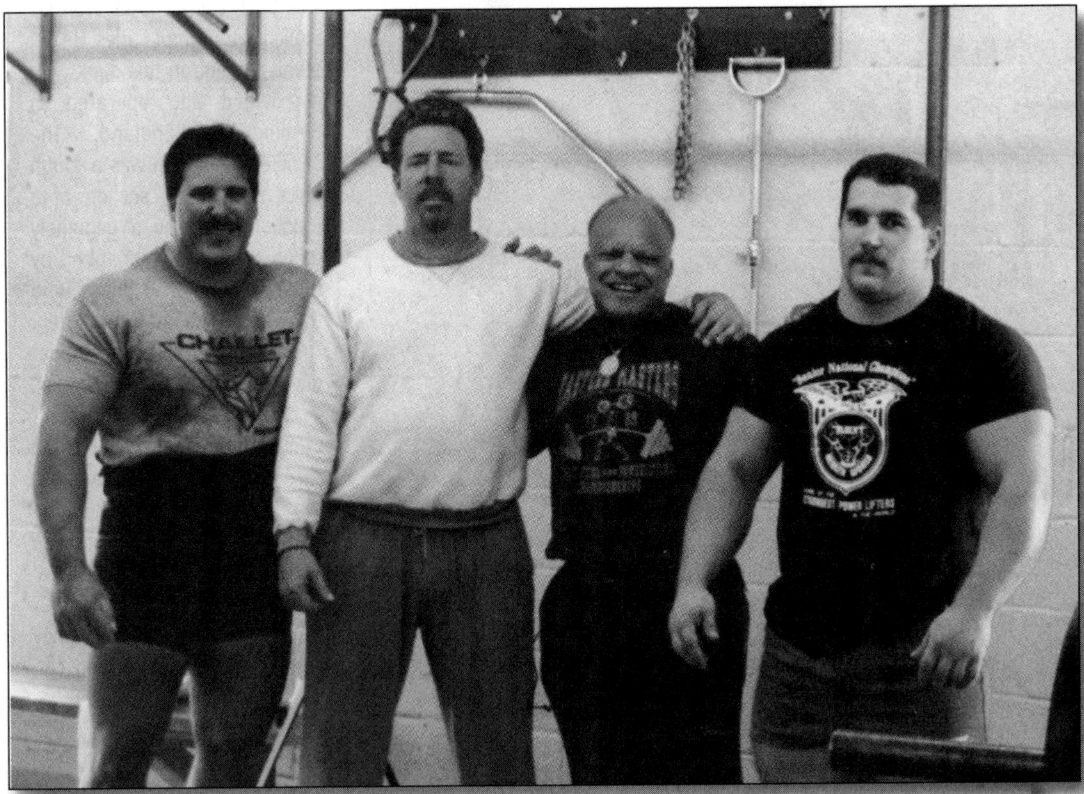

Good Group: World Champion Mark Chaillet, me, 6-time IPF World Master's Champion Don Mills and World Champion Kirk Karwoski. I was in bad shape at the time: on crutches seven months after suffering a compound fracture of my left leg. I was still undergoing corrective surgeries. Don Mills was a holy lifting terror with a beatific, beaming, magnetic personality. He squatted and deadlifted 700 and bench pressed 500 weighing 218 at age 55! Don was never beaten as a master lifter.

After 45 to 60 minutes, for someone in reasonably good condition, energy starts to fade quickly, strength plummets and performance begins to suffer so badly that logic dictates that the session should be ended.

Those in better physical condition might be able to prolong the point when the muscular fatigue curtain falls. Those in poor physical condition might only last 10-15 minutes before running up the white flag.

Hypertrophy-triggering resistance training is a body shocking, muscle fatiguing experience that obeys its own dictates and has zero respect for your puny preconceptions. Trainees new to hardcore resistance training come to an initial session crammed full of preconceptions and bright ideas and the grim reality is shocking—like an ice-cold shower or a hard slap across the face. Real resistance training, the kind that actually strengthens and grows muscle tissue is all about *effort*...teeth-grinding, pants-splitting, eye-popping, ball-busting effort. We push and pull on heavy objects with all our might, using every bit of available strength. This kind of effort saps strength and energy at a rapid rate.

Traditionally we take a few warm up sets using sub-maximal poundage before the all out effort(s.) Preliminary sets serve a variety of purposes: they raise the core temperature of the target muscle and grease nerve synapses and neurological pathways. Warm-ups are critical. A proper warm-up ensures specific muscle motor pathways are greased and opened and crisp technical execution is ingrained before the main event: the Top Set or Work Set. Everything prior to the top set is exercise foreplay; necessary to maximize top set performance, but on their own the preliminary sets do not cause growth. These sets lay the technical, physiological and psychological groundwork for the real work: the hypertrophy-triggering, strength-infusing top set.

In order to perform a top set at maximum capacity, the warm-up sets need to be done with real concentration. One easily observable difference between a real Iron Pro (regardless their discipline) and rookie trainees, is how the elite handle warm-up sets. Rookies will slap-dash their way through the warm-ups using sloppy technique and piss-poor form. Pros "pretend" the warm-up sets are maximally heavy and treat the lightest poundage with maximum respect. Though they might be going to hit 755 for 5 in the deadlift, they will handle 135 and 255 as if it were 755. This is a lesson lost on beginners.

Once proper warm-up sets are dispatched in the correct fashion, as true dress rehearsals, the top set should be, needs to be, *must* be a stone bitch to complete! Purposefully difficult, we seek to stretch the lip of the limit envelope in some manner or fashion every time we train. The physiological aftereffects of all out physical effort are devastating. There are only so many top sets an individual can perform during a workout before physical disintegration occurs. When this happens, the uninformed continue the workout and the informed call it a day.

Novice resistance trainees, stuffed full of platitudes and preconceptions, try and apply chronological boundaries to an organic undertaking. "I weight train for two hours per session six times a week." The novice might boast. The experienced man hearing this goes, "Well if that's the case, you can't be handling *jack shit* in terms of poundage."

A powerlifter, Olympic lifter or strongman competitor does not think in terms of time. His body will *tell him* when it's had enough. The tip off is performance: when strength nosedives and poundage plummets, when reps regress and performance cannot come within a country mile of capacity when fresh, it is then time for the weight trainer to cease weight training. If a man is capable of 350x10 in a particular lift when fresh and rested and when he gets around to that exercise, deep into the session, he can only push or tug 310x10 or 340x6, that man is crispy fried and should pack it in.

There is no hypertrophy to be triggered or strength to be gained wrestling with poundage or reps 30% less than what the individual is capable of when muscles are fresh. If a fatigued trainee insists on handling big poundage in a weakened state, there is a real risk of catastrophic injury. I've seen a man's trembling arms collapse while holding 550 at arms length and the leftovers of that wipeout ain't a pretty sight. It's "Someone call 911!" time. Being a tough guy and insisting on manning-up when no one is asking you to man-up is asking for trouble. I've seen biceps ripped on a bounced deadlifts (a ripped biceps rolls up like a Venetian blind) and I've seen legs collapse with 800 on a man's back. Each accident was attributable to pushing too long and too hard.

Experience teaches us if you are in reasonably good shape and really blast away in the gym, going hard and heavy the way you're supposed to with enough training intensity to grow muscle and amass strength gains, after 40-60 minutes strength starts to flee fast. Fit guys can go a little longer; overweight, out-of-shape or anemic types won't make it much more than 20 minutes before hitting the wall.

Generally there are two types of trainees: those who generate the requisite intensity and reap results and those who train in a not-so-intense fashion and reap nothing of any real significance. 90% of all weight trainers fail to train intensely enough to trip the hypertrophy switch that triggers muscle growth. Most trainees are genuinely unaware of the sheer physical effort required to trigger tangible results. No one has ever taken them aside and said, "Look—unless you *really* extend yourself—I mean REALLY extend yourself—unless you press the effort accelerator to the floorboard, unless you take it to the limit and beyond, consistently and repeatedly—nothing of any real physical significance is going to occur.

Capacity is a Shifting Target

If you train with the requisite effort, you *can't* go very long. If you *can*, you're not going hard enough.

Going through the motions, i.e., using the same poundage in the same exercises for the same number of sets and same number of repetitions, week after week, doing the same things in the same ways, is going to net zero results. Only by pushing the body *past* current capacity, only through dogged struggle, only by attempting to equal or exceed your previous best, will anything of muscular significance occur.

Keep in mind that capacity is a shifting target. On an "off" day, capacity might be 15% less than when you have an "on" day. That's okay and needs to be taken into account. Trying to hit or exceed 100% of maximum capacity on an "off" day is dangerous. Capacity can be breached using different strategies. Look around when you go to the gym. If by simply performing the same number of reps using the same poundage in the same exercises triggered the adaptive response, the gym would be crawling with muscle monsters.

The human body does not favorably reconfigure itself in response to ease and sameness. The body only grows new muscle and becomes stronger when pushed into new territory. Those who go through the motions (staying within their comfort zone) can train for a long time. Those who train intensely enough to trigger hypertrophy have between 30 and 75 minutes before the sheer intensity of the effort causes them to run out of energy. Super hard and super heavy training drains physical energy and also drains psychic energy. Only the trained, experienced individual, a member of the athletic elite, can train hard longer than an hour.

Science has shown that serum testosterone levels plummet when the body is pushed past a certain point. The Bulgarian Olympic lifters put their medical people on the case and they recommended that training sessions be limited to 45 minutes. Before you get too excited about that particular training time limitation, be aware that Bulgarian National Coach, Ivan "The Butcher" Abadjiev, said, "Fine. We'll limit national team lifting sessions to 45 minutes per session—but we'll have *six* sessions per day."

Exercises done at the beginning of the session are attacked hardest because energy levels are at their peak. Exercises done at the end of a long hard session inevitably and invariably suffer. Energy is a finite substance and is depleted by all-out effort. Attack the most important exercises first, while energy is high and always start with the big, sweeping, compound, multi-joint exercises. Then follow up with the less intense isolation exercises.

The Purposeful Primitive knows the energy clock is always running, the sands in the hour glass are shifting and sliding downward, imperceptibly, inevitably, and time is not on our side. Never compromise on expending *intense effort* in order to artificially extend the length of the session. Get through the important compound movements before the endurance gas tank runs dry. A good rule of thumb: train hard enough to trip the hypertrophy switch; energy is going to start heading south at about the 40 minute mark. An insider trick-of-the-trade: drink a "smart bomb" shake during the workout (combination of protein and carb powder). Come to grips with the physiological fact that if you train correctly, hard and intense, you only have about an hour!

PROGRESS MULTIPLIER: THE TRAINING PARTNER

The Only Thing Better Than a Hardcore Training Partner ...Is a Group of Hardcore Training Partners

Any athlete that has played for a winning team knows that a group of athletes can develop a collective synergy that needs to be experienced to be truly appreciated. The optimal group dynamic creates a hurricane of momentum as players play over their heads and exceed realistic expectations on a routine basis. As a result of athletic synergy the grand total exceeds the logical sum of the combined individual parts. Team synergy

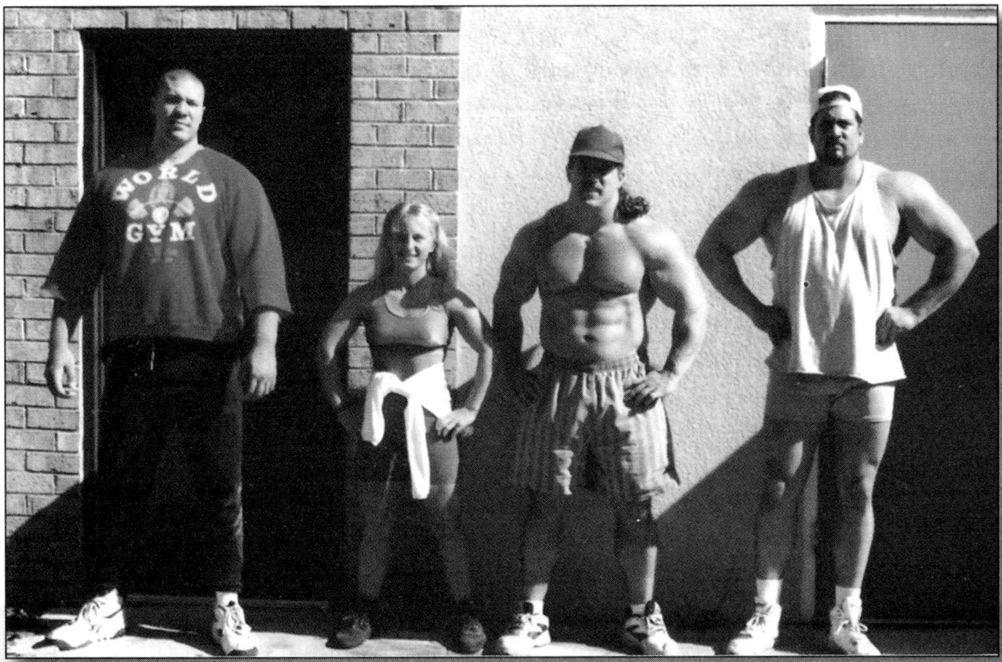

Out back of MAC: These were my training partners at Maryland Athletic Club circa 1995. Run by a notorious, poisonous dwarf named Ian Burgess, MAC was home to lots of great athletes. Left to right: Big Bullet, a 375 pound ex-pro ball monster man; Sioux-Z Hartwig, multi-time National and IPF World Powerlifting Champ at 123 pounds; Karwoski sports a fake pony tail weighing a plutonium-dense 280. Bob "Nacho Del Grande" Myers tips the beam at 320. Bob took second at the USPF Nationals that year. I took the photo. We'd finished deadlifting and were pooling money for a beer run.

can be replicated in resistance training by lifting with like-minded, highly motivated individuals regularly and repeatedly. A training partner, or better yet, a group of training partners, accelerates gains way past your wildest imaginings.

If the chemistry is right, if the person or persons pushes you and demands the best from you, if they do so without being reckless or hurtful, if they inspire you to do more than you would on your own, and do so without veering into injurious training practices—you are in for the most productive physical training period of your entire life. It is a predictable phenomenon and for this reason the athletic elite cluster together to train. It's only natural for the strong and capable to seek each other out.

The elite know that loafing or giving less than 100% effort is less likely when training in front of individuals who are your athletic equal or preferably better than you. If possible or given a choice, seek to train with individuals stronger and more knowledgeable than you as they will drag your game upward. When it comes to stimulating your own physical progress, it is far better to be the small fish in the Big Pond than the Big Fish in the small pond. Nothing seems to make that insurmountable 400 pound squat barrier (your personal best) seem slight and insignificant as when training with people who squat double that poundage for reps.

At first glance it might appear intimidating but once you swallow your ego, training with better athletes is a real advantage. If you live in a tiny pond where everyone is in awe of you because you squat 400, it is a lot harder psychologically to view 400 as just a step and not an ultimate destination. Ever wonder why so many times the youngest brother in a large family becomes the best athlete? This is an example of the benefits of playing with athletes bigger and better than you. It forces the little ones to "up their game" in order to hang. In the end that is a good thing, athletically speaking.

When you have a larger frame of physiological and psychological reference, you come to understand that by striving, by continually and unrelentingly pushing yourself in order to keep apace with your betters, you improve—or you break down, physically or psychologically. A good training partner has a responsibility to himself and to his partners. You are required to show up on time at the designated training venue, ready, willing and able to blast the living dog-shit out of some muscle, lift or body part.

Muscle growth and additional strength lies in those reps barely made, the stuff you'd be crazy to try on your own.

Practicing primitive free weight barbell and dumbbell exercises collectively, each in turn stepping into the spotlight to lift as the others watch, critiquing each other immediately after the set, is an intimidating, daunting and exhilarating experience. Your ego is flattened when more experienced training partners tear you to shreds with blistering critique before rebuilding you with constructive criticism prior to the next set. To have someone "spot you" on the potentially dangerous lifts allows you—inspires you—to give 110%. We all pick up our game when another person or persons are watching us do something and watching us intently. The attention makes us perform at a different level, a higher level.

A spotter allows you to extend yourself. Lifting by yourself when bench pressing or squatting, requires you to leave a rep or two "in the bank"—you need some reserve strength left at the end of each set. You cannot afford to get pinned under a heavy weight and that means you never try that questionable rep. With a spotter you are now liberated to try that extra growth or strength producing rep that safety and sanity won't allow when training solo. Muscle growth and additional strength lies in those reps barely made, the stuff you'd be crazy to try on your own.

With spotters the dangerous reps become plausible and beneficial. You don't need a spotter for a 40 pound leg curl or a 15 pound triceps kickback, but you damned sure need them when you are attempting to handle 405x6 when the most you've ever done is 405x5. Spotters allow you to go where no timid man should venture: into the productive danger zone of extended reps and increased poundage.

Purposeful Primitives instinctively push against the limits of the poundage and rep envelope: that is where the gains reside. Anyone performs better when all eyes are riveted on them during a heavy lift. As my old Zen power coach once said, "You only think you're training hard until you get sucked into a training group, a group way smarter and way stronger than you." Better to train in a dump with Supermen than in a posh palace surrounded by low-pain tolerance politically-correct metro-sexual sissies.

How Simple can the Physical Renovation Process be made Without Losing Effectiveness?

Recently I've had to do something I hadn't done in decades: introduce folks who've never lifted weights in their entire lives to my peculiar ways and methods.

Working with clinically obese folks caused me to undertake an unexpected reexamination of my own Purposefully Primitive methods and procedures. Could I break the basics of an already ultra-basic system down even further? Was it possible to create a framework sparser than the spare template already in place? Could I create a skeletal framework so limited that it could be used effectively by the untrained; people who work full time jobs, people with large families and lots of responsibilities? How simple can you make the physical renovation process without losing effectiveness?

My back-to-basics immersion caused me to deeply reconsider procedures and philosophies done for so long and so regularly that, in some cases, I'd forgotten *why* I do things the way I do them. I've lifted weights since the age of

Mark and Buck Chaillet: There was no more super-simplistic trainer than Mark. You couldn't do much less than Mark, yet he became one of the best in the World.

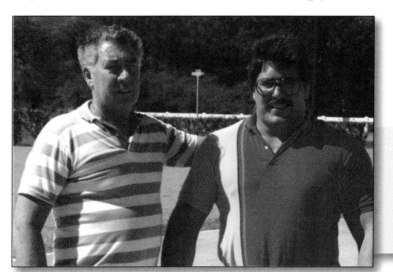

twelve and at age 57, I've accumulated 45 years of hands-on, in-the-trenches experience. That's good and bad. Anytime a person does something for that long they tend to get pretty damned good at it. On the downside they tend to become a bit dogmatic, automatic and pedantic. Elemental modes and procedures should not be taken for granted. It had been a long time since I'd pondered *how*, *what* and *why* I do what I do in the way that I do.

When I started explaining to the stone-cold beginners why I wanted them to do things in a certain way, I noted that I could rattle off reasons and rationales like an auctioneer at a cattle sale. But it somehow seemed hollow to me. I was being superficial and rote. I said things without thinking and decided that I needed to reevaluate *how* and *why*. Dealing with total beginners, something I had never done, caused me to rethink much of what I'd taken for granted for so long.

It was as if someone had opened a window in a room full of stale cigar smoke and a fresh breeze had blown in: hard, cold, chilly and bracing. It felt good to reexamine my treasured orthodoxies. Normally I only work with elite weight trainers. These are very experienced athletes who without exception have a tremendous amount of progressive resistance training under their belts before they seek me out. I'm purposefully obscure, hard to find and off the beaten track. When an ardent lifter or athlete makes their way up to the mountains to see me, they are looking for fresh direction on a journey already long underway. I see these seekers for four or five hours then they head back to their world. I'm sort of a one-man Iron Finishing School: a guy who might be able to alert an elite athlete to some heretofore unconsidered offbeat angle or progress-stimulating approach.

This time it was different. This time I'd decided to work with complete beginners with zero fitness experience. These were local folks from right in my neighborhood. To compound complexity, I was looking to extract maximum results in a relatively short timeframe. I'd worked hard and diligently to remove myself from society. I purposefully constructed a rural, isolated lifestyle in order to get really good at my many solitary pursuits. Now life suddenly took a sharp left turn. Circumstance presented me with an opportunity to give something of value to folks who could really use some assistance. This required I reenter the societal world I purposefully left.

Fitness folks that come to me for advice are a savvy lot. I don't spend time going over *why* I do the things I do. Like a celebrity chef I have my particular style of cuisine and my very own repertoire of signature dishes. A certain segment of the public loves what I do. All was right with my relationship to the world insofar as maintaining my comfort groove.

Then along comes a gaggle of stone cold beginners that have no freaking idea who I am; people that have never ever touched a weight; and now I'm put in charge of maximizing physical progress of a little gang of totally untrained regular people.

All of my beginners were clinically obese, i.e. carrying a 30% or greater body fat percentile. Some of my new clients had 50% body fat percentiles. My goal was to see if it was possible to spark a substantive physical makeover in obese individuals using minimalist methods. The process would take ninety days and I would stay true to my Purposeful Primitive philosophy. That these methods worked for elite athletes was beyond dispute; grounded in biology, the methodological effectiveness is rooted in scientific "cause and effect," do *this* and *that must* happen. I believe in biological imperatives. Lift weights in the proscribed fashion and muscles are required to grow. Perform cardiovascular exercise as instructed and organ function and caloric oxidation must improve. Eat with precision and discipline and stored body fat must be preferentially oxidized. Put all three modes together and the human body *must* reconfigure itself. Subjected to proper procedures executed in the prescribed sequence the human body has no physiological choice other than to build muscle and oxidize excess body fat.

With four decades of empirical experience under my belt, I know what works. I also know what procedures are a waste of time. My self-imposed challenge was, could an already sparse methodology be pruned and pared, trimmed and reduced, without losing the essential essence? This was a challenge that excited me in a way that I hadn't been excited in a long time. It has proven to be a literal lifesaver for people whose bodyweight was jeopardizing their health and threatening to prematurely kill them.

Was there a way to reduce Purposefully Primitive methods to an *irreducible core essence* that could be used by obese individuals to solve their bodyweight dilemma? Could I create a user-friendly, time-efficient training and nutritional method for use by untrained obese folks that would provide maximum bang for minimum time investment?

The Self-Imposed Rules

I wanted to make my test as tough as possible. Again, how *little* could we do and still elicit results? I wanted to train them as little as possible using only a barbell and the fewest number of exercises possible. I wanted cardio exercise to be limited in duration and confined to walking. I wanted to use only foods available at the grocery store. No pills, potions or supplements. No more than five cumulative hours per week would be dedicated to training. I broke this out into three weekly weight training sessions of 30 minutes each. Weight training would consist of three exercises done three times a week. Three sets of 10 reps in the squat, bench press and deadlift. Seven weekly cardiovascular sessions of 30 minute duration would be the sole aerobic activity. Cardio exercise was outdoor walking. Insofar as diet, they would eat only food purchased from the grocery store. No nutritional supplements. I showed them how to cook delicious lean protein dishes and fiber carb dishes. None of the participants had *ever* lifted weights or participated in a serious fitness program.

Ron

Started off weighing 241 pounds standing 5'9." This 48 year old Mack Truck factory worker was able to squat 95, bench press 95 and deadlift 135 for reps on day one. On day 88 Ron squatted 245, bench pressed 225 and deadlifted 400 weighing 175 pounds. Ron took 3rd place in his age and weight division at the 2005 AAU World Powerlifting Championships.

Betty

Started off weighing 305 pounds standing 5'2." This 61 year old grandmother was unable to walk 50 steps without stopping to catch her breath for 15 minutes. She was unable to perform a single squat with zero weight. She could perform one incline pushup with no weight and was unable to squat down to grab a deadlift bar. On day 88 she won her age group at the AAU World Powerlifting Championships with a 205 pound squat, a 100 pound bench press and a 195 pound deadlift. She was able to walk the circumference of a 154 acre farm without stopping and weighed 264 pounds.

Connie

Started off weighing 183 pounds standing 5'3." This 39 year old mother of five boys was able to squat and deadlift 75 pounds on day one and bench press 40 pounds. On day 88 Connie won the AAU World Powerlifting title weighing 148 pounds. She squatted 185, bench pressed 145 and deadlifted 185. In training she had bench pressed 95 for 10 reps.

Jen

Started off weighing 305 pounds standing 5'8." This 33 year old computer programmer on day one was able to do 10 incline pushups with no weight. She was able to perform one full squat with no weight and one deadlift with the empty 45 pound barbell. On day 88 Jen won her weight class at the AAU Championship squatting 200, bench pressing 105 and deadlifting 280 before barely missing 300. She weighed 271.

All final lifts were done under the strict scrutiny of three judges in high level powerlifting competition. No suits, belts, wraps or bench shirts were used in training or competition and no one ever did any lift other than the squat, bench press or deadlift. Sessions were done thrice weekly and everyone walked outdoors everyday for 30 minutes. Ron made the most gains and I think this was attributable to his sticking the closest to the diet. Ron opted for a Parrillo-style multiple-meal eating schedule. He lost 65 pounds of bodyweight in 90 days. In fact his progress was even more astounding in that he added 12 pounds of muscle. Using the add-back equation reveals that Ron lost 78 pounds of fat and added 12 pounds of muscle to end up at a scale weight of 175 pounds. At the competition he missed a 3rd attempt squat with 275 pounds. Betty's progress in some ways was more astounding. While she didn't lose the bodyweight that Ron did, her health went from feeble and life-threatening to strong and empowered.

Ebb and Flow

Progress is Difficult to Generate, Tough to Keep Going and Sure to End…

Physical progress is an ebb and flow proposition. The only surefire bet in the world of fitness-related pursuits is that all progress eventually grinds to a halt, no matter how sophisticated the program or how great the individual effort.

Progress Booster: The boys watch the video playback of Don Mill's 635x5 squat weighing 211. Left to right, Pat Brooks rolls his wraps, Ray Evans, Joe Ferry (700 deadlift, 500 bench press @ 198) Don, Marshall Peck leans forward. I stand on the far right getting ready.

The video playback was deservedly popular among lifters. Why depend on someone else's 'opinion' about how your just completed lift looked—watch it yourself 30 seconds after completion and make the appropriate in-flight adjustments. We had the squat camera set up at parallel height looking at depth. The bench camera was set high looking down. The deadlift camera was straight ahead at bellybutton height.

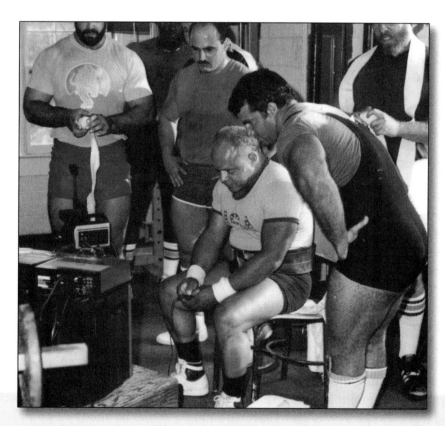

Any untrained individual who suddenly subjects themselves to an intense progressive resistance program will generate substantial progress—for a while. The trick is recognizing when progress ceases and knowing what to do about it when the inevitable stagnation arrives. The real pros have a veritable arsenal of exercise routines and diets ready to roll out when the proverbial well runs dry. The real pros are so physically attuned that they actually *anticipate* stagnation before it takes root and have new modes and methods all ready for inclusion and rotation whenever the current approach plays out. Progress is difficult to generate, tough to keep going and sure to end.

Regardless the sophistication of your approach, regardless the amount of workout intensity you are able to generate, regardless the sheer amount of time you devote to the pursuit of physical training, eventually all routines and all diets cease delivering results.

Repeating the same eating and exercise procedures creates a habit pattern and the Soft Machine will eventually figure out the habitual pattern and produce a physical antidote. The human body is a miraculous organism and given time and exposure to a particular mode or method, it always finds a way to neutralize the training effect.

The trick is to not allow the body to generate the antidote; change modes and methods before the body solves the puzzle. Human beings are creatures of habit. Legislating periodic change runs contrary to basic human nature.

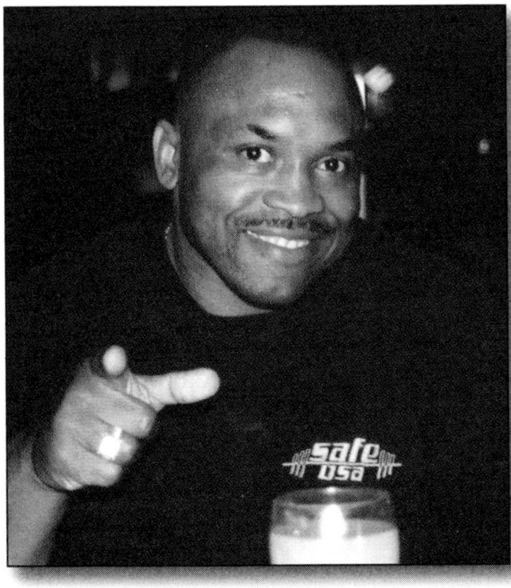

Change Master: Gene "The Machine" Bell was one of the top five lifters of all-time. He was a study in contrasts. Here he is at lunch with me: intelligent, soft spoken, a career military man, somewhat of a Clark Kent, at least at casual glance. On the lifting platform he morphed into a powerlift Terminator. They called Gene "The Machine" because of the methodical, systematic fashion in which he destroyed opponents.

Thesis, Antithesis, Synthesis
Embrace Change, Legislate Contrast

Proper training and effective eating favorably alters the shape and composition of the human body. It does so by imposing *biological imperatives*. Do *this* and that *will* happen: simple scientific cause and effect. The biological imperative is the physical expression of the Hegelian Dialectic: thesis, antithesis, synthesis. The status quo *thesis* (your body as it is) is impacted by something radically different, the *antithesis* (a new system of training/nutrition.) Eventually that which was once radical and different morphs into the new status quo and becomes the *synthesis*. The synthesis becomes the new thesis and the process repeats itself.

If we are to keep the progress ball rolling, new modes need to be periodically rolled out. "New" is no guarantor of better. As Krishnamurti points out in an appropriate analogy, "Just because the window is open there is no guarantee the breeze will blow in. However if the window remains shut—there is no possibility the breeze will enter." Recognizing stagnation is terrific, embracing change is noble, but that in and of itself is no guarantee the changes selected will be the correct ones that will stimulate new progress. Effort is no substitute for success.

To trigger progress, consistently and consciously examine the current status quo and assess if progress is proceeding apace. When a radical new procedure is implemented it needs to create dramatic *contrast* to the current status quo. If the contrast is sufficient the organism will undergo an *adaptive response*. Slight variations in current procedures are insufficient to trigger the adaptive response. Rearranging the contents of the box is not enough. To create contrast sufficiently contrary to the current status quo requires stepping outside the box entirely. Radically new exercise and/or eating procedures are needed. The antithesis needs to possess significant contrast to the thesis.

New and different stresses need to be imposed and once the new and different stresses are no longer new and different, once the contrasting procedures are no longer innovative and shocking, measurable physical improvement is *over*! The theory of the adaptive response also applies to nutrition. We need to periodically institute radically new and different dietary procedures. Perhaps changing the *amount* of food consumed, or changing the *type* of foods selected or changing *when* we eat. Once the body becomes used to nutritional or training procedures progress peters out. The truly attuned continually rotate in new protocols and procedures.

No One System, Mode or Method Trumps All Others

No single exercise routine or system, no single dietary approach or eating protocol, trumps all others. There is no such thing as a single exercise or eating strategy that is so effective that it can be used forever. Yet those who make fitness devices and market fitness products would have you believe that they have invented a product or a system that beats all others and will deliver incredible results endlessly. This is another fitness myth.

Here is a fitness truth of the first magnitude: no one system trumps all others and no one system can deliver progress ad infinitum. That is a fitness fact-of-life. Progress must be nurtured and stagnation recognized. Savvy transformation masters know that periodically the body needs to be jolted out of its complacency. Pablo Picasso once said, "Occasionally a man needs to be jerked out of his torpor." These are words to live by in life and in all fitness and nutrition-related pursuits.

When those protocols once shocking, jarring and exhilarating morph into old and familiar, when what was once radical has now become tired, it is time to institute radical change: thesis, antithesis, synthesis. Learn to embrace change and cultivate continual contrast. Most fitness devotees labor under the illusion that once they stumble upon a system or mode that delivers substantive change, that system can and should be used on an exclusionary basis ad infinitum. After all, "I know it works for me." The devotee develops a rabid allegiance to that initial mode or method that provided that initial burst of physical progress.

Here is a salient point grounded in fact: when *any* untrained individual suddenly subjects themselves to a 'serious' training regimen (or a radical diet) virtually *any* system will deliver results—for a while. An appropriate fitness cliché is..."It's not so much *what* you do as *how hard* you do it." Any untrained individual suddenly subjecting themselves to an intense resistance program will trigger gains for a period of time.

The trick is not in generating progress initially—but rather how to revive progress once that initial burst subsides.

Better To Use a Lousy System with Great Intensity Than A Sophisticated System Halfheartedly

When an individual suddenly and consistently trains the body intensely using new methods the body responds. I've seen people obtain incredible results from lousy exercise systems by generating incredible training intensity and applying Herculean physical effort. I've seen other people obtain terrible results using incredibly effective exercise strategies as a direct result of sub-maximal effort and piss-poor application. The best of both worlds is to combine a superior training regimen with gut-busting effort and consistent application.

Result-producing exercise routines and effective diets need to be rotated on a regularly reoccurring basis. Using a favored mode, method or tactic exclusively and ceaselessly, is stagnation-on-a-stick. Sameness is the progress killer and the athletic elite accept the inevitability of becoming stagnant. They actually anticipate stagnation ahead of time and figure its arrival into future plans. They know that when stagnation arrives the best way to rekindle momentum is to construct a new exercise or dietary approach that *contrasts dramatically* with what they have been doing.

One mistake repeatedly made by fitness buffs (too clever by half) is to alter the current effective approach ever-so-slightly. They do not understand the need for a dramatic alteration. Dramatic contrast jolts the body and stagnation morphs into momentum. Slight modifications are easily neutralized by a body that has figured out the status quo antidote. It is a relatively easy thing for the organism to adjust to a slight change in the current status quo. It takes guts to jettison a program that has been proven effective. It is psychologically difficult to toss a system we've grown to love. But we don't throw it away forever: categorize it as effective and simply set it back on the shelf for future use. The athletic elite have an arsenal of proven effective training and eating regimens, hung in their philosophic closets like a row of clean shirts on hangers.

Don't Turn a Once Effective System into a Religion

People fall into a reoccurring trap: they obtain spectacular results from a particular resistance, nutrition or cardio program and attempt to turn the effective regimen into a *religion.* They become acolytes and adherents and feel compelled to use the precise regimen that worked for them at one time in the past. They develop an unhealthy allegiance that often veers into religious zealotry—this despite the mathematical fact that any meaningful results have long since dried up. They refuse to change, or if they do change, the changes are so minor, so cosmetic and minute that the antithesis remains virtually indistinguishable from the original thesis. This rearranging of the deck chairs never works.

Periodically institute a complete and total overhaul of what you are doing. To trigger results requires *significant deviation* from current protocol. Real results require real change. At best, continued usage maintains the status quo. Someone said stupidity is repeating the same behavior over and over while expecting different results. Stimulating progress requires the institution of a new regimen that significantly contrasts to the current status quo.

Legislating Contrast

Activity	Status Quo Thesis	Contrasting Antithesis Prescription
Weight Training	10 rep sets	5 rep sets
	5 weekly sessions	3 weekly sessions
	60 minute sessions	30 minute sessions
	Fast pace	Slower pace
	Moderate speed reps	Purposefully explosive rep speed
Aerobic Training	Treadmill	Outdoor power-walk
	4 weekly sessions	6 weekly sessions
	30 minute sessions	60 minute sessions
	Moderate pace	longer session
	80% of age-related HR	70% of age-related HR
	Done at night	Done 1st thing in the morning
Diet/ Nutrition	Hi-protein/low carb	Low fat/moderate carb & protein
	2,000 calories/day	4,000 calories/day
	1 meal	7 mini-meals
	High protein	Moderate protein
	Low carbohydrate	Moderate carbohydrate
	High fat	Low fat
	Warrior Diet	Saturated fat kept to 10% of calories

Contrast Is King

Generally speaking most exercise and diet routines lose effectiveness after 4-6 weeks, but this can vary. Knowing when to change comes with experience.

The more training cycles you have under your belt, the better you'll be at identifying the signs of stagnation. Don't use change as an excuse to change every thing every week. Three to four weeks is the absolute minimum to stay on a selected course. Anything less and you can be accused of not giving the approach a decent tryout. Humans are creatures of habit and when left to their own devices prefer to follow a path they know. The iron elite are attuned to the body's subtle rhythms and patterns and they know that blind allegiance to a particular system, mode, methodology or approach is progress suicide.

The Purposeful Primitive understands that while anyone can design an *initially* effective training or eating regimen, the real secret to prolonged physical success is in knowing what to do when the initial burst of progress ceases. After a while the trainee becomes aware of the natural ebb and flow of training and eating and gravitates naturally towards a holistic system that provides a reinvigorating change of pace every 4-6 weeks.

Embracing change eventually becomes something we look forward to: it becomes exciting to try radically different modes and methods. The journey of self discovery positively impacts the physique in ways you never thought possible. Embrace change and become comfortable with the fact that Contrast is King. Over time come to understand that there's a natural ebb and flow to training and eating—and life itself.

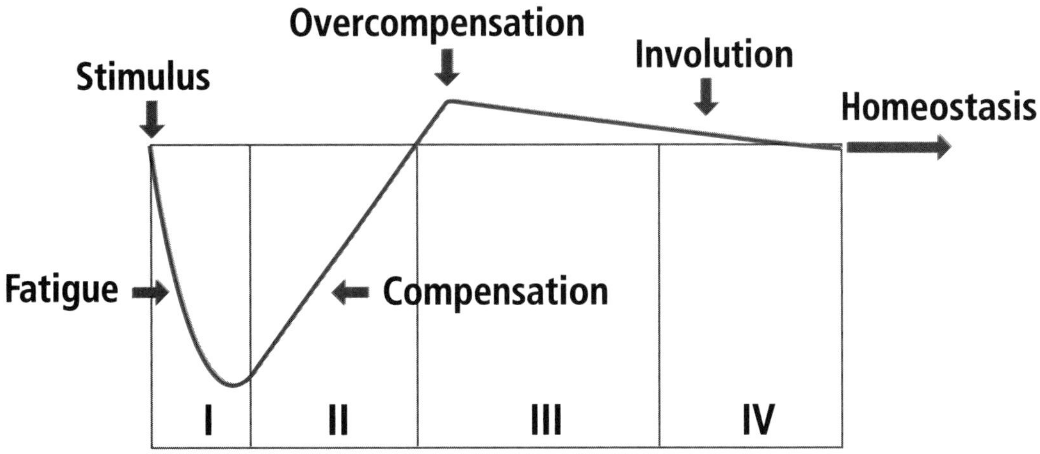

This graph by Iron Curtain genius, Tudor Bompa, is the snapshot blueprint of my life. In Phase I the cycle starts: coming off a vicious, result-producing workout, the human body is fatigued and needs time to heal and recuperate. Once the body is rested and regenerated, hit it again, hard! This is represented by the rocket-ride that starts in Phase I and ends in Phase III. Think of 'Overcompensation' as '10 steps forward' and 'Involultion' as 'two steps backward.' Theoretically the net gain is physical progress with the 'homeostasis' finale ending at a higher level than the initial 'stimulus' jumping off point in Phase I. This peak and valley linear chart is not just about lifting weights. It is inexorably intertwined with cardio activity, nutrition and state-of-mind. None of this matters if the training effort is of insufficient intensity.

Direct Muscle Soreness and Deep Muscle Fatigue

In my experience there are two distinct types of post-weight training aftershock: *Direct muscle soreness* (DMS) and *deep muscle fatigue* (DMF.) Both are the result of training intensely enough to trigger muscle hypertrophy. High repetition training is the culprit for DMS: I have never experienced "sore to the touch" muscle trauma using low rep sets, even when using multiple sets. Direct muscle soreness is fiber trauma related to high repetition training. DMS is caused by performing high rep sets that equal or exceed capacity in some fashion. This type of training creates intense muscle soreness that is a result of cellular micro-trauma.

Are the cells torn apart or pressurized? Forcibly expanded? Forcibly contracted? Ripped or shredded? The medical people can't seem to agree, but one thing is for sure, some sort of micro-cellular calamity is occurring. Deep muscle fatigue, DMF, occurs when a particular muscle or muscle group is hit so hard using low reps and heavy poundage, that the entire body is engulfed in waves of fatigue. For days afterwards the afflicted athlete feels as if their limbs are made of lead or that they are moving through mud or water. Overcoming DMS and DMF requires sleep, food and avoidance of further weight training until the sore to the touch or leaden feeling subsides.

Sometimes the intensity of DMS/DMF becomes so severe that it debilitates the athlete. The muscles are traumatized to such an extent that the athlete actually experiences mild forms of paralysis. In both cases nutrients, rest and often therapeutic remedies such as heat, water and massage can accelerate recovery. Traumatized muscles and fatigued muscles need to heal, repair and regenerate before subjecting them to any further weight training.

I first crossed swords with the debilitating effects of direct muscle soreness when as a 13 year old man-child I found a 10 pound solid dumbbell (talk about a life omen) on my grandmother's hardscrabble Arkansas farm. I just found it in the burn pile one day. It was black and solid. Being a dumb kid who was already reading *Strength & Health* magazine,

I proceeded to do 50 repetitions of one-arm curls for each arm every hour on the hour for something like 10 straight hours. It seemed like a cool and potentially productive idea. I wanted to build big guns in the worst way and in my young, innocent mind this seemed like a hell of a good idea. I loved the arm pump I was getting every hour on the hour. I would run to the bedroom to pose in a small mirror. My little guns would swell and I loved the way the veins appeared.

The exhilaration on Monday went out the window Tuesday morning when I awoke in intense pain. Something was terribly wrong. I sat up in bed with both fists involuntarily clenched next to my face. My arms had locked up; each arm had frozen in the contracted position. The biceps would not, could not relax. Flex your biceps with your fist next to your cheek as hard as humanly possible as you read this: now imagine this extremis flexion lasting for two days. My trauma was so complete and intense that both biceps remained involuntarily contracted for 48 straight hours.

Any attempt to straighten my arms even a few inches resulted in excruciating pain. Nothing could be done for me and I tried to hide the fact that I had racked myself from my 80 year old grandma and my needlessly cruel brother and hillbilly cousins. That was easy as her eyesight was bad and she was kindly and not suspicious. My brother and cousins sniffed out my dilemma like a pack of wolves separating a young caribou from the herd for a kill. They used the occasion to pay me back for what they mistakenly perceived as the horrible things I, the oldest and strongest, did to them on a regularly reoccurring basis.

The easiest payback was to simply grab my hands and tug them downward. This sent spasms of intense pain shooting up my arms and spasms of glee across their satanic little faces. It was oppressed sibling payback time. The inmates had rioted and taken control of the prison camp capturing the commandant. They sincerely hoped my condition would last for the rest of my life.

My grandmother kept asking what my periodic screams were all about. My male pride kept me from saying anything and the gleeful torturers weren't about to fess up. On day three I awoke and the pain was gone. I lay in bed and plotted. I slipped away to the woods before anyone arose and set up an elaborate payback scheme. I pre-positioned garden tools I swiped from the shed. I returned and pretended to still be asleep and debilitated. I faked pain for the first couple times they pulled on my arms and pretended to run away to avoid them. I ran into the woods behind the farm. They ran after me like a lynch mob.

They were quite shocked when after getting out of earshot of the farm I ambushed them and beat them bloody. I stacked them up like cordwood and tied them up. While roped together at the ankles like a chain gang, I made them dig a shallow hole in the sandbank next to the creek with a shovel I'd stashed there earlier. I then buried them up to their necks.

Only their heads protruded above ground. I told them I was going to run over their heads with a lawnmower. They screamed like sissies when I fired up the mower. My tools of mayhem were pre-positioned and I took several close mower passes by their heads. I made them cry. One actually pissed his pants. They ran home bawling and sandy. I told my grandmother that they had ruined their clothes and soiled their britches. They told her outlandish tales of beatings and burial and lawnmowers that sounded so ridiculous that she dismissed them as lies.

I laughed as they got whippings. Good clean kid fun.

I had to ride out my muscle soreness until my shattered biceps eventually relaxed. This taught me a lesson about resistance training that has lasted me a lifetime.

I use milder versions of muscle soreness to determine if the exercise used is targeting and isolating the intended muscle in the way I want. Muscle soreness tells me two things: did I train intensely enough to generate soreness, and if so, is the soreness where it should be? I will often perform a single resistance exercise and wait and see if, when the muscle soreness arrives, it is centered on the targeted muscle. If I do barbell rows does the exercise generate soreness? If not, I am disappointed. Secondly, if there is soreness, is it located on the targeted lat muscles? Has the exercise totally missed the target muscle? Perhaps I feel the soreness in the traps or rear deltoids.

Before every set of every resistance exercise I identify the target muscle and strive to make a mind/muscle connection. Soreness is the targeting report card issued later. Soreness determines if the muscle targeting has been accurate. If I become sore in other than the target area, that means I need to change the technical execution of the exercise. If there is zero soreness then I know I need to train harder. I will tell myself that perhaps the mind/muscle connection was ill-defined, unrefined or not focused enough. The Iron Elite understand that soreness is a natural part of the resistance landscape. The modern "split routine' was born as a direct result of the soreness phenomena. With both types (soreness/deep fatigue) I have found that light to moderate cardio exercise helps flush toxins and waste products out of afflicted muscles.

Accelerating circulation within a sore muscle stimulates recovery. If deep fatigue prevents me from blasting away, moderate intensity power walking super-oxygenates the body and, along with food, accelerates fatigue recovery. Use your common sense and be aware that Purposeful Primitives pay heed to fatigue and soreness. You can actually use it to your advantage.

Progressive Pulls

Old School Method for Total Back Decimation

Compound multi-joint progressive resistance movements done with a barbell or a pair of dumbbells are without question the most effective exercises ever devised for building muscle. No system of exercise produces the muscle growth free weight progressive resistance training delivers. This is a flat statement of undeniable scientific fact.

In my opinion the most effective single progressive resistance routine ever devised specifically for building the muscles of the *back* are *progressive pulls*. I was exposed to this routine around 1965 in an article in *Strength & Health* magazine. In the interceding decades I've added a few subtle twists. Anyone that I've gotten to use this program the way it is supposed to be used has gotten fabulous results.

Progressive Pulls will grow back muscle on a steel post and nothing more is needed than a barbell and a big pile of plates. This is hard and heavy work and if done correctly (regardless your current degree of fitness) builds and strengthens every muscle on the human posterior. The sheer effort and intensity should knock the tar out of you physically. If it doesn't you're not doing the various pulls hard enough or heavy enough.

The human back is a complex conglomeration of large, medium and small muscles. Over time, nature and biomechanics have taught us unconsciously to allow the back muscles to act in a synchronized fashion in order to accomplish whatever muscular task is undertaken. To build a massive powerful back requires compound movements that take advantage of this naturally coordinated synchronization.

Ironically, nearly every 'expert' recommends isolation exercises for the back. This common mistake ignores the back's biomechanical strengths and panders to its biomechanical weakness. The best way to blast the back is as a unit, and all at once, not piecemeal.

Let's examine the component parts:

- The ***trapezius*** muscles sit atop the collar bones and run downward to mid-back
- The ***rear deltoids*** lie behind the anterior deltoids
- The ***rhomboids*** and ***teres*** are nestled in and around the shoulder blades
- The ***latissimus dorsi*** starts at the armpits and end at the buttock muscles
- The ***spinal erectors*** run from traps to tailbone and are shaped like twin Anacondas

The back muscles need to be shock-blasted using big, raw, sweeping, free weight exercises that cause the back muscles to work explosively and in sequential fashion. We pick movements done with two hands that require you to move a heavy object over a maximum range-of-motion (ROM) pulling and tugging *upwardly*. This stimulates back muscles with a thoroughness that needs to be experienced. This is a timeless routine and all of us, regardless our level, need to perform this routine identically. The poundage used varies according to ability, but technique does not.

A concentrated dose of Progressive Pulls does physiological wonders. This is a "Big Man" routine and as my comrade Kirk Karwoski might say, "Time to put away the pretty pink plastic Barbie dumbbells and get freaking *serious*!" Obviously a Purposeful Primitive will routinely perform the Progressive Pulls. If done with the requisite gusto this routine should only be done once a week. The idea is to establish initial poundage baselines in each exercise using crisp correct technique. Over time you increase poundage with no erosion or degradation of technique.

Increase poundage or reps on the top set of each exercise for six straight weeks (or longer). Avoid technical disintegration: if execution gets sloppy and you persist in continuing, nasty injury awaits you. Welcome to the Thunderdome. Are you ready to bite into something substantial? Can you wean yourself away from all that happy-time, cotton-candy machine-centric back training? Can we toss the lat pulldowns? Do you want to take a seat at the adult table? To make dramatic physical progress you will have to stroll into the pain zone. Actually the pain zone should more accurately be called the discomfort zone. Pain, real pain, is the indicator to immediately stop what you're doing.

You cannot trigger muscle hypertrophy (the irreducible root-core goal of progressive resistance exercise) by training sub-maximally. Unless you brush up against the lip of the limit envelope you can forget all about altering the shape of your body. The body does not favorably reconfigure itself in response to sub-maximal effort. Each day is different and limit capacity might differ significantly day to day, week to week. Regardless the limit of capacity on a particular day, if the stress imposed is not significant, nothing of significance will occur.

Limits can take many forms: reps, number of work sets, rest interval between sets, speed of the individual rep...all could be used as stress inducers and stress benchmarks. Do you have to go to failure or use forced reps on the top set of every single exercise? No, absolutely not. There are no forced reps in this routine. Establish baseline benchmarks in each exercise and consciously and continually seek to improve. Plan ahead; project future performance using periodization principles. Here is a hypothetical poundage scenario for an "average" person. If you are stronger or weaker, alter the baseline benchmarks.

Six Week Progressive Pull Periodization Cycle

Week	Reps	Power Clean Poundage	High Pull Poundage	Deadlift Poundage	Stiff-leg Deadlift Poundage	Row Poundage
1	10	65	85	135	85	65
2	10	70	90	145	90	70
3	8	75	95	155	95	75
4	8	80	100	165	100	80
5	5	85	105	175	105	85
6	5	90	110	185	110	90

Our hypothetical beginner performs five exercises. The poundage climbs upward, peaking with the deadlifts then back down again, culminating in the rows—hence the moniker Progressive Pulls. For the first two weeks, work up to a top set of 10 reps in each exercise. In Week 1 all 10 rep sets should be completed explosively. If you struggle to complete the final reps in week one, you're too ambitious and need to dramatically scale back the poundage starting point. Each week use slightly heavier poundage. Reps are dropped from 10 to 8 in weeks 2 & 3; from 8 reps down to 5 reps in weeks 4 & 5. Adept Big Men might want to start off with 7 rep sets, then 5's and finally finish with triples. We start off below capacity and end up above capacity.

Over the life of the six week periodization cycle, reps are dropped and poundage increases. This routine peaks power and strength and triggers a concurrent increase in muscular size and is best used during a mass building phase. Taking in extra calories is highly advised. I would also advise average size men push their bodyweight up one pound a week in order to ensure positive nitrogen balance. Power training combined with ample calories and sufficient rest is the ticket for amassing massive back muscles.

Once you've built some muscle to work with, something worthy of defining, double back and "lean out" using a periodization program designed to melt off body fat. Let's acquire some muscle before we get hung up on ripped abs and shredded deltoids. Who cares about seeing ripped abs on some guy who looks like he just broke out of a Viet Cong Prison Camp after being held in a tiger cage for six months? Who cares about defining a 14 inch arm? Here's the technical rundown on the lifts and their proper running order. Keep them in this sequence and on every rep of every set, strive for total technical perfection.

Exercise	Description	
Power Clean (PC) ➲ 2-3 Sets	The starting position of the 1st four exercises is identical. In the PC, the bar is pulled to pec height before snapping over the wrists. For full description of Power Clean, see page 125.	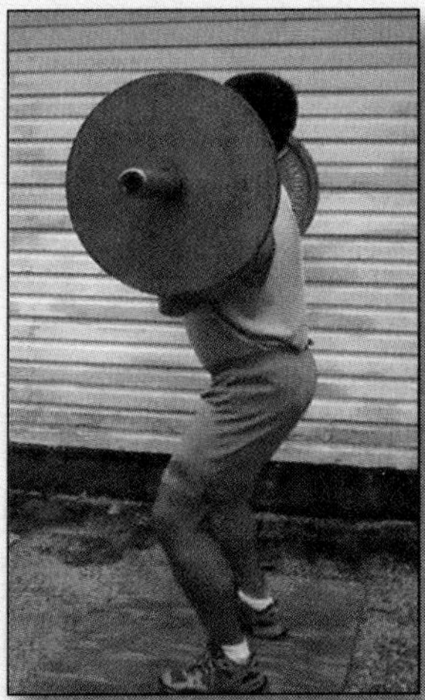
High Pull ➲ Increase poundage from Power Clean ➲ 2-3 Sets	Do not jerk the weight to get it moving. In all lifts the bar travels upward in a straight line! Pull the hi-pull to the belly button.	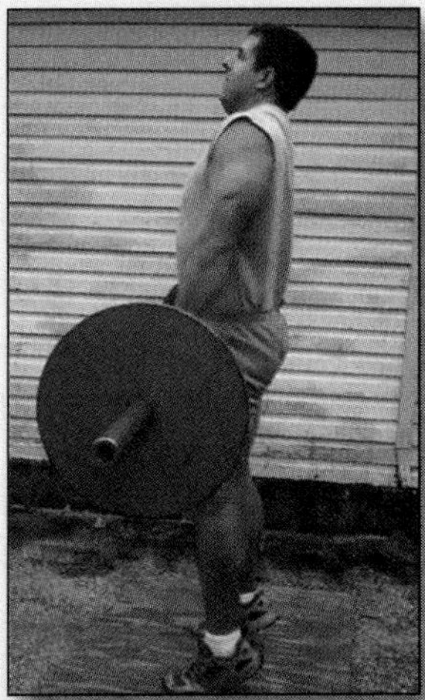

Exercise	Description
Conventional Deadlift (DL) ➲ Increase poundage from High Pull ➲ 2-3 Sets	Smooth, straight pull with knees, back, and shins vertical. Bar stays in contact with the legs at all times. Pull the dead to above the knees. No bouncing. For full description of Dead Lift, see pages 113-114
Stiff-Legged Deadlift (DL) ➲ Decrease poundage by 35-50% from Conventional DL ➲ 2-3 Sets	With a tight torso and semi-straight rigid knees the hip is the hinge. Allow hips to move back as you lower. Feel it in the hamstrings. No bouncing
Barbell Row (not shown) ➲ Decrease poundage by 25% from Stiff-Legged DL ➲ 2-3 Sets	Back is parallel to the floor. Pull to just below the pecs using lats, not arms. Elbows lead the action. Lower the weight to a dead-hang. For full description of Barbell Row, see page 126.

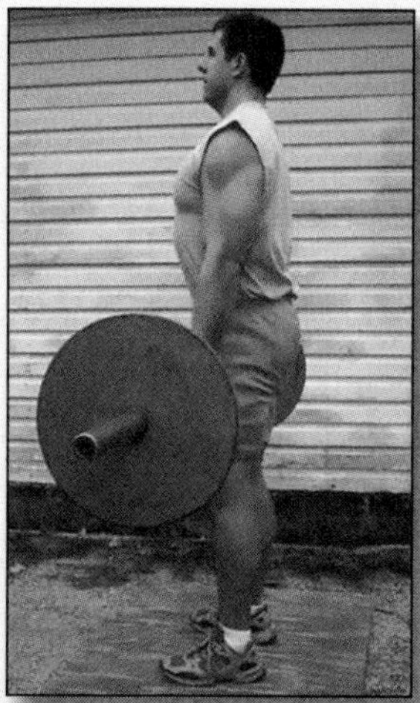

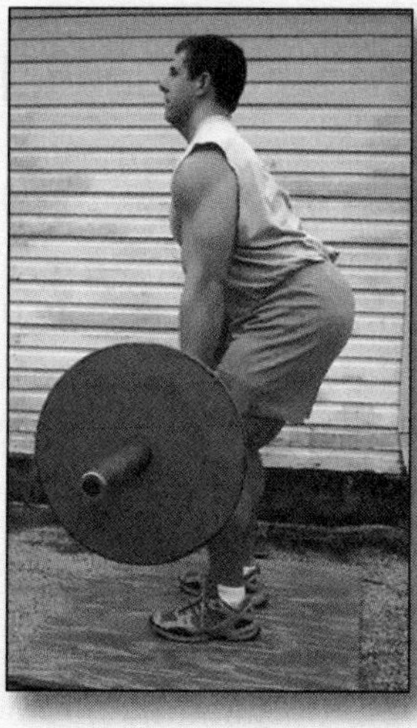

You will find detailed exercise descriptions for the power clean, deadlift and row earlier in this chapter. For high pulls and stiff-legged deadlifts we offer the following descriptions...keep in mind that in the broadest sense *all* progressive pulls are identical—regardless the height to which the barbell is pulled, regardless the configuration of the body as the pull is being done—the barbell moves (or should move) upward in an absolutely straight line. Here are exercise descriptions of two exercises not explained previously...

High Pulls

After finishing power cleans, we add poundage and continue onward into high pulls for 2-3 successive sets. A high pull is identical to a power clean. The difference being that the barbell is not being pulled high enough to wrist-snap and rack. Pull the barbell to belly button height or higher on each rep. Add poundage for each subsequent set. If the bar can only be pulled to crotch height—bag it! High pulls hit the erectors, rhomboids, teres and upper and lower lats. Try and go up on your toes and shrug your shoulders at the top. The poundage should be too heavy to arm pull. The arms should be thought of as hooks that hold the poundage, not arms that lift the poundage. Use the legs to start the weight moving and keep the arms straight and extended throughout—don't bend the elbows. Pull straight up with a tight, arched back.

Stiff-Legged Deadlift

You have gone upward in poundage from power cleans to high pulls to deadlifts. Now it's time to strip some weight off the bar and head back down in weight. A stiff-legged deadlift is a lower back and hamstring developer without peer. I would reduce the conventional deadlift weight by 35 to 50%. If you deadlift 400 x 5 perform stiff-legs with 200-250 x 5. Pull the first SL rep to completion using standard deadlift technique. Stand erect with the bar in deadlift fashion on the 1st rep. Now lower the barbell downward on semi-straight yet rigid knees, allowing the bar to break away from the body. Lower slowly with straight arms until it touches the floor, gently. No bouncing the plates off the floor to create rebound.

Upon touching the floor, quietly, begin an immediate rising up using a tight arched back. Pull to complete lockout. As you lower, pay attention and push the hips push rearward. At the turn-around, where descent becomes ascent, use the hamstrings and lower back to power you erect. I think of the stiff-leg dead as a "hip hinge" exercise. Everything below the hip hinge stays rigid and tight (the legs) and everything above the hip-hinge stays rigid and tight (the torso.) The hip joint is the fulcrum. Strip weight *off* the bar between the first and second set. This exercise done right is a hamstring and erector developer without peer.

After 2-3 sets of power cleans, 2 sets of high pulls, 2-3 sets of deadlifts, 2 sets of stiff-leg deadlifts and 2 sets of bent-over barbell rows, you should feel physically *decimated.* If you aren't exhausted, drained, battered and ready for a nap, I would strongly suspect you're not handling enough poundage. Done correctly and completely this routine will lay low the mightiest of Iron Warriors.

You must Smart Bomb immediately after training in this fashion. Your battered back muscles are screaming out for regenerating nutrients. Drink a protein/carb liquefied shake to amplify workout results. This is not an option. I consume my shake after the deadlifts to forestall energy nosedives on stiffs and rows. So there you go…a brutal back training program that works every single time it is performed in the way in which it was designed. If you want to build a powerful back you need to perform powerful exercises. Avoid the seductive traps of performing a few sets of lat pulldowns and seated cable rows, perhaps some effete machine pullovers and congratulating yourself on a "great" back workout—that's sissy stuff appropriate for 12-year old boys brand new to the resistance training game. If you are a man then train like one!

Base Strength

I once received a lesson in power and strength that lasted less than 15 seconds and provided me mental fuel that has burned for twenty years. In the mid-1980's I was at a powerlift competition coaching a friend. Coaching another lifter was George Hechter, the number one ranked heavyweight lifter in the world at the time. He was a smart, sharp guy and a protégé of iron icon Bill Starr.

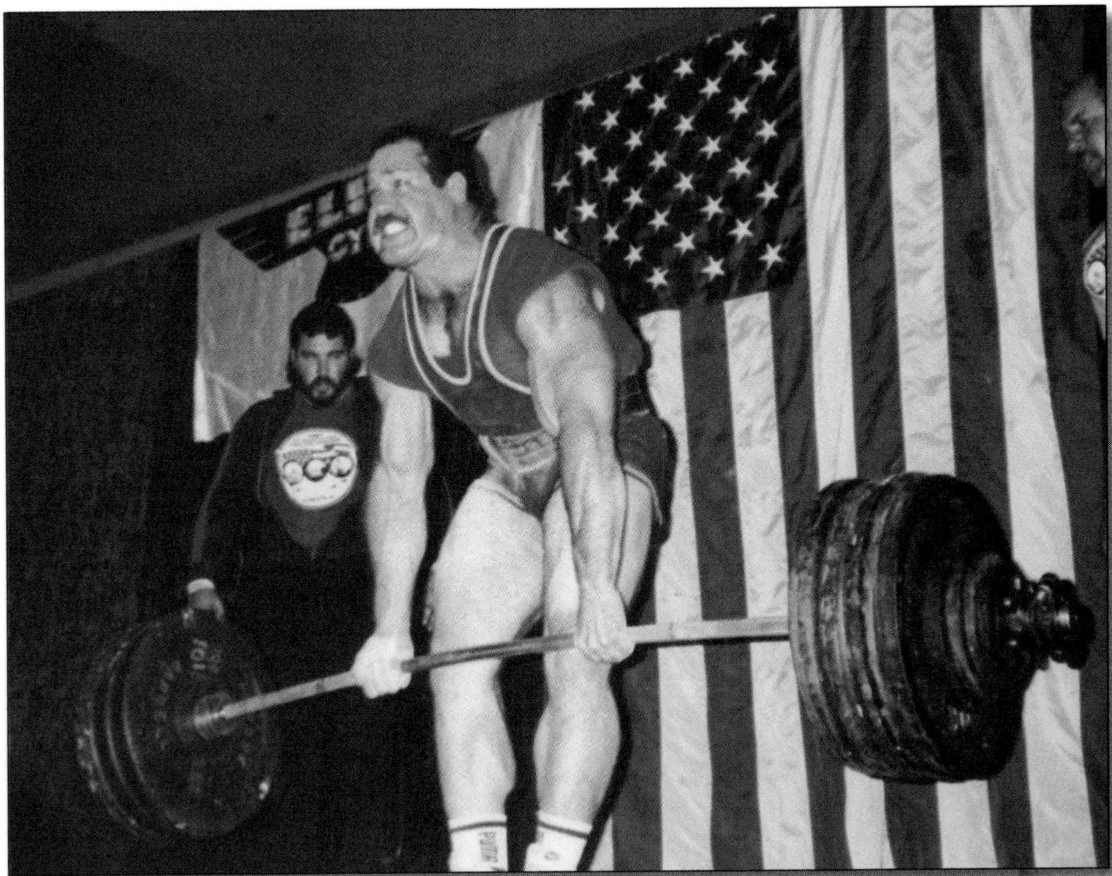

The mythical George Hechter in a rare photo: George totaled 2400 and took second at the IPF World Championships in the 80's. He squatted 975, benched 600 and deadlifted 830 weighing 360 pounds. He was 5'10". He reduced down to 239 pounds (pictured) and squatted 880, bench pressed 550 and deadlifted 840. Plus he looked absolutely incredible. I handled him at this APF meet where he got in trouble on the squat and took second place to Willie 'The Hammer' Bell.

Dozens of athletes and coaches were backstage scurrying around getting lifters ready. George and I had just gotten our two lifters through the emotional rollercoaster of the squats and now done, we were filtering backstage. George and his athlete were walking ahead of me. As we passed the warm-up area, a squat bar still sat on the racks loaded to 505 pounds. It had been the last weight one of the lifters had used to warm-up. George walked over to the loaded bar, dipped under it, stood erect, took a step backwards and did ten perfect, no sweat reps. He wore street clothes. No belt, no warm-up, no spotters, no knee wraps, no dramatic psyche up and no big deal. He repped the weight and replaced it before anyone noticed. I noticed and as he fell back in step to catch up to his lifter I said, "You could have asked for a spot George. Shouldn't you have warmed up a bit?" I prodded. He was dismissive, "It was *only* 500 pounds Marty." That hit me like the old Zen joke: "What is the sound of one hand clapping? The answer? "A slap across someone's face"

A few weeks later I saw George squat 975 pounds at the Potomac Open as if it were 500. He was good for at least 50 pounds additional pounds on that day. In the intervening years I've replayed that 500 squat set in my brain, so casual, so easy, so effortless—still it was 500 pounds for ten reps! The lesson I took from it was this: George had built his *absolute strength* upward to such an astounding level that 500 was "only" 50% of his single repetition maximum. To put that in context, I myself could squat 50% of what I am capable of at any point in time without any warm-up or drama. I would not need spotters nor would I be in any great danger with 50%. So what's the lesson? I wonder if, over a protracted period of time, rather than attempt to raise the *absolute strength* ceiling, the 1 rep max, what if you sought to raise the 50% base strength level? Would this reverse approach, over time, allow you to increase the absolute 1 rep maximum? If you could squat 400x1 and could squat 50% 200 for say 20 reps, could you increase the 400x1 limit by working the 50% 200x20 limit to say 200x25 or 250x20 over time? Would tweaking the 50% poundage translate into increased absolute strength? I've deliberated on this Zen Koan for decades and it's provided me with mental fodder I *still* ponder. I eventually would like to try this approach out on some crazed young athlete who is gutsy and game to try something completely bizarre. If a man increases his 50% weight by 50 pounds would that push his absolute poundage upward by 50 pounds?

The Seductive Siren Song of Machine Exercise

Don't Lie Down In That Field Of Fragrant Poppies… You Might Never Wake Up!

They say that variety is the spice of life. In the world of resistance training this old cliché is often used as an excuse to avoid mastering tried and proven ultra-basic free weight exercises. Training with barbells and dumbbells using compound multi-joint exercises remains the most effective way ever devised for growing and strengthening muscles.

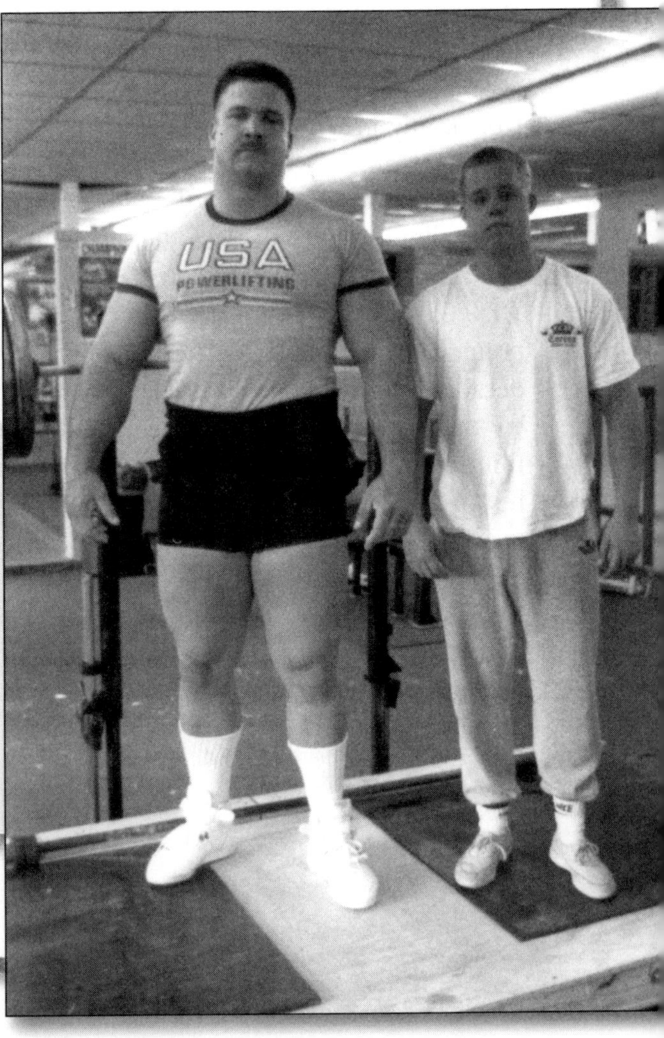

The guy on the right stands 5'7" and weighs 170, so how big is that dude on the left? Elliot Smith weighing 325. You don't build this kind of size doing nautilus pullovers or machine curls. Use barbells and dumbbells. Use full range of motion and compound multi-joint exercises. Follow the big sweeping exercises with an isolation exercise or two. Never eat desert (isolation exercises) before the meat & potatoes (compound exercises) and if you are full, skip the desert.

Thematically, mastering basic free weight exercise is the foundation on which all future resistance training efforts need to be constructed. Yet most young fitness devotees labor under the mythical illusion that using machines that mimic the basic free weight exercises are just as effective as the free weight exercises they mimic. This is a muscle myth of the first magnitude. There are a whole host of physiological reasons why free weights trump machines: the human body has to work harder, much harder, to keep a barbell or a dumbbell locked into a specific motor-pathway. Free weights force the user to cut their own rep-stroke groove through time and space. Machines eliminate what I term The Third Dimension of Tension: side-to-side resistance control. By removing the need for muscle stabilizers to activate in order to control the *third dimension of tension*, results are reduced 20 to 30%.

This critical distinction, elimination of muscle stabilizer activation, creates vastly different results for what appear to be (superficially anyway) identical efforts. A mimicking machine has a predetermined groove frozen into place and the user's only job is to keep the resistance moving either up or down; no side-to-side control is necessary. Having to work hard to keep the weight confined within a groove is a *good thing* when it comes to building muscle.

Easier is not better in the world of muscle building and muscle strengthening. This is why free weights trump mimicking machines every single time. Machines have become so popular that many should require you purchase a ticket beforehand, like an amusement park ride.

> ***"Wow! Smell that rich Corinthian leather; feel the exquisite way the resistance travels up and down on the ball-bearing expressway to a powerful lock-out! Wow! That was 400 pounds? That was so easy! I must be getting so much stronger! When I use this machine the poundage feels so much lighter and the reps are so much smoother and easier! I love using this machine and I hate doing the same exercise using those cumbersome, antiquated, stone-aged barbells!"***

Hey! Dude! Wake up! You've fallen asleep in a field of fragrant opium-infused poppies and you now need to stagger to your feet and get moving over to the free weight section of the gym. Otherwise you might become a hopeless exercise machine addict. The reason machine repetitions are so smooth and easy and light is because they are *smooth* and *easy* and *light*! The actual poundage is literally lighter than advertised; all as a result of modern technology, superb mechanical efficiency and precision engineering. When resistance travels over a super-efficient ball-bearing pathway, 100% of your available strength and energy can be allotted to pushing or pulling. No effort whatsoever is required in order to control bothersome side-to-side movement and things are made a hell-of-a-lot easier.

Easier is not better in resistance training. Optimally resistance should be rough, tough and heavy. If all things were equal machines would surely be the way to go: no fuss, no muss, no mess, no plates to load or unload, no need of spotters, no danger, safe as drinking warm milk. Expensive machines certainly keep the user safe and fear of injury is a big concern to timid civilians. If safety is your biggest concern, perhaps bowling or golf might be a more appropriate use of your time.

Machines are sultry seductresses...you get to sit down or lie down when you use a machine and people love to sit down, or better yet, lie down when they exercise. If all things were equal people would pick machines over free weights every single time. Hell I would too! But all things *aren't* equal, not even close! And that is the point. Accept the irrefutable biological fact that free weights are physiologically superior to machines. Understand that the vast majority of our training time *must* be spent doing basic free-weight exercise. The typical beginner or intermediate trainee often complains, "I'm burnt out doing the same free-weight exercises over and over; I use machines in order to get some variety into my training." Nice try Gilligan.

An entire Cosmos of exercise variety exists within the basic, barbell/dumbbell compound multi-joint exercise universe. By varying foot stance (we *love* free-weight exercises done standing on two feet) or by altering grip width, by making slight technical changes in specific exercise techniques, by altering velocity, rep speed, range-of-motion and rest time between sets, we can create enough variation to provide the trainee unlimited variety. There are enough variations in the free weight squat alone to keep a serious athlete busy for years. It took me a *decade* to perfect my conventional deadlift technique.

All this and we haven't even touched on modulating training volume or session frequency or exercise placement. Something as simple as consciously altering the speed with which we push or pull a repetition drastically changes the muscular effect. Muscle fiber is stimulated in a totally different way when we alter the variables. Combine subtle and overt technical alterations with rep-speed and volume alterations. There is a universe of free weight possibilities. Put it all together and you have a mind-blowing menu of variation within the free weight world. If you are inventive, clever and determined, you can inject an amazing degree of variety into standard barbell and dumbbell exercises. Variety is limited only by imagination.

Too often trainees fall into a rut and perform the same basic barbell and dumbbell exercises in the same identical fashion all the time. A serious fitness acolyte should seek to elicit different physiological effects by modifying base techniques. Don't be seduced by sultry exercise machines with their lotus-eater seats and pads, all things *are not* equal in the wide wonderful world of resistance training and as the old saying goes, "If something seems too good to be true, likely it is." Harsh, hard and difficult are the way to go when it comes to maximizing results from resistance training. Thomas Hobbes once quipped, "Life is nasty, brutish and short." I would expropriate this dictum and say "effective resistance training sessions should be nasty, brutish and short."

> ***Some machines are not machines at all: cables and pulleys, used for lat pulldowns, cable crossovers, triceps pushdowns, etc., are not machines under my elastic definition. Cables allow you to cut your own groove through space and therefore cable exercises are exempt. Ditto dip apparatus, ditto pull-up or chin bars, ditto incline sit-up boards, power racks or prone hyperextension benches. These are devices that allow you to perform an exercise, but don't confine you to a precise and exact pathway. Plus these devices allow for tons of technical variation.***

Whenever I hear some rookie complain how *bored* they are doing basic barbell and dumbbell exercises I just shake my head and muse about the ignorant folly of youth. George Bernard Shaw said, "Youth is wasted on the young." And I sometimes have to agree; so please, if you are a weight trainer bored to tears doing the same old exercises in the same old way—blame yourself! You can infuse as much variety as needed into your very next free weight workout and the only thing stopping you is your imagination. Stop the clinging adherence to tired old ways and methods. Be on the continual prowl for new and better modes and methods; those who are semi-serious whine and complain, clinging to old comfortable ineffectual methods, they gaze longingly at those shiny exercise machines that beckon seductively, "Come hither! Sit on me…come lie down on me…push or pull half-heartedly…I'm just as effective as those nasty old barbells and dumbbells...Meow!"

Those who allow themselves to be seduced by machines are doomed to fall asleep in the fragrant poppy field of eternal exercise sameness. Those who find ways to inject new techniques into Old School free weight exercises will bust through to the next level of physical development. The choice is yours.

SPAWNING SEASON

The Names Have Been Changed to Protect the Guilty

As told to Marty Gallagher by GRILLMAN

While one who sings with his tongue on fire,
Gargles in the rat race choir,
Bent out of shape by societies' pliers,
Cares not to come up any higher,
But rather get you down in hole he's in!
—Dylan

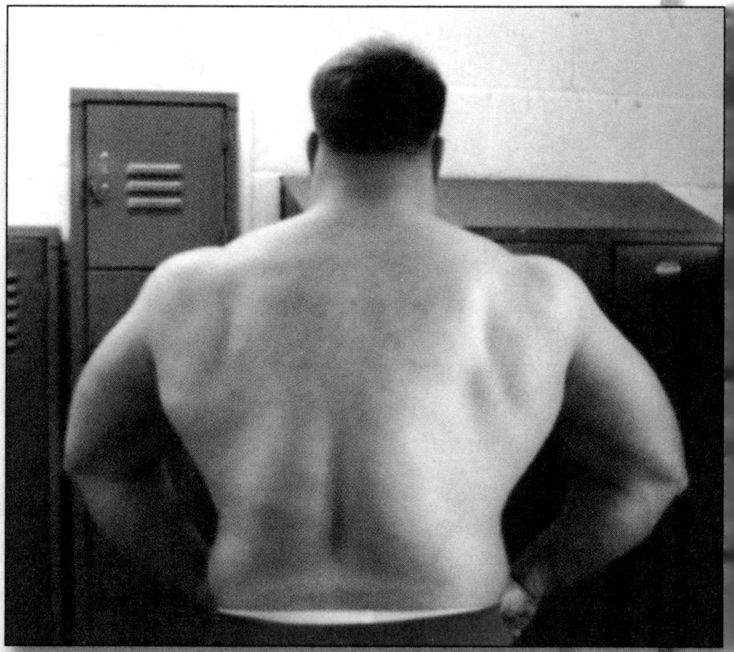

Behold the Grill Man, 6"2" 350: Gym Mullet / noun: American slang term describing a peculiar type of land-based, quad-limbed fitness enthusiast that travel in schools or herds and invades, infests and inhabits gymnasiums commencing January 2nd of each year. Weaker species of gym aquarium mullets last 2 to 14 days before disappearing while some stronger member of the species have been known to infest weight rooms for up to six weeks before evaporating back to the nether-regions. Exuding negative energy and exerting parasitical strength-sucking powers, they are genetically encoded to subvert excellence whenever confronted with it. Mullets possess zombie-like subconscious primordial urges that compel them to destroy any productive process. Psychologically, mullets are conflicted: obsessive-compulsive, underachievers cursed with inflated egos compounded by low self-esteem, a deadly psychological cocktail, as any competent psychiatrist will attest. The following is a harrowing account of one man's encounter with "The Swarm." His real name is disguised in order to avoid blood vendettas and legal entanglements.

My name is Grill so they call me Grill Man. I'm 6'2" and weigh 350 pounds. I have a 14% body fat percentile and can dunk a basketball with either hand. My goal is to deadlift 800 in a powerlifting competition. I have done 771 officially and 780 in training. So I'm close. I'm serious as a heart attack when I walk into the gym. I go to the local Steel House at the same time of day every day five days a week and have done so for 15 straight years.

All through the Christmas Holidays my training had gone splendidly. I was preparing for the Mountaineer Open Powerlifting Championships in March. I always put a big red circle around January 2nd on my training calendar because I need to prepare myself mentally for the onslaught of the Mullet influx that strikes my gym. I have come to expect the migration and try to make allowances in advance. I was determined this year *not to allow* the annual mullet infestation to derail my Mountaineer Open training efforts. I'm an Iron Pro and can rise above just about anything. I need to train and I need to train hard. Each training week is critical and I cannot afford to lose three or four weeks of effort dicking around with mullet-mania. I will not allow these Lilliputian slackers to prevent me or hinder me from achieving my goal. Deadlifting 800 pounds is no freaking joke! Distractions are the enemy of progress and I hate enemies.

This year's infestation was particularly gruesome and horrific. As I parked my monster truck in the parking lot, I knew *they* had arrived. The parking lot, normally half full, was stuffed to capacity with Volvos, Hybrids, Mercedes Benz station wagons and other assorted weenie-mobiles. As I walked through the front door of the gym on the day after New Year's, the cacophony was ear splitting. I stood at the front desk trying to get my bearings; three days ago the joint was deserted. Now it was *packed* with dweebs moving about frantically, emitting a collective high pitched hum. They flittered about like a swarm of mosquitoes on crystal meth.

As I stood slack jawed, a mullet face-dancer actually bumped into me. Of course he didn't bother excusing himself. He just looked up at me with those vacant, hollow eyes (think 'Children of the Corn') before he rebounded off me and spun off in another direction. I can go an entire year without being bumped into by *anyone*—yet here on my home turf, my home away from home, I suddenly have some dork bump into me inside of sixty seconds of walking through the door.

I felt soiled and defiled.

In my mind's eye I envisioned a water buffalo about to be swarmed and eaten by a horde of ravenous fire ants or perhaps attacked by a school of Piranha. Mullets attack fitness facilities every year, ostensibly in search of building muscle, but I know better. They supposedly seek to become big and strong because they are weak and small. Since they are incapable and unwilling to exert themselves in the slightest, they seek to drag everyone else down into the hole they are in...as Dylan prophesized back in the 60's. Dylan's my man. "Don't follow leaders, watch your parking meters." I've lived by that code for decades.

I surveyed the gym and *they* were everywhere, a herd, a school, a tribe, a freaking *army*...It was *go time*! Blank-faced mullets gathered everywhere: sitting or lying on top of every exercise machine and bench in the facility. I actually trembled a little and got a hot flash walking to the squat rack. I wanted to lash out and attack—this was *my house* and these irreverent punks were desecrating the sacred Steel House. The swarm was abuzz; each one in frantic motion, using pathetic pee-wee poundage and ridiculous, goofy exercise techniques that I've never seen before or since. I could only compare the maelstrom to an army of muscle-less drum majorettes twirling batons, but instead of batons they were frantically waving teeny dumbbells. Normally during the annual January frenzy, the Tribe represents a small percentage of the gym population: not this year, this year the school had swelled to alarming levels. I suppose it's attributable to the upturn in the economy.

This year the population had multiplied with astonishing rapidity. Compared to last year, the clan had quadrupled. The ancient Greeks postulated that the ideal physical proportion was *sameness* and the Grecian ideal was based upon geometrical perfection: the neck, arm and calf, the Grecians mused, should be identical in girth.

"Measure and proportion always pass into beauty and excellence"

Plato said that in Philibus. But Plato was flat freaking wrong Holmes! Plato never saw a modern gym mullet stroll in sporting the supposed ideal identical:11 inch neck, 11 inch arms and 11 inch calves; a 34 inch chest perfectly matched with a 34 inch waistline. Plus mullets all have outsized heads and tiny hands and feet. If Plato saw a modern mullet in all his resplendent glory, Plato would be forced to add lots of asterisks and provisos to his original thought about 'measure and proportion always pass into beauty.'

To make matters worse, the flock is no longer demur and frightened as in the good old days of yore. Nowadays Mullets have *rights*! Back in ancient times, when I was coming up "beat downs" did not end in lawsuits. The modern *uppity* mullets are a different breed: now they have freaking Mullet Rights Groups! The stigma of being branded as a murderer, or worse, a "mullet-a-phobic" makes us predators reluctant to *act* for fear of legal retaliation. Guys like me do not fear other men. We only fear The Man and The System. Few are now willing to beat a mullet senseless and toss the limp carcass into the gym dumpster or out onto the parking lot as an ominous symbol for other mullets, as was once commonly practiced. In olden times, a mullet ass-whipping was our way of saying, "Danger! Little People! Danger! Stay Away!"

Now real men are even afraid to speak nasty talk to a mullet on account of Hate Speech

Laws. I for one will not be silenced even if my speaking out results in being branded as a hater. Sure I hate, *I hate* mullets. But my bigotry is rooted in commonsense and self preservation. It's damned difficult in this day and age for a human predator (like me) to be up on what identifiable segment of the population has been granted protection under the 1965 Civil Rights Act. If you are prone to violent encounters, nowadays you need a lawyer riding shotgun with you everywhere you go: to the gym, to the strip club, to the Chinese buffet, to the Blockbuster, to work and to the movie theater. My life morphed from restful to stressful all on account of litigious mullets.

Their credo is: do less, go lighter, quit sooner and use the recovered training time to *talk* about training. To a true Mullet, a seasoned and mature mullet, the credo is pure perfection: 99% of available training time should be spent *talking* about lifting and 1% of the time should be spent actually lifting. Regular gym mullets are normally manageable, but annually the pack gets augmented by "resolution" acolyte mullets. These newcomers spring into half-ass action and act out their fitness resolution fantasies in the weeks immediately after New Year's Eve. Swarms of mullets attack gyms nationwide. It makes you want to quit the commercial gym scene altogether.

Is it any wonder there is a resurgence of home gym training among the Iron Elite? I was scheduled to squat with Mongo, Joe Don, Mandigo, Tex and Sonny last Tuesday, January 6th. As I made my way to the squat rack, I found five mullets clustered around the holy and sacred squat rack, defiling it, placing upon it a 5 pound aluminum bar loaded with 2.5 pound plates on each side. *Sacrilege! This cannot stand! The line must be drawn somewhere*! Tex was already there and before I could stop him, he took action. The Mullets were taking turns doing cheat curls. Placing a curl bar on the squat rack allows them to not have to bend down and pick the bar up off the floor, thereby wasting valuable mullet strength that could be used for the real work: the post-set *conversation* about how great that set of just completed curls was. Mullet gab between sets can last for upwards of 30 minutes. No sense wasting valuable conversation strength bending over to pick the bar off the floor. That would be stupid.

Since murder is wrong and maiming, even accidentally, is out of the question, (even if you beat the criminal charges, then there's civil court to deal with) my kind have to watch our Ps and Qs. Tex was quivering. I tried to calm him down. I suggested he take some of the powerful narcotics I knew he always kept handy. He should have listened to me.

Gym owners, once our allies, now insist we must learn to peacefully coexist with mullets. When we complain, gym owners throw in our face things like, "Mullets are prompt payers whose checks don't bounce." The Iron Elite, gym owners are quick to point out, are actually more trouble than they are worth. The owners are always chasing the muscle men down for dues in arrears, while mullets pay in full for the whole year in advance and often in cash. Management loves mullet business: their checks clear the first time and they don't bend up bars and curse and scream obscenities, scaring the shit out of other customers. Best of all, after a mullet pays for a full year in advance, they disappear after two or three weeks. They don't reappear until the following January.

All in all, mullets are the perfect gym member insofar as management is concerned. When they appear, whatever mullet members want, mullet members can have. Mullets are easily insulted and will take their business elsewhere at the drop of a hat. They are litigious. Big Tex is a Hell's Angel and was visiting with us until things cooled down back in Oakland. On this particular squat day, despite being heavily sedated, he lost control and made the mistake of slapping the taste out of the mouth of a smart-mouthed mullet. He made a bad thing worse by choke-slamming the mullet, launching him backwards at the speed of sound over a flat bench. This occurred after the head mini-me mullet made some smart-ass comment about our cursing. Until then, Tex was willing to limit his outrage to screaming. The mullet curl club was creeping through ten sets of curls taking twenty minutes between each set. Things spun badly out of control. Tex leapt up and with one hand tossed the tiny curl barbell twenty feet across the room, barely missing a small mullet herd clustered around the water cooler.

The head dumb-ass mullet just had to bait Tex, "Hey, you oafish *goon*!" said Dennis the tribal chief of this particular herd, "You can't do that! You muscle-headed dreadnought!" Dennis hissed at Tex like a viper. "You *better* pick that barbell up and bring it back over here *right now*! Apologize before I call the manager over and have you banned from the club! You and your type are gene-deficient mongoloid imbeciles and if you touch me I'll sue!" That's when the choke-slam occurred. Tex has been sued before, plenty of times. What Dennis had overlooked is that when you have *nothing* (other than a Harley and a bunch of Lynard Skynard 8 track tapes) being sued is an empty threat.

Tex has been shot before. He's been stabbed a few times in prison. He was once hit with a taser on an episode of *Cops*. He carries around taped copies of the show and he will autograph and sell you a copy for $20. Tex left before the paramedics and cops arrived and put Dennis on the straight board so as to not further injure his neck. Dennis the Mullet, it turns out, is a senior partner at a local ambulance-chasing law firm. Once they catch him, Tex will be headed back to San Quentin to serve out the remainder of his sentence. Since "the incident" my Mountaineer Open Plans are disintegrating before my eyes. Pray for me. I am a bundle of nerves and fear my deadlift goal is flying off the rails.

If it were physically possible, I would kick my own ass.

Back in the Day

Life at the Muscle Factory

Symbiosis is defined as the close union of two dissimilar organisms. I have always thought that there was a symbiotic relationship between a really good, authentic BBQ shack and a really good, authentic hardcore training facility. It is about as difficult to find a really good BBQ joint as it is to find a really good hardcore gym...I can't quite put my finger on the exact nature of the symbiosis. I am a true aficionado of both and have spent a lifetime searching for both exquisite BBQ joins and Hardcore gyms. I feel deeply qualified to expand upon my semi-incoherent thesis by relating a true tale of finding a truly hardcore gym...

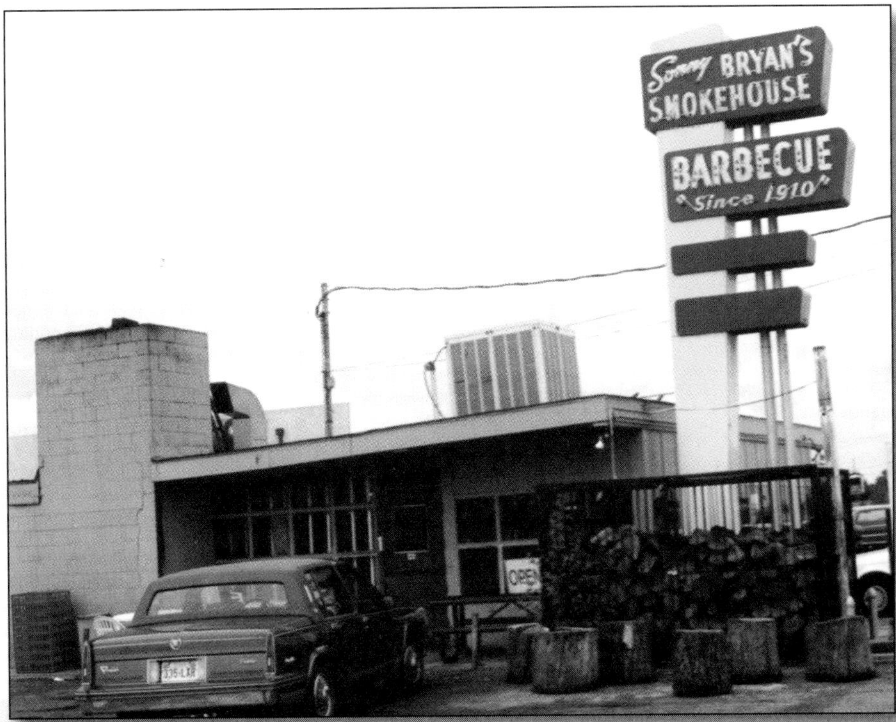

Sonny Bryan's in Dallas has been in business since 1910—longevity is a quality clue. Note the stack of hickory in the front and the plaintive, run down ambiance. Another tip-off is aroma: the smell of hickory-infused meat emanating from the smokestacks serves as a macho honing device. Texas "Q" is all about beef brisket. Funky ambiance is 'BBQ' critical: Ditto for hardcore gyms.

Back in the late eighties I ended up taking a job in Bridgeport, Connecticut. Anyone from Connecticut knows Bridgeport was one rough freaking place. Incongruously a yacht club had sprung up next to a waste recycling plant in the heart of Bridgeport, right next to a notorious ghetto housing project. My friend Bobby relocated to Connecticut to take a job working for his brother's import/export firm. He asked me to help crew his 28 foot, twin-screw Sea Ray from Deal, Maryland to its new home at the Bridgeport Marina. It was a terrific trip and as it turned out, it was a ploy by the brothers to lure me into taking a job with their firm. They enticed me by paying me way more than I was worth to do way less than I was capable of. On the first day at the new job Bobby walked into my office. I was nervously unpacking my stuff and trying to get my bearings.

"You look tense—let's go get a drink!" This was 10am on Monday. But hey what the hell, he *was* my new boss. "Meet the new boss—not the same as the old boss." We drove to the Bridgeport Marina in his new red Corvette. We arrived and parked. We walked towards the brand new complex of shops that lined a mini-boardwalk. The shops and boardwalk bordered a long line of docks that housed hundreds of boats. Suddenly a smell, make that a stench, hit me. It was putrid and overpowering. "Bobby, what in the hell is that god-awful smell?" Bobby, a rail-thin bon vivant with a wicked Jack Nicholson smile, gestured towards a sewage reprocessing plant next to the marina; it loomed like a building in Blade Runner. "That *smell* is the reason the son-of-a-bitches that built this marina bought the property for so *freaking cheap*!" He laughed.

The shops and bars that lined the boardwalk were shiny, new and impressive. He led me to the centerpiece building, a massive bar/restaurant. We went inside and it was impressive: a huge replica of the Titanic hung over a four sided bar. Since it was 11am, Bobby ordered us a brace of Bloody Marys. The place was packed. "Welcome to your first day of work!" We clinked glasses and surveyed the decadence. I munched on the celery stalk and noted how strong and properly peppery the Bloody Mary was. I was mystified. The bar was full, the crowd boisterous and it was all happening at such an early hour. I asked semi-rhetorically, "What in the hell are all these people doing here at 11am on a Monday morning? Why are they getting crocked at a beautiful bar located in place that smells like shit?" I was serious.

Bob ogled the attractive women. "We could be back at work doing something mindless. Besides I thought you were a writer. Didn't you ever read *The Great Gatsby*? We are hanging out with the idle elite. Egg Harbor is just a hop skip and jump down the road. These are the chuckleheaded parasitical offspring of Tom and Daisy Buchanan. This is the local aristocracy shaking off the effects of their fabulous weekend and starting the new week off on just the right foot. Everyone's having a few belts before firing up their boats and heading out to sunbathe. C'mon! Get in stride and go with the flow!" He leered at a passing senorita. The June breeze whipped through the open doors and windows and would have been perfect—had it not smelled like a dead squirrel left in the sun for three days.

He pushed his way through the crowd and beckoned me to follow. We made our way out onto a huge wooden deck overlooking the marina. The sun blazed and the deck was packed. A Caribbean Steel Band mounted an elevated bandstand and started working their way through a hopped-up version of Jimmy Cliff's "The harder they come." The crowd whopped and the well-heeled revelers began to shimmy and bop to the infectious calypso beat. The sun was warm and the dancers moved in weird white person syncopation. A patron wearing a red beret began banging on a cow bell with a single drumstick. He appeared to be a member of the audience.

Bobby caught my fascination with this strange character: squat and stout, he was a dead ringer for Leon Trotsky. "That's Rhythm Ray." Bobby yelled over the cacophony, "He's an institution. He shows up to every live band performance at the marina and plays along on his cowbell from the audience. The management lets him do it. He used to drum for Three Dog Night or some such shit." Rhythm Ray was stealing the band's thunder and the bass player and drummer were scowling. The band morphed into Bob Marley's, "Lively up your self."

Bobby disappeared and returned with two more fresh drinks. We clicked glasses. He smiled his devil grin and scanned the crowd as he lit up another Marlboro Light. He was a bachelor and a smooth-talking, good looking guy with a warped sense of humor. He jabbed me hard in the ribs and yelled, "Hey! Look at *that* huge bastard! You *must* know that guy!" How ridiculous; I thought. Here I am in a new city, first day on the job, half in the bag by noon. I'm somewhere I've never been to before in my life and my new boss tells me I must know some guy.

Naturally I did. Bobby Bagalino stood 6'2", weighed 300 and was a powerlifting champion. He was known as Bobby Bag-of-Donuts. Bobby had competed at the APF National Powerlifting Championships in Tampa, Florida the previous spring and one of my athletes had barely edged out Bobby. My guy took second place and Bobby took third. I never saw Bobby Bag-of-Donuts before or since. In Florida, after the competition, we'd struck up an extended conversation at the post-meet beach beer bash. A group of lifters sat outside and drank a lot of beer clustered around a keg until midnight.

Now, eight months later and 1,000 miles from the city in Florida where I met some guy for the first and only time, fate had brought us back together. With 300 million people in the United States what were the chances of me running into him at this time and place? Big Bobby Bag-of-Donuts was wearing Ray Bans and holding court: a couple of rich dudes in shorts, expensive silk shirts and penny loafers stood around Bobby Bags. Three extremely attractive, skimpily clad women, no doubt the rich guys' dates, appeared completely enthralled by the giant Italian's speed rap.

I made my way over to where Bobby stood. He looked massive and thick. He was a good looking *Man* with a capital "M." He oozed power. For a giant he had an amazingly streamlined body. Though he weighed way over 300 pounds he was shapely, proportional and a gawd-awful gargantuan. I later learned that he was heir to a mobbed-up trash collection firm that had offices in the waste treatment sewage plant. He glanced my way as I pushed through the crowd. I saw the look on his face morph from puzzlement to tension to vague recollection to recognition. As I pierced the inner circle he said. "Mar-tee...half-man, half par-tee! What the f#@* are you *doing here*!" He enveloped me with arms that must have weighed 100 pound apiece. I smiled as the gaggle of sycophants appraised me. I whispered into his ear conspiratorially, "So Bobby—where do the *boys* train in this neck of the woods?" He got all solemn: we were now talking the secret language of the elite Iron powerlifting brotherhood.

"There ain't but one place...Kenny Fantano's Muscle Factory in West Haven."

Ken Fantano was a legendary character and for good reason. He had exploits galore and his lifting accomplishments were world class. His bench press methodology, from what I'd heard, was revolutionary. He was Old School with some new twists and I was eager to meet him. From Cassidy to Coan to Furnas, all my mentors stressed a similar message: get as strong as humanly possible in the three powerlifts using as little supportive gear as possible. As it turned out, Ken would affirm and amplify that same message.

Elite power men tend to be obsessed. Everything else in life was secondary: wives, families, jobs, responsibilities, only kids trumped powerlifting in the world of the elite brute. Fantano's Muscle Factory was an oasis for the obsessed. I asked Bag-of-Donuts if he would be so kind as to make a formal introduction on my behalf to Ken. This was power etiquette; the equivalent of Samurai formalism in feudal Japan. He was the local Major Domo and I was a newcomer to his fiefdom. I was requesting an audience. I heard back from Bag-of-Donuts later that same week that yes, I would be most welcome and could I be at the Muscle Factory at 4 pm the following Monday. Please come alone.

I rolled into The Muscle Factory in West Haven on the appointed day at precisely the appointed time. Ken sat on a sturdy iron stool behind a homemade wooden counter. Kenny was huge and shapely, he weighed 360 pounds and with a goatee, balding head and soft eyes, he looked like a dead ringer for the legendary turn-of-the century Canadian strongman, Louis Cyr. He sat stoically on his stool behind the counter watching the comings and goings outside the gym while keeping an eye on the lone room that comprised the business section of the Muscle Factory.

Stuffed with every conceivable piece of resistance equipment, there was not a single cardio machine of any type. This "joint" was the epitome of a hardcore lifting establishment, and the clientele the polar opposite of the Egg Harbor crowd at the marina. I strode to the counter and introduced myself. He knew of me as I knew of him. I sat down and we began comparing notes. We'd each been in the game for decades so our list of mutual powerlifting acquaintances went on and on. He appeared sullen because he was sullen. But once he knew you were one of the hardcore he allowed his sense of humor to emerge. Within twenty minutes it was as if we'd known each other for years.

We'd been talking for a few hours when a dapper gentleman of say 45, dressed in a $1,000 business suit, complete with silk tie, cuff links and a diamond stick pin, walked through the door and approached the counter. I sat in front of the counter and Ken sat behind it. Kenny glanced over to the approaching dandy and said in a flat, but loud voice.

"Not for you—take off."

"I beg your pardon?" The business-type strode closer, "I wanted to talk to someone about joining your gym and engaging the services of a personal trainer...." He might have been a professor from nearby Yale, or a business tycoon or a doctor.

"Not for you – this gym is not for you."

This business exec promptly identified him self by name. He was used to getting his way and he was used to being treated deferentially; he could not believe his ears.

"Is the owner around? I wish to speak with the owner." To this man's way of thinking it was an impossibility that this hulking behemoth behind the counter could be anything more than an 8 dollar an hour staff person holding down the desk while the owner was out getting diner.

"I am the f#*king owner F#*k face!...and I needs *YOU* to *take off* right now! NOT FOR YOU!"

Fantano stood up and the dapper man got a full view of the massive Italian for the first time. Ken's mood was menacing and I stepped down off my stool. Was Fantano going to body slam this guy? Would I be a witness in a manslaughter case? What if he asked me to participate in the beat down and then be asked to help dispose of the body? "Help me drag his corpse to the bathtub—we'll cut the body into little parts and dump them into the Long Island Sound." It all ran through my head...I didn't know Ken from Adam. Would Fantano "off" a rich guy seeking to join the gym? I was baffled and disoriented. The exec was also disoriented and his face went from indignant to the look a person gets when they find themselves alone in the woods and suddenly confronted by an enraged grizzly bear. He began back peddling towards the door. He then went into full panic mode, wheeled and ran through the door. Ken sat back down, I sat back down. The atmosphere was electric with hostility.

"Damn Kenny, you got a nice touch with the general public." I said. He shook his head; opened the refrigerator; and took out two bottles of Miller beer. Twisting off the tops and tossing them in the trash, he sat one in front of me. "See—the problem with those types is they come in and plop down a lot of dough. Then they pay up for a year in advance and $300 bucks to them is like walking around money…we got lots of Yale type guys around here. The money is great at the time and I take it and spend it inside a week. Then I have to put up with the asshole for an entire year. They demand I drop every freaking thing from the moment they walk through the door until they leave. They bitch and complain because they aren't making any progress, but they can't make any progress on account of they have the pain tolerance of a 9 year old girl! They run their yaps all the time until one day I blow up and someone gets physically ejected. Then I got a lawsuit on my hands. Half of them are lawyers." Ken, I later learned, was big on physical ejections.

Mic Golden was a USA assistant coach to Sean Scully. Mic was a Fantano protégé and had once respectfully asked Kenny to devise a bench press routine for him. Mic was maybe 20 years old at the time. On one occasion the bench poundage scheduled for that particular day and training session was 220-pounds for whatever combination of sets and reps Ken had predetermined. Mic was hitting his bench presses when suddenly Ken comes roaring out from behind the counter. He was mad as a hornet and off his iron stool waving a huge sausage finger in Mic's face.

Ken says, "What was on the F%King bench press schedule today?"*

"220!" Says Mic.

"So why is there <u>225</u> on the bar?"

"Because with 220 I got to load up two 45s then two 35-pound plates, then two 5-pound plates then two 2.5 pound plates—with 225 I just load up four 45-pound plates!"

"The schedule says 220—NOT 225!" Ken is yelling and suddenly with snake strike quickness, he grabs Mic by the hair and spins him around like a rag doll into a neck-wrenching headlock. Mic whelps in pain, protestation and embarrassment and with 60 gym members watching, Ken wrangles Mic to the front door and flings him outside into a snow bank. Ken walks back inside and locks the front door. Mic ended up walking home that day in gym clothes.

Ken was "client selective" and refused to allow "normal people" to train at his facility. "The Muscle Factory was more of a private club than a gym for civilians off the street. "All I need is to rough up some vicious lawyer who causes me to go off. Then I get my ass sued and lose the gym. All on account of way back when, in a moment of weakness, I took 300 bucks in cash." He looked at me with a look that said this man knew that of which he spoke. I shrugged my shoulders and said, "Well you weren't weak-minded today." As he was about to respond, a weird sound started coming from the left rear section of the gym. It sounded like someone was torturing a cat. Ken moaned. "Oh Jesus— this is all I need— Brucie! Knock it off!" I turned and saw that the high pitched squealing was coming from an oversized goon doing triceps pushdowns. He was wearing a cassette music player with headphones and singing at the top of his lungs. Singing would be a stretch; it was more like Neil Young being subjected to some hideous torture involving water, 220 volt raw electrical power and a blowtorch.

He was oblivious, lost in the endorphin rush of the pushdowns. He couldn't hear because music was blasting through his headphones. Ken turned back to me, "So, anyway, I am looking to enter the APF National Championships in July. I think I got a good shot at a 950 squat. My bench press training...." The singer/squealer cranked his vocal volume up a notch, "*Jeeeeezus God! Shut the hell up Bruce!*" Fantano was standing up now and his face had turned beet red.

"It's the chorus from Hey Jude." I said.

"WHAT?!" Ken yelled at me; he looked flustered.

"The chorus from Hey Jude—Naaah nah nah na na na nah! Nah na na nah! Hey Jude!"

"WHAT THE HELL!" Bruce was repping the entire stack with all his might and singing with all his might at a volume that could only be matched by a Marshall amp stack set at 10. Ken spun around to the product shelf behind the counter, looking, looking, looking...until he found what he was looking for. He wanted a throwing implement, a projectile. For the first time I noted he was left handed. He ripped a two pound canister of protein powder off the display case behind the glass counter and in one motion spun and threw a fireball that would have done a major league pitcher proud. The protein canister sailed twenty feet through the air across the gym floor towards Brucie.

"NAH! NAH! NAH! NAH! NA! NA! NAH!"

This is the god's honest truth: the can hit Big Brucie square in the side of the head and exploded. A cloud of anthrax-like powder swirled around his head. He let go of the handle, the weight stack zoomed downward as the pushdown handle flew upward. The headphones flew off his head. An airborne powder cloud settled on his sweat-drenched torso: his shaven head, his pig-like face, his 20-inch neck—everything covered in white protein powder. He looked as if he'd thrust his sweat-soaked head into a bag of flour, like Curly in some prank gone awry in a Three Stooges episode. Big Brucie growled and crouched down; he swiveled looking for someone to bust up. He looked as if he had lots of ass-kicking experience; perhaps today he would commit his first murder. He'd calculated the trajectory and looked in my direction: he caught my eye and stared with black-death eyes through a layer of white powder. He growled loudly and dropped further into his crouched stance. He was about to attack me, maul me, perhaps even kill me; the stranger. Likely he'd rip out my throat out with his teeth. I took my right finger and pointed left. Kenny was scowling, standing right next to me. As soon as the powder-dredged maniac saw Fantano, the killer went limp. Like a dog who'd been caught stealing the turkey off the Thanksgiving table. From enraged psycho killer into submissive puppy ready to pee himself all inside of ten seconds.

It was, what I would later learn, was what the boys called, "The Fantano Effect." Ken yelled to Bruce. "One more time with the singing Brucie and You are OUT of HERE! FOREVER! Capiche?!" Brucie said nothing. Ken was insistent: "Are you HEARING ME! Cause I 'shore was hearing YOU!" The monster nodded. Bruce was submissive and chastised. He gathered his tape player off the floor and headed to the bathroom to towel off. Being a good sport, he cleaned up and came back out to finish his workout. Ken yelled from his seat, "And you owe me 14 bucks for the protein powder!" Brucie nodded and everything returned to "normal." It was just another day in Ken World.

What Not To Do How Not To Train

Fitness-Themed Reality TV Strikes Out

Whenever I think fitness-themed reality TV cannot possibly sink lower or become any lamer, I am proven wrong. Who would have thought the sheer cruelty of the "Biggest Loser" or the idiocy of "Celebrity Fit Club" could possibly be topped? Yet now we are presented with a new contender for the frivolity title: *Workout!* (On Bravo, Tuesday night at 9 pm EST) The show's protagonist, Jackie, claims to possess a 3% body fat percentile. She doesn't come close: try 13%. She professes to have "97% Attitude" (chutzpah) and trust me she doesn't. She is a gawky, giraffe-limbed woman with a muscle-less, albeit lean, physique. In one ad she perches spider-like atop a man doing a pushup. At the end of the TV ad she strides boldly towards the camera, flings her arms wide while wearing a skintight outfit as if to say "HEY! TAKE A LOOK AT THIS! WILL YA!" The weird part is there is no "there" there. This 39 year old couldn't take 12th place in the easiest class of any local female bodybuilding competition held at the local high school in the gym auditorium.

Mysteriously, Jackie is a fitness superstar; unfathomably successful, she is the in-your-face Queen of Mean. She lives in a million dollar home and works her "magic" at a trendy Hollywood muscle emporium called *Skysport & Spa*. Jackie preposterously portrays herself and her modest gym as "The finest fitness facility in the city staffed with the top fitness trainers in LA." Her fitness pronouncements, profoundly arrogant and at the same time aggressive and challenging in tone and timbre, roll off her tongue with astonishing ease. Her claims have no basis in reality and one is left wondering if perhaps she is afflicted with some deep-seated delusional psychosis.

One would also hope she was being purposefully outrageous in the same way a highly paid professional wrestler rants into the microphone during a *Smack Down* interview. One gets the strong impression that Jackie actually *believes* her bravado and rootless claims. In the through-the-looking-glass world of commercial fitness, a parallel universe exists wherein glitz, flash, fast footwork, fluff and filler are easily and repeatedly mistaken for substantive, tangible, measurable results.

But I put too somber a point on this unintentionally humorous show. Workout! is sublimely funny, a regular fitness *Fawlty Towers* with Jackie as Basil Fawlty. The Skysport Spa resembles any weight room in any local-yokel racquet and health club found anywhere across the United States. Nothing special. Neanderthal powerlifters (of whom, in the interest of full disclosure, I admit to being a tribal member) would call Skysport a "Fern Spa." Unimaginable, unintentional, laugh-out-loud lows are repeatedly achieved by Jackie and her squad of sycophant minions.

Antics abound as Jackie and her touchy-feely trainers interact with the dazed-and-confused clientele…there is the girlfriend who bites and leaves marks, the eternal after-hour booze consumption, the limos, the never-ending litany of pompous platitudes and fuzzy fitness philosophies screamed with a harshness reminiscent of a Stalinist-era political commissar; it all combines to create unintentional slap-stick of the highest order. To put a finer point on it, clients are under-trained in the weight room with ineffectual soft-ball routines; then over-trained in cardio with mindless 'boot camp' enduros. All clients are then starved to within an inch of dying.

I had thought the Nazi prison guard female trainer on *The Biggest Loser* was the benchmark for incompetent sadists masquerading as competent personal trainers. Jackie makes a determined run for the arrogant ignoramus title. What can you say about a woman so obviously ignorant yet incongruously successful? As Oscar Wilde once quipped, "She speaks with the easy assurance of the blissfully ignorant." The setting is Beverly Hills; specifically a private training studio perched atop a 12 story office building. High jinks ensue. Jackie continually refers to her squad of adolescent-acting sycophant trainers as "the best personal trainers in Los Angles." Again, this is mystifying: none of the group appears to have any muscle whatsoever nor are any of them particularly lean. Jackie's muscle manifesto consists of mindlessly beating the piss out of any client unfortunate enough to cross her path.

Her motto should be, "Do as I say not as I do." Don't hold your breath waiting to see her participate in the mindless boot camp exercise sequences she loves to dish out. "I'm going to break them down. I am going to see who really *want this*!" Wants *what* Jackie? She periodically intones profound asides to the camera while in the background an obese woman cries and writhes in pain. She never ever joins in any of the pain-train exercise routines she dishes out. She barks fitness platitudes interspersed with ridiculous exhortations. Her stated goal is to "run them until they fall down or throw up." How easy is that? I could have Reilly, a 5 year old neighborhood kid, sit on his little plastic yellow chair and put adults through the most grueling "Mother-May-I" boot camp imaginable: "Mother says do 100 jumps on your left leg. Mother says jump in the air and touch the sky 50 times! Mother says do 100 pushups!" Jackie's Boot Camp enduros ("It's the wave of the future!") are endless and excruciating, pure cruelty, mindless motion mistakenly labeled as effective fitness training.

Jackie tells boot camp participants that the medicine is good for them and will transform their pathetic physiques. She mistakes inducing fatigue and inflicting pain for triggering transformation. Her smug assertions are ludicrous; as if repeatedly stating something makes it true. By any measurable benchmark, Jackie and her team are weak as kittens, technically ignorant, psychologically challenged and factually wrong at every turn. It's the "Emperor has no clothes" come to life. Empress Jackie struts down the boulevard proclaiming loudly for all to hear that she and her minute minions are the *grand maestros* of the art and science of physical renovation. Her grandiose posturing is groundless, her methodology mistakes effort for success; she is the antithesis of training smart. Smart training, for Jackie, appears to be an irresolvable contradiction in terms.

All of Jackie's squad of incompetents masquerading as personal trainers feels the need to *touch* their clients as they train. Apparently the "PT Touch" infuses clients with extra power and strength. There appears to be a touching correlation: the better looking the client, the more the touching occurs. The Sky Spa might be "the finest facility in the city" if the city were perhaps Kampala, Uganda or Bear Claw in the Yukon. Being located in a city generally considered the epicenter of worldwide body worship makes Jackie's claim akin to a 12 year old, 100 pound high school cheerleader proclaiming she could whip the piss out of a 240 pound, 10 year Navy SEAL vet with two tours in Iraq under his belt.

Jackie is demonstrably lame as a personal trainer. Her technical instruction is riddled with flaws, akin to watching a young child attempt to play Mozart's *Requiem* on a violin in front of the school assembly. Now imagine if after butchering the piece the 10 year old strode to the front of the embarrassed (for her) audience and said, "There you go you pack of morons! The greatest interpretation of Mozart ever heard!" Jackie unconsciously personifies Karl Marx's declaration that "Audacity is 99% of the battle." If you are feeling dreary and need a dose of laughter to cut through the quiet desperation of day to day life, I would suggest watching Jackie and her fraud-squad of simpleton sycophants. What better tonic than uproarious laughter to counteract life's pain?

Watch as goofy immature girls are presented as expert personal trainers and then turned loose to beat up or baby ignorant clients charged $300 per hour. Watch another Jackie PT, "The Peeler" (nicknamed for his ability to "peel off fat." Incongruously his physique is smooth as a baby's ass) speak in an unintentionally comedic drawl appropriate for a Lynyrd Skynyrd roadie. He proclaims that his physical transformational abilities approximate that of a master sculpture. "These hands are like Michelangelo!" He dramatically intones, offering up for camera inspection the hands touched by God. It is highly doubtful Peeler could name a single work the 14th century master ever produced. It is also highly likely you could stand atop the roof of The Sky Spa and throw a medium size rock in any direction and hit another facility that has someone capable of bench pressing 300 or someone possessing less than 10% body fat. No one has either at Jackie's Sky Spa.

I have a suggestion for the Bravo TV programmers: if they want a real fitness reality show with some substance, grit and guts, have personal trainers *compete* against each other using untrained individuals for 30 days. Let's see who can generate real results for regular people using regulated amounts of training and only foods available at the local grocery store. No supplements of any type. Limit the total amount of training to say 4-6 hours per week and use real people, living real lives, working real jobs, with real responsibilities. Let's see who can obtain the best results; success would be defined as quantifiable muscle mass increases and body fat decreases.

Establish a level playing field. Bring on the yoga instructors and Pilates proponents, bring on Jackie and her chuckle-heads; bring on the Biggest Loser prison guard. Let's get some head-to-head fitness combat going and highlight what works and what doesn't. Let's expose lurking charlatans and identify effective trainers and effective methods. The ultimate winner would be the confused public. I won't hold my breath.

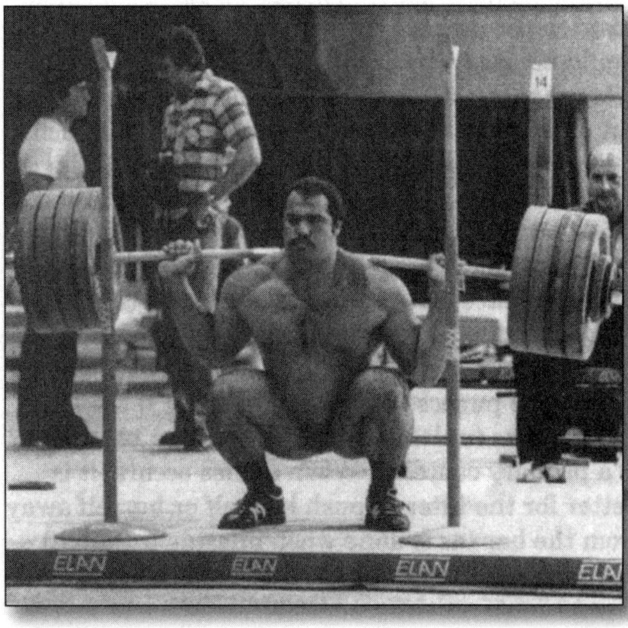

THE Anti-Jackie: What is the polar opposite of a surface skimming fitness poseur? I nominate multi-time Russian world Olympic lift champion Anatoli Piserenko. Taken from the greatest book on Olympic lifting ever written, Art Drechler's "Weight Lifting Encyclopedia." This photo shows absolute squat perfection: high bar, narrow stance, super deep—I tear up just looking at this! This is technical art!!

REMEMBRANCES OF DAYS PAST

Coaching Team USA

The picture on the last page is of the World Champion American Powerlifting Team after we captured the World Team Championships in Orebo, Sweden in 1991. I was one of three coaches for the US squad. I became a coach after my own powerlifting career was cut short.

In 1983 I had a horrific power accident at age 33: I was squatting with 700 for reps on a light day without spotters. After all it was *only* 700. Anyway, it was a hot and sticky day and my T-shirt was soaked. The bar slipped down my back. I was about to toss it backward and leap forward when a well-intentioned buddy saw what was happening and leapt to my assistance. It was a nice gesture at precisely the wrong time. He tried to wrestle the barbell while standing behind me. He wanted to save me. There is no way anyone is going to prevent gravity from taking 700 exactly where it wants to go: straight down. He and I got tangled up and I took the full brunt of 700 pounds dropped from four feet across my left lower leg. It snapped like a match stick.

I had squatted 840 the previous week weighing 250 and thought I had a real shot at breaking Danny Wohleber's 871 world record in four weeks at the nationals. That accident effectively ended up my career as a powerlifter, at least for the next decade. I made a comeback as a master lifter (over 40 years of age) at age 42, but I never hit the heights I'd achieved before the injury.

After the accident I wanted to keep my hand in the game and rather than become an official or an administrator (never my style) I decided to coach. At the local level I helped Mark Chailliet and Kirk Karwoski rise to international prominence and as a result I was 'drafted' by John Black to help Coach Black's Gym at national competitions. We captured three National Team titles in five years.

Our main competition was, always and forever, the mighty United States Armed Forces squad coached by my old Irish buddy, fighter pilot/instructor, Air Force Academy graduate, 500 pound bench presser, Sean 'Slim' Scully. Our team tussles were epic and over a five year period Black's captured three team titles and the Armed Forces two.

I remember at the 1991 National Championships when Bob Fortenbaugh and I squeezed together on the top rung of the victory podium to receive the humongous 1st place team award, the much taller Scully stood on the 2nd place pedestal. Right before the anthem played I looked down and nudged Sean, "Scully, you wouldn't *believe* the view from up here! It's *incredible*! Maybe someday after Bob and I retire you'll be able to stand up here once again. By the way Sean, you look as if your hair is getting real thin on top." Sean instinctually ran his hand on his crown to check and Bob and I laughed so hard (Sean too) that we almost toppled off the podium.

As a result of coaching Black's I was able to work with Eric Arnold, Dan Austin, Joe Ladiner, Incredible Eddie Coan, Mike Hall, Dave Jacoby, Phil Hile, Bob Bridges, (Mike's brother) Kirk, Mark, Bob Dempsey, Dan Wolheber, Lamar Gant and a host of others who's names escape me. Working with the very best, up close and personal in the white hot heat of national and international competition is one of the most frightening and exhilarating experiences imaginable. Six months of back-busting work are on the line and some athletes rise to the competitive occasion while others wilt in the glare. I am no fan of international travel, but when I was asked to be a coach for the Team USA. I agreed.

In 1990 my protégé Karwoski had lost the World Title to The Fearsome Finn, three times World Champion, Kroyosto Vilmi, by a miniscule 4.4 pounds. It was Kirk's first IPF World Championships. Vilmi pulled his final deadlift of 788 to eek out the win. I kicked myself in the ass for not having gone as I am quite sure that my presence would have been good for that additional five pounds Kirk needed for victory.

The next year Kirk and I traveled to Europe looking for blood. Back then the US Team would always arrive at World Championship competitions in Europe or Asia ten days ahead of time so the athletes could adjust to the jet lag and time changes. This particular trip was a travel nightmare...buses, planes, connecting flights, more buses, dead time in terminals, more long bus rides; all this effort to arrive in a modest Swedish town in November. All the locals were sour and dour and an average lunch in an average Chinese restaurant cost $40. (I'd say $60-$70 today) I remember a group of us going to the McDonalds. I paid $22 for two Big Macs, an order of fries and a shake—shocking!

The local Swedes rode bikes or drove Volvos and seemed depressed. Even in the bars things were somber. "Who died? What is *up* with these square-ass people?" Kirk summarized when he and I got a beer (or ten) at a local tavern one night. Any squad of American athletes on an overseas trip is boisterous, raucous, profane and good-natured. Our squad appeared barbaric contrasted to the somber Swedes. It seemed that in this particular culture smiling was frowned upon and laughing out loud in public was considered very bad manners indeed. Well here came the American Barbarians and you'd have thought we were Jack Palance in Shane. Maybe we were. Every one wanted to see the cocky Americans whipped: unfortunately for them the only whippings administered were administered by us.

The competition was run with precision and great care...I coached Phil Hile, a dwarf PhD who at 114 pound bodyweight could squat 520. He took 4th. I then had the honor of coaching Dan Austin in the 148 pound class. Dan was the strength coach at UNLV at the time and was so dominant that the foreign guys were moving to other weight classes to avoid him. He did not disappoint. Dan not only won, but set a World Record Deadlift (688) and captured the 'Champion of Champions' award given to the single most outstanding lifter amongst the eleven weight classes.

We didn't have a 165 pound lifter since we had decided to double up our entries in the 242 pound class. I remember seeing Karlo Virtanan (Jarmo's younger brother) warming up back stage. He did a series of standing broad jumps that were incredible...he would squat down and then leap forward three times in a row...bang, bang, bang! A good athlete can perform a standing broad jump of 10 feet and I swear this guy covered 40 feet in three leaps...he did five "three-jump reps" as he felt it helped his explosiveness in the squat and deadlift. He was the deadlift World Record holder so maybe there was something to it.

In the 181 pound class Dan Wagman, an army Ranger/Paratrooper with a PhD, took 4th in his 1st World Championships. Dan later became the health and science editor at *Muscle & Fitness* magazine after some hard lobbying on my part. Jim Wright had left Weider to go to work for Scott Connelly at MetRx and Tom Deters, the editor in chief at Weider, was ringing his hands and agonizing, unsure if Ranger Dan would fit in with the fem-man staff at M&F. Dan got the job and had a great long run at Weider before moving on. George Herring won the 198 pound class, going nine-for-nine, nine attempts and nine successes. George was a free thinker and didn't believe in the jet-lag theory: "Foreign food sucks and I lose strength by showing up a week ahead of time—the hell with all that!" Herring showed up less than 24 hours beforehand and proceeded to lift perfectly at what would have been 3 AM for him back home in Georgia. He did a fabulous job.

At 242 Steve Goggins bombed out when he insisted on opening his squats at 832. We tried to warn him how strict the IPF judging was, but he was beyond coaching. Bip, Bang, Boom...he was out of the competition. I worked with Dave 'Superman' Jacoby, the defending World Champion. Sean made a rare coaching mistake by jumping Dave from an 804 second attempt squat success to a third attempt with 832. He had a close miss. Sean called the lift without consulting Dave or I and I will never forget the look of surprise/anger/shock on Dave's face when Sean told him his 3rd squat would be 832, "Damn that's a BIG jump Sean! Can you change it to 819 or 826?" Too late. Dave's close miss would later come back to haunt us. Dave tore a pectoral muscle on his opening attempt bench press and came off the platform holding his limp arm, "We got a problem." He said. Our team doctor, Dick Herrick, looked him over and the prognosis was not good. I remember the tense huddle with myself, Dave, Doctor Dick and Sean.

Scully looked at Dave and said, "Can you lift or not? Tell me yes or no right now." Dave thought for a minute and said, "Yeah, let's do it." The doc said, "Are you sure?" He was immediately cut off by Sean, "The man said he can go – so we're f#@*ing going to GO!" No deadlift warm ups. I dropped Dave's opening deadlift to 704 and he pulled it with great pain. As soon as he came off (in agony) we iced the pec and inched him up to 733. He made that lift, but a Norwegian, who couldn't touch him with a ten foot pole on a good day, seized the lead. Every time Dave pulled a weight this guy would pull 4.4 more to maintain his lead. After Dave made 733 the other guy made 738 to take the lead again. Dave went out for his third and final lift in front of a packed house.

Dave went out for his third and final lift in front of a packed house. The Europeans were mad/crazy with their cowbells and air horns. They'd whistle at us, their form of booing, and clap in syncopated fashion for their Scandinavian golden boy who was about to upset the Seven Time World Champ. Dave pulled 744 pounds 7/8's of the way to completion before it fell to the platform. No lift. I remember seeing the Norwegian jump five feet straight up in the air and yelling in ecstasy when Dave failed. The auditorium, packed to the rafters, exploded with joy. The heavy favorites, Goggins and Jacoby, had been upset. I glared at the guy. Dave was upset and in real pain as he held his damaged arm. I didn't know what to say so I hugged him. Paybacks are hell and the next year a righteous and vengeful Jacoby lifted at the World Championships in England. He decimated the field one final time. He retired on top.

In the 275 pound class my protégé Kirk Karwoski destroyed the best competition the world had to offer. He dispatched the others with such ridiculous ease it was anticlimactic. This would be the 1st of ten straight IPF Titles for him. It was fitting that I was there: his win was the culmination of six years working together. We truly collaborated over the years: he was the ideal student. Engaged and inquisitive, he was never defensive or entrenched. Karwoski was always receptive and willing to try new things. His home brewed training had taken him to a certain level, a high level to be sure, but he knew that if he were to leap into the Big Leagues he would need to up his game to an entirely new level. The methodology needed to accomplish that lay outside his knowledge base.

I told him upfront that all his exercise techniques would need to be revamped, his training template would be tossed in the trash can and his nutrition would need to be "squared up." He wanted it bad enough to comply. I started him off on what I would call "Modified

Cassidy" training and over time morphed his training template into a mirror of the methodology used by Ed Coan and Doug Furnas. At the time I was conversing with Ed weekly and I would continually share with "The Great One" how "The Kid" was doing. I would alert Ed on how Kirk's training had gone the previous week and seek Ed's thoughts. I'd relate the glitches and potholes we encountered and Coan was magnificent. He would ponder with me about what had happened and would continually make incredibly insightful suggestions about how to up Kirk's game.

Ed's core advice was oddly resonant with my own discoveries when I first began training. John McCallum, my first Iron Mentor, had repeatedly stressed the importance of the 5-rep set. Later when I trained with Hugh, he too stressed we should get as strong as possible using 5-rep sets. My introduction to Ed and Doug's training template was old home week when Ed indicated that the backbone of his strength philosophy was "getting as strong as possible in the 5-rep set." Ed encapsulated the rationale: "The 5-rep set strikes the best balance between low 1-3 rep power-building sets and 8-12 rep tissue-building sets." I anchored Kirk's training template around the 5-rep set and he took to it with a vengeance.

The last piece to the Karwoski puzzle fell into place when he ventured to West Haven Connecticut at my beckon to learn "The Fantano Bench Press." For some reason, structurally or psychologically, Kirk absorbed this complex method effortlessly. While it took most lifters years to master and incorporate all the subtle, interrelated complexities, Kirk picked it up in no time. It was like handing a boy who had never touched a football the ball and having him throw a 70 yard "frozen rope" bullet pass on his first effort.

Nutritionally he needed help. He was massive but fat and eventually we hooked him up with a monstrous bodybuilder named Anthony D'Arrezo (RIP). Anthony got Kirk squared away on a big man nutritional regimen that dropped Karwoski's body fat percentile from 20% to 10% without any degradation in muscle mass. Karwoski morphed into a power Terminator and just as I had been there when he commenced his national domination, it was fitting that I was there when he began his world domination. We captured the world team title with ease.

At the awards banquet afterwards, the greatest non-USA powerlifter in the World, the Finnish 181 pound World Champion, Jarmo Virtanen, came up to Dan Austin immediately after Dan came offstage after being awarded the Champion of Champion's award. Virtanen had his Finn posse with him and these genuine bad asses sauntered over to Dan and I. Jarmo looked like Charles Bronson and was in a confrontational mood. He swilled a double vodka with one hand while he chain smoked Marlboros with the other. I thought he was going to offer congratulations; instead he ignored our handshakes and glared at Dan, "So, Don, I see you have *my* Champion of Champions award; be a *good* boy and hand it over!"

Silence...I didn't know if I had heard him right or if Virtanen was aware of the racial insensitivity he was displaying towards my African-American comrade, but he spoke good English and he knew our swear words and slang so I always suspected he knew what he was saying. I instinctively settled into a back-loaded fighting stance as I really thought these nasty, inebriated Finns were going to throw down on us. One of our young team managers innocently wandered into our midst, drunk, laughing and began poking the stock still Austin with a playful finger, this distracted him enough to break the deadly mood. I've always wondered if Virtanen's real intention was to pick a fight at the awards banquet. That would have been one hell of a Pier Nine bench-clearing brawl. There was no love lost between the Finns and us.

The Russians would have loved a reason to mix it up with their Finnish northern neighbors. Whereas the Russians and the Ukrainian's were fierce competitors, they were good guys immediately after the competition. The Finns and the Russians had some serious differences of opinion about everything. The US lifters were hated because we always stood between the Finns and the World Team Title. Too bad! I drank hard with Kirk and the Russians (what a combination) and the next day was a hangover blur. We had to commence our god-awful trip home, this time exhausted and with exploding heads. It was a terrible way to end a successful trip.

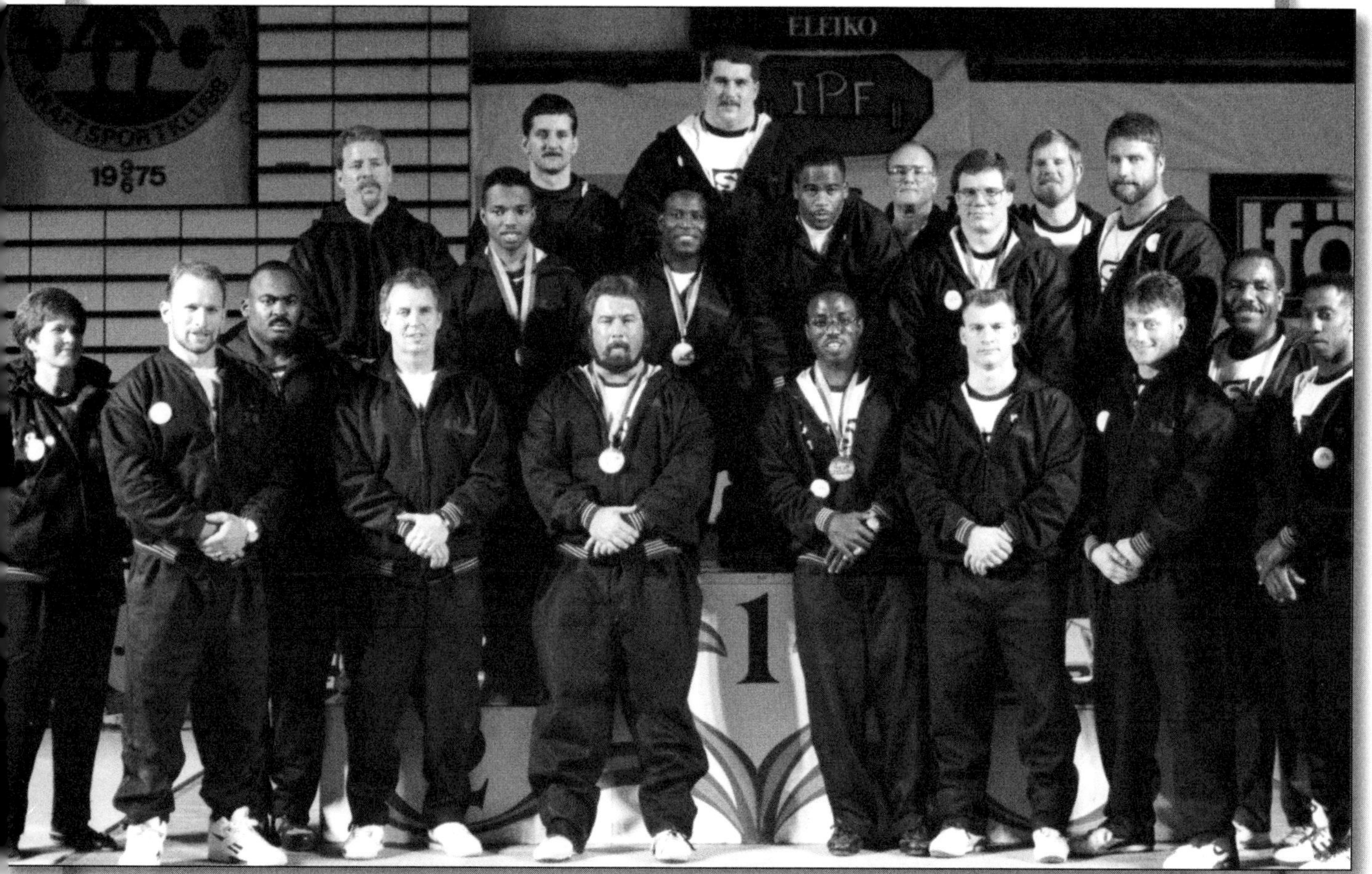

The 1991 World Champion United States Power Lifting Team
Karwoski and I flank Sean Scully. Dan Austin leans forward on Kirk's left.

Mind Masters

"The cessation of thought is the awakening of intelligence."

—Krishnamurti

"When an athlete imagines certain movements, a specific system of neural connections is activated. When the image is repeated over and over, the tenuous system of these nerve connections is strengthened and thus improves the physical execution of the movement. If the student imagines the correct execution of a particular movement, the correct system of nerve connections will be strengthened."

—Dr. Aladar Kogler

Mental Mentors

Cognitive	Intuitive
Thought	No thought
Rational	Artistic
Left Brain	Right Brain
Western	Eastern
KOGLER	KRISHNAMURTI

Two psychological geniuses have crossed my path during my life journey: Jiddu Krishnamurti and Aladar Kogler. Each man stakes out one extreme of the Brain Train conundrum. Iron Mentor Bill Pearl was once asked what is the single most difficult muscle to develop? "The brain." He said only half joking.

People seeking physical transformation think the process is strictly about the training and nutrition. While it is true that proper training and nutrition are the *tools* we use for eliciting gains, unless the individual is *motivated* to wield these tools consistently and persistently, the tools are worthless. Motivation, consistency and persistence are critical mental attributes; each is needed in ample amounts if we are to be successful in our physical renovation efforts.

The important first battle in the war to transform is motivating oneself to begin the process. Training and nutrition are critical and must be properly instituted and implemented. Simultaneously a monumental battle is fought on a parallel playing field over force of habit. Ingrained bad habits must be modified or the effort to morph the body is doomed to failure. If the trainee is successful in their efforts to mentally recalibrate, detrimental habits can be overcome. Modification of ingrained habits is accomplished by maneuvering the mind: willpower can be used initially to gain a toehold (as we shall discuss) but willpower only takes you so far.

Experience teaches us that for those seeking to change existing detrimental habits into beneficial new habits, the first fourteen days are critical. The first two weeks usually determine success or failure. The phantom precursor needed to ignite physical progress is mental recalibration.

Willpower is the ability to force yourself into doing something that you don't want to do. Willpower is not the key to triggering a true transformation. Willpower is *initially* used to jump start the process. The transformative process must eventually be powered by *enthusiasm* if it is to succeed.

There are three transformative tools: weight training, cardiovascular training and nutrition. Initially the Purposefully Primitive template may seem complicated, confusing and cumbersome. You do what you are supposed to do and settle in. At first we use willpower to power the process. After a few days things become clear. The individual *feels* better. This is critical both physiologically and psychologically. By performing cardio, lifting weights and cleaning up the diet, very real biological changes occur within a matter of days. The trainee develops more energy and vitality. If the process is executed as it should be, at the end of fourteen days, tangible biologic and physical changes are visibly apparent. Nothing motivates a person more than losing body fat, adding muscle and feeling flat better; more energy, more endurance, more vibrancy. The individual thinks, wow! If I can look, act and feel this much better in just fourteen days—imagine my improvement after fourteen weeks! At this juncture enthusiasm takes over from willpower in powering the process.

When enthusiasm enters the picture, enthusiasm generated by irrefutable physical change, discipline becomes *effortless*. This is a predictable and expected phenomenon that occurs every single time an individual commits totally to the Purposefully Primitive process. We use willpower for a few days or weeks until tangible change becomes apparent. This triggers enthusiasm. Transformation of the human body originates in the mind of the trainee. When real results appear, the trainee comes to enjoy, look forward to, and crave the intense training and regimented eating. Once the trainee develops a love for the process, a real corner is turned and the person never again looks at fitness, training and diet in the same way.

The battle to recalibrate the brain is a riddle wrapped in an enigma tucked neatly inside a paradox. What we seek is *effortlessness*. Entrenched habits die a quick death when the mind is presented with better options. Those who succeed are those who initially use willpower to commence the process, yet understand the finiteness of Will as a mental propellant. We use willpower in those critical first days and weeks to overcome force of habit, knowing that when willpower exhausts itself, another mental propellant comes online to carry the process forward; a mental propellant that is self-regenerating, the mental equivalent of solar power: enthusiasm.

Is it possible to make hard training and disciplined eating fun and enjoyable? Absolutely. How do we get to a place where we actually derive primordial joy from training and look forward to eating foods that help instead of foods that harm? We use our brain to set up effective training and eating regimens that actually work. We train with passion and eat with gusto and zeal. Intense training triggers the release of endorphins, a powerful hormonal cocktail that transforms intense physical training into a joyful experience. In a week or two very real, very tangible physical and psychological changes appear. Now the process gains real traction.

- Hard and intense weight training causes the release of *endorphins* into the bloodstream. This narcotic-like substance creates a sense of wellbeing that has to be experienced to be understood. The feeling is pleasantly addictive; a legal high and unlike other altered states this high is beneficial, not detrimental, desirous not toxic.

- Hard and intense cardio training creates this same physiological phenomenon. The endorphin rush associated with intense aerobic activity is called "runner's high." The runner's high can be acquired using any cardio mode, even walking. Intensity is the trigger.

- Another source of real enthusiasm comes from tracking progress. The use of training logs creates a sense of momentum. Weight training and cardiovascular training both lend themselves to numeric report cards. Those new to the process are able to see very real, substantive, mathematical, tangible progress on a consistent basis. I have had beginners make uninterrupted progress in every single training session for three straight months. This type of improvement is not difficult for untrained and out-of-shape people. It is easy for a beginner to create skyrocket progress in lifting and cardio if they are lucky enough to find the right training and eating tactics. Elite athletes review progress weekly.

- This feeling of gaining real traction generates something the untrained and out-of-shape person has never experienced: a genuine enthusiasm for physical training. The fact that they are understanding the process, the fact that they are seeing real progress, progress in their poundage handling ability, progress in their cardio efforts, progress in how they feel and act, progress in terms of their weekly report cards…it all adds up and creates an enthusiastic feeling. "Finally! I am onto a system and a method that makes sense, a system that is delivering what is promised; a system that I understand and feel good about doing. I now don't dread intense workouts—I look forward to intense workouts!"

- All this can occur within fourteen days; fourteen days that can change the direction of a person's life.

The most difficult mind battle is overcoming *nutritional habit-force.* Food habits are ingrained from childhood and the battle to overcome taste addiction requires subtlety and tact. We all have certain foods that we like to eat and that are perfectly acceptable in our new Performance Eating regimen. Psychologically, we seek to identify those healthy and acceptable foods we like to eat and make them the backbone of our new relationship with food. We understand the futility in trying to suppress the chokehold that taste has on us. Instead of suppression and repression we utilize taste to our advantage. We recalibrate our relationship with food. Once we are able to develop a repertoire of foods that we like to eat and are beneficial; once we learn how to prepare these beneficial foods quickly and easily; once we discover how to infuse great taste into foods that are good for us; dieting ceases to become a battle. By using taste to our advantage food becomes our biggest ally instead of our main impediment.

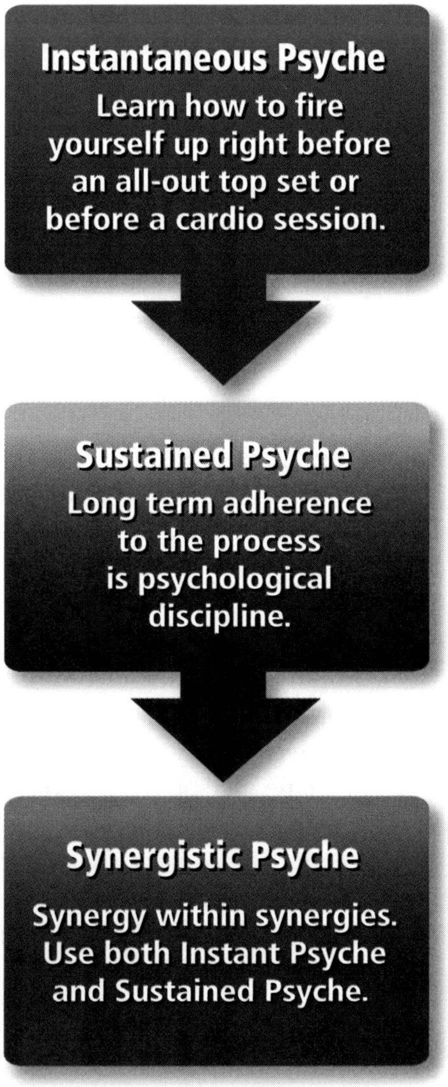
Instantaneous Psyche
Learn how to fire yourself up right before an all-out top set or before a cardio session.
Sustained Psyche
Long term adherence to the process is psychological discipline.
Synergistic Psyche
Synergy within synergies. Use both Instant Psyche and Sustained Psyche.

Two men have helped me immensely in understanding how and why we think the way we do. These two men taught me how to change how I think. Each man has provided me an immediately applicable, usable mental template. Too often nowadays the psychological approach towards fitness is either touchy-feely New Age garbage or Brusque Brutes spouting Hitlerian fitness platitudes, invoking willpower and discipline. The first approach is couched in fuzzy, furry, friendly phrases and feel-good bon mots about "getting in touch with ourselves." At the other ridiculous extreme are fitness Brown Shirts, morons that scream "No Pain No Gain!" and "You just don't want it bad enough!" We reject these psychological surface skimmers.

A passionate and recalibrated Mindset elevates the individual's performance during the workout session. When we learn to love the sweat and exhilaration of hard training, a dramatic corner has been turned. A recalibrated Mindset provides us with that infinite mental propellant: genuine enthusiasm.

So who are these two mental masters and what do they have to say that might be relevant to our particular quest? Krishnamurti is the master of the intuitive. He stresses that we need to access a wordless state of vibrant, electric alertness. This state of mind emerges out of profound mental silence. Aladar Kogler is the cognitive genius. He uses rational thinking and organized thought to create structures of extreme logic.

The Functions of the Human Brain

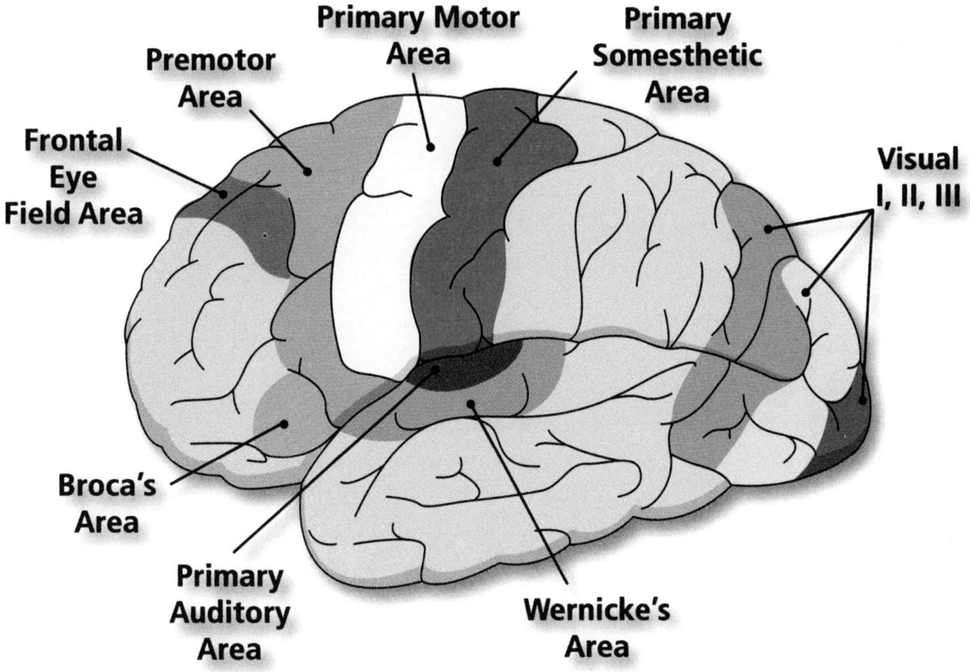

Recalibrating the Five "Sense Gates"

When you train with great intensity, you achieve a Samadhi-like state. Athletes wax poetic about accessing "The Zone." This is a Western slant on a psychological phenomenon that has been understood in Japanese Budo for centuries. Truly intense physical activity causes the five "sense gates" to fall into perfect alignment. Hearing, seeing, sense of smell, tactile touch and taste are independent subcontractors. When the body is subjected to taxing physical effort, sensory input is unified and amplified.

Taxing physical effort short circuits the "thinker." Cognitive function becomes laser-like and easily focused on the athletic task at hand. This is sport-induced meditative Samadhi.

JIDDU KRISHNAMURTI

Intuitive Primitive

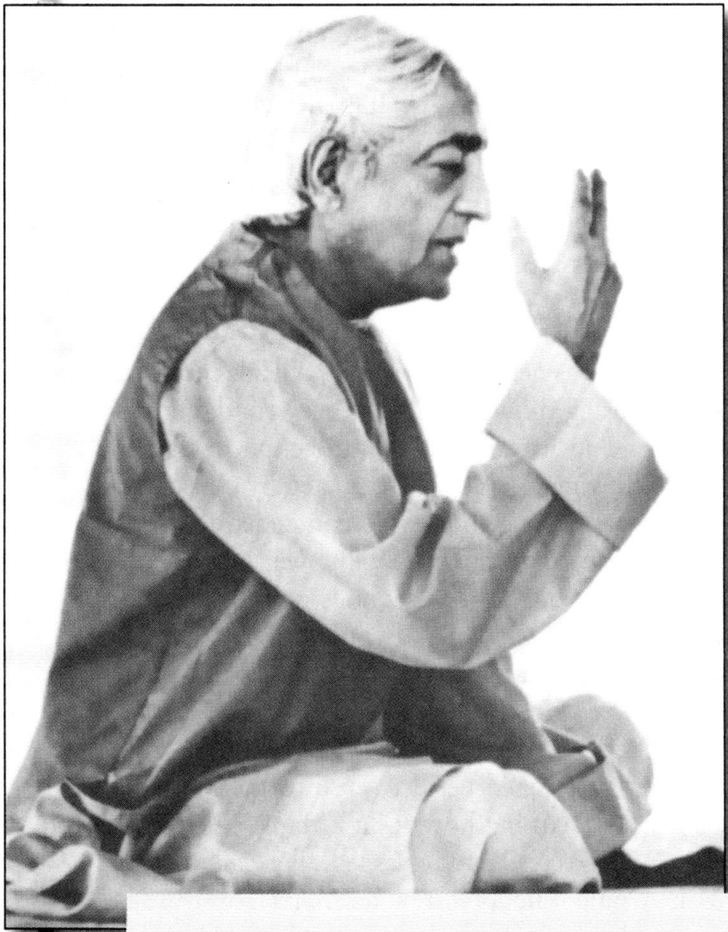

I was fortunate enough to attend several Krishnamurti talks, including one at Constitution Hall on his last lecture tour, shortly before he died. He was still lucid, candid and funny as hell, even at age 90. I had the good fortune to talk with him in a small group years earlier. He was witty, insightful and self depreciating. I was always impressed with his ability to guide you into a non-verbal state using words. He used negation and logic and verbal creeping incrementalism to arrive at a state-of-being that was profoundly silent—yet your senses were fully engaged, heightened and ultra-alert. He championed an intuitive, non-verbal artistic frame of mind that I myself had experienced in athletics.

Other mentors taught me how to train, how to eat, how to improve athletic performance, how to write—Krishnamurti taught me how to *think*. Or more accurately he taught me how *not to think*. I had noticed during my long and extensive athletic career that at times of peak athletic performance, I was mentally silent. I was super-alert, acting and reacting. Whether thundering off-tackle or pushing upwards underneath a limit squat or overhead press, I was *not* thinking, I was *doing*! I might have been thinking up until the ball was snapped or up until the barbell was in motion, but once the deal was on, I was not thinking about how to do what it was I was doing. I certainly wasn't preoccupied with thinking about totally unrelated matters. I long noted that during intense athletic moments I wasn't consciously thinking about *anything* yet I was aware of *everything*.

In the middle of furious athletic battle, be it with an opponent or a barbell, things unfold too fast for the conscious, rational mind to participate. You come to rely on ingrained training and intuition. In the 70's I was introduced to yoga, Zen, Hinduism and Taoism and was struck that meditating monks sought a state of 'no mind' wherein internal dialogue ceased, allowing 'original mind' to emerge. That synced up with my own no-mind athletic experiences and I wondered if athletic no-mind should or could be carried over into everyday life.

Those athletes able to access The Zone (the Americanized phrase for no-mind) sought The Zone because they recognized that they performed better when in its throes. I waded through all the methods and modes used by the mystics and seers and eventually came to a man that used 'no-system' to arrive at 'no-mind.' To say I was intrigued would be an understatement. Krishnamurti was a no-nonsense iconoclast that punched holes in everything I'd learned to that point. It was his contention that all systems used to quiet the mind were inherently flawed. How do you resolve the inherent contradiction of using a mechanical, rote system, devised by the conscious mind, as a doorway to true mental silence? Riddle me that Batman!

He irreverently pointed out that ritualistic methods were merely mental tricks. You were still playing within the box of the mind when what was needed was to step outside the box. The mind could not be quieted—truly quieted—using thought. All systems were the product of conscious thought. By definition this was an irresolvable contradiction in terms. How could true mental silence be arrived at following a system constructed by conscious thought? What a paradox! This was subtle and appealing to me. He contended that the mind could never be forced or subjugated into silence. You can't use willpower to suppress thought. Only through 'negation,' only by sorting through the falsehoods would we eventually arrive at 'real truth,' *Wu Wei*, as the Taoists called it, The Way of Emptiness. It was, and is, an intriguing concept, enthralling me for thirty years.

His contention, that "the cessation of thought is the awakening of intelligence" synced up perfectly with my own peak athletic experiences. It made perfect sense to me that the human brain, like any other muscle, needs rest. By learning how to 'not think,' the brain muscle would be given a much needed respite. When rested and refreshed, then called back into action, the fresh brain, like a fresh muscle, would function far better than an over-used, over-heated brain. The dilemma of 'not thinking' can not be forced; methods that dull the mind or beat the mind into submission are mental wolves hidden in sheep's clothing. To arrive at real mental silence, he suggested, was a matter of being able to be in the absolute, instantaneous present.

I continually experienced being in the present in the middle of a savage workout. Become completely and utterly involved in what it is you are currently doing and the mind falls silent. This synced up with my own rudimentary discoveries. Being in the mindless present was a grand and addictive feeling. I sensed the truth of what he said. I repeatedly lost all sense of self in intense training and craved it. I asked him about this and he smiled and told me to "Carry this lack of center over into day to day life." That single sentence response has given me enough to work on for over twenty years.

He was always insightful and fierce; even at the very end, as his body was failing him his insight and power of reasoning were awesome and inspirational. He moved me as few men have. He taught me to become immersed in the immediate present. Be aware that the eternal chatterbox, the thinker, the observer, needs to be silent if the brain is to rest itself and revive. Ceaseless internal commentary prevents us from perceiving reality. Reality *always* unfolds in the absolute immediate present. If you are thinking, you are unable to perceive reality: you are preoccupied and distracted by the intrusive internal commentator. When thought falls silent you experience a vibrant, electric, hypersensitive alertness and aliveness. Intense physical training is the surest way I know to quiet the mind, experience the present and access The Zone.

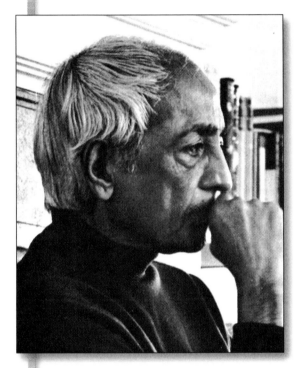

ALADAR KOGLER

Iron Curtain Brain Train Grand Maestro

Aladar Kogler is a mysterious Hungarian largely responsible for formulating the Iron Curtain Brain Train methodology used for applied athletics. Kogler and his cohorts were the Mind Masters behind the Big Red Machine back in the halcyon days when communist athletes were routinely decimating and dominating opponents at World Championships and the Olympic Games with yawning regularity. With the full weight of state sponsorship behind their sport's apparatus, no expense was spared to produce showcase athletes that could and would demonstrate to the World the superiority of totalitarian societies.

Of course we now understand that this system had a slimy underbelly: athletes were treated as patients, jacked up on steroids and testosterone then discarded like human rubbish when the first flaw or performance decline was detected. The rest of the athletic world was suspicious yet ignorant when robotic communist athletes, stuffed to the gills with the finest performance enhancing drugs known to man, beat the rest of the naïve world stupid. Later, when the advent of drug testing came to pass in the early 1970's, the Red Medical people created designer drugs that were stealthy and undetectable. The state supported sports machines resorted to every illegal trick in the book. The Reds created an army of paid professionals to compete against pathetic amateurs, real people that had to hold down day jobs in order to survive. It was the most un-level of playing fields.

Dr. Kogler didn't deal in dark-side black arts. He took psychiatry and psychology and molded them into a systematized Brain Train program that became universally used behind the Iron Curtain. He immigrated to the United States in 1981. A Czechoslovakian native, he lived in Hungry and over time developed a mental system that was honed and refined and battle-tested for decades. I interviewed him on numerous occasions for magazine articles and became enamored with his cerebral approach. His book, *Clearing the Path to Victory; Self-guided Mental Training Programs for Athletes* was largely ignored in this country. This was criminal: *Clearing the Path* was a benchmark book, a no-nonsense treatise about state of the art Brain Train for applied athletics. He presents his comprehensive approach in clear-speak language that spells out exactly what needs to be done and exactly how to do it...

"Imagery and visualization are one of the most important means for improving {sport} performance. The key is the effective control of imagery. The Eastern European term for this type of imagery utilization in sport is called ideomotor training (IT). Ideomotor Training is the imagining of action, recalling of action in the mind, or practice in the mind applying the use of imagery. IT is a process by which the athlete recalls an image of a certain movement, skill or action in order to improve it. It is a method designed to supplement learning through movement—referred to as motor-learning. The use of IT speeds the learning, perfecting and retention of movement skills. It stems from autogenic techniques and is especially significant in sports that require a high degree of movement coordination, but is effective for all sports."

This was no abstract theory. Kogler and his cohorts were entrusted with producing concrete results that improved athletic performance by those athletes who used his system. In the world of state supported sport, everything was viewed through a prism of suspicion and skepticism. The only things that counted were World Records, World Championship wins and Olympic Medals.

Dr. Kogler produced results so profound that his procedural practices became tightly held state secrets. The Iron Curtain sports aristocracies shared Kogler's system with sister Iron Bloc countries on a 'need to know' basis.

Soon the superstars of Russia, East Germany, Bulgaria and the Slavic states were requiring that their National and International level coaches and athletes become acquainted and adept at Kogler's comprehensive mental approach. By utilizing certain codified mental tactics, sport performance improved dramatically.

"The goal of IT training is to recall and practice in the mind an accurate, detailed image of movement skill, including all its components. The three physical components of movement skill are...

1. The space component: the direction and range of movement
2. The time component: the speed of the movement
3. The strength component: the degree of muscle tension

> *The scientific basis for Ideomotor Training is the principle of ideomotor reactions. A mental image of physical movement produces involuntary muscle contractions. The scientific rationale for the use of mental processes in physical performance dates back to Jacobson's studies of electrophysiology. When an athlete imagines certain movements, a specific system of neural connections is activated. When the image is repeated over and over, the tenuous system of these nerve connections is strengthened and thus improves the physical execution of the movement. If the student imagines the correct execution of a particular movement, the correct system of nerve connections will be strengthened."*

Have you ever seen a Russian weightlifter standing over a barbell, motionless, lost in thought immediately before lifting? He is practicing Ideomotor/Autogenic Training (AT) in the form of vivid imagery. The lifter is viewing a movie in his mind. Over and over, the weightlifter runs the internal movie in which he is lifting the barbell overhead in flawless fashion. When he is ready, he opens his eyes and attacks the real barbell.

As a result of his IT/AT training, the lifter has a 15% greater chance of success.

Mind Methods

The way of knowing, the Master says, depends on subtle adjustments that occur with constant mindful repetition of form and a consciousness that tells us when *rather than* how *to do something. The intuitive faculty—although innate—must be trained and organized if it is to become reliable.*
—Neil Claremon, Zen in Motion

A centered, focused mind allows a man
to exceed the sum of his psychological parts.
—Katsuki Sekida, Zen Training

THE TAO OF FITNESS

Mental Amalgamation: Proven Psyche-Up Procedures

The Master's arrow penetrates deeper than that of the student.
—18th century Korean Zen Archery Master, Li Pak

Regardless your level of athletic proficiency, psychological recalibration of your mental state for the purpose of performance enhancement will dramatically improve your training and competitive placing. **Brain Train** is the most overlooked and underutilized aspect of fitness as it relates to the common man and his Sisyphean effort to transform from geek into god.

I work with all levels of the athletic strata and one obvious difference between the athletically ordained and the athletically ordinary is the elite have an (innate?) ability to

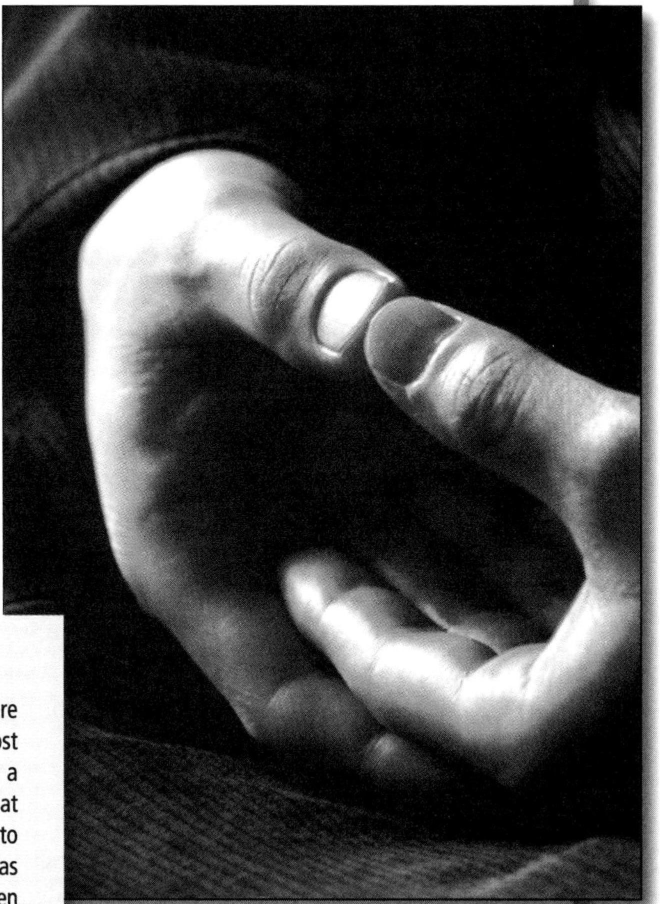

Human Biofeedback Device:
The Dhyani Mudra is one of ten 'seal signs.' This hand posture enables the meditator to tell if they are focused or have lost focus. Optimally the thumbs lightly touch, as if holding a sheet of paper between them. If the meditator notices that the thumbs have drifted apart or that they are squashing into one another, this is a surefire indicator that the mind has either drifted into a nen (unit of thought) chain or has fallen into a somnolent sleep state.

center and focus the mind on the athletic task at hand, whereas the civilian, the normal person, attacks weight training with the same approximate level of mental commitment they muster for watering the lawn or brushing their teeth. Training to the mortal is a chore, a bore, a bother, manual labor without compensation; whereas for the elite, training is a transcendental experience and mind prep an indispensable ingredient in the quest to excel.

Regardless the athletic battleground—ordinary training session or head-to-head competition—the elite effortlessly access the mythological Zone, a beatific mental state wherein athletic performance exceeds all realistic expectations. You can do the same.

There exist specific procedures used by Zen Masters to establish concentration and focus and specific procedures used by Iron Curtain athletes to peak the psyche immediately prior to a limit attempt. Our suggestion is to learn each and then link them. Our Mental Amalgamation uses the Zen procedure to achieve a quiet alertness, then gently segues into an intense visualization process designed to peak the psyche and pre-program you for immediate athletic success. Best of all, the techniques we relate are simple and battle-proven. These are mental tactics that obtain quantifiable results; results that separate 1st place from 9th place, or transform the ordinary, mundane training session into a mind-boggling, muscle-expanding, result-producing *event.*

Some applied mental fire and brimstone, as it relates to fitness training, could make a world of difference for you in terms of results; assuming you buy into the seemingly obvious conclusion that a focused, concentrated, fired-up mind is conducive to superior physical performance. The path has been blazed by Zen Masters, martial art monks, elite power men and Iron Curtain Olympic Champions. The first order of business, to echo the Zen Archery Master, is to understand *when* and then *how* to use Brain Train as it applies specifically to weight training.

The optimal time for the bodybuilder or serious fitness trainee to jack-up their psyche, to enter into what Arnold Schwarzenegger labeled the "maximal arousal mode" (hush-up your dirty minds) is just prior to performing a limit set. Before you become maximally aroused, you need to become maximally quiet. First we calm the mind then we focus the mind, we strip away extemporaneous thoughts and eliminate external distractions. This is accomplished by taking conscious control of the breathing process and applying particular techniques and tactics.

Within two minutes of commencement (using our procedure) you will achieve maximum chill: alert, centered, focused and quiet. When Stage I is complete, we rip a page out of the training logs of top Communist athletes from a bygone era and get fired-up using *auto-visualization (AV).*

AV teaches you to vividly imagine yourself hoisting the ponderous poundage using exquisite technique while projecting ease, power and precision. The idea is to picture oneself performing the limit lift. Imagine in your mind's eye a movie, repeatedly shown with an ever increasing degree of detail, played in real time.

The elite use some type of psyche-up procedure and they do it for practical reasons: a proper psyche (not too over-the-top, or conversely not too reserved) will add 10% to your top set poundage. Over time this proves profoundly beneficial. Hoist bigger poundage and/or squeeze out more reps and reap maximum muscle growth. Strength simultaneously skyrockets; all by harnessing the mind.

Allow yourself a few minutes to familiarize yourself with a specific breathing procedure known in Zen meditation as *Shikantaza*. Understanding and implementing this technical procedure is deceptively simple; yet mastery is elusive and requires repeated and systematic practice for a protracted period of time. Use this simple and straightforward mind-centering technique to instill clarity, centeredness and quietude. Avoid a somnambulant, sleepy, groggy, dreamy state-of-mind, and instead seek a vibrant, electric, crackling alertness.

Using Shikantaza the athlete becomes wordlessly focused, internally and externally silent. Inevitably and invariably this procedure alone produces superior training results. This Zen concentration technique serves as the perfect launch pad for Iron Curtain auto-suggestive techniques, the type used by elite Communist athletes prior to World Record attempts. We link these two classical mind meld tactics together in a one-two, brain train punch. After two minutes using this procedure, open your eyes, stand up, walk to your battle station and turn internal fantasy into external reality.

Shikantaza Checklist

1. Count from one to ten in a rhythmic fashion, syncopate counting with breathing. Sit on the floor or position yourself on the end of an exercise bench keeping the spine straight with head erect and eyes looking straight ahead. Don't let your chin drift upward as this denotes a lack of attention. Avoid the dreamy unfocused mindset of dream sleep. Strive for razor-sharp, super-alertness. Eyes may be left open or shut; if open-eyed, fix on a particular spot and don't let the eyes wander.

2. Inhale lightly through the nose and silently say the word "one…" When you have a full breath, mindfully hold the breath for a split second (the turnaround) before exhaling slowly through the nose. Try and sync the slow, steady breath exhalation to coincide with a slow and silently uttered "two…" At complete exhalation, pause for a split-second at the turnaround. This completes one cycle, or repetition.

3. Continue in this fashion for ten complete breath reps. A complete breath pattern has four parts: inhale, turnaround, exhalation and final turnaround. We mindfully pause at each turnaround. Often the mind wanders in the instant between in and out: these are the "gaps."

4. Two types of thought arise during our 4 part Shikantaza breathing process: *passing thoughts* and *clinging thoughts*. Passing thoughts are just that, little unrelated mind-snippets that pop into your head and vanish as quickly as they arise. Ignored, the passing thought passes and does not interrupt or disrupt our breath counting. A passing thought appears and disappears in an instant without taking root. It doesn't "cling" and turn into a "nen," in Zen lingo.

5. A clinging thought is one that "takes root" and leads to further internal dialogue. The initial clinging thought hatches a whole succession of subsequent thought chains known as "nens." When nens cling together and start to stack up, you lose count; concentration is broken and the Shikantaza breath pattern disrupted. When this occurs go back to "one' and start over.

6. The idea is maintain an electric alertness without any internal commentary, without any internal dialogue. Just count the breaths, observe the mini-pause at the turnaround, go from 1 to 10 without allowing any clinging thoughts to take root and don't turn passing thoughts into clinging thoughts. Sounds easy?

7. Optional: The Cosmic Mudra. Zen practitioners hold the two hands in a specific pattern, palms placed face up in the lap of the sitting practitioner, left fingers on top of the right fingers, the two thumb tips are held aloft and touch ever so lightly. If the thumbs drift apart or mash together, you've lost concentration. The two lightly touching thumb tips serve as a Zen biofeedback device. This is optional.

8. Inhalation starts in the pit of the stomach and expands the waist before lower lungs and finally the upper lungs fill at breath's conclusion. Exhale using the exact opposite procedure. Deflate sequentially: upper chest, lungs, waist and navel area.

9. Rinzai Zen adherents will breathe so subtly that they make no sound inhaling or exhaling—try it—this is a lot tougher then it sounds.

10. Shoot for two uninterrupted, successful Shikantaza rounds. Then without moving or changing position or breathing pattern (cease breath counting) shift wordlessly into the Iron Curtain auto-visualization procedure.

Psychological Segue: Shikantaza leaves you are alert, centered and focused. The mind is extremely susceptible to *autogenic* techniques using imagery, self-visualization and auto-suggestion. The Shikantaza breath control procedure provides the perfect foundation for segue into Phase II

Auto-Visualization Ideo-Motor Checklist

1. With eyes closed imagine the gym. Detail and accuracy are all important. The more accurate your visualization the more intense and effective the result. View the scene as if you were looking at yourself through a movie camera and the camera is head on from about 10 feet away. Picture yourself sitting and visualize your current posture and surroundings. What color are your clothes? Mentally zoom in on the exercise equipment. We set the visual scene.

2. Assume you are doing squats and have already completed 2-3 warm up sets and are about to attempt a new personal record in the squat: 375x8 with collars. Where is the squat rack? Picture the loaded bar: six 45 pound plates, two 25's and collars.

3. Imagine standing up and moving to the bar. Crisp details please! Place your imaginary left hand on the bar, then your right hand. Dip underneath and center the bar on your back. Feel the knurling dig into your traps. Take a huge breath and break the barbell from the squat rack. Sense how incredibly *light* the weight feels.

4. Imagine yourself as you step backwards; right foot, left foot and adjustment step. Picture yourself sucking in a massive breath of air in final preparation for the first rep. Imagine the exhortations of your training partners. What are they wearing? How are you feeling?

5. Visualize yourself unlocking your knees and descending to correct squat depth utilizing perfect technique and incredible control. Imagine squatting super deep, then firing the weight back to lockout without hesitation. Imagine each subsequent repetition...don't rush through this mentally! Pay particular attention to the speed and propulsion of the final rep.

6. If the auto-visualization is detailed and realistic, upon opening your eyes there should be some sort of physical manifestation: increased heart rate or increased breathing, goose bumps might appear. Mentally, you should feel fired-up! Coach Cassidy manifested goose bumps.

7. Try one or two visualizations prior to a top set of an exercise. As with anything else in life, practice improves performance. Once you've completed the final visualization (the last "movie" should be far more intense and focused then the first) open your eyes and recreate your waking dream; turn internal vision into external reality.

8. Pitfalls: if you are interrupted during the psych-up procedure, the process will be demolished. The delicate mental image you were constructing is smashed to bits. Many champion athletes listen to music as they go through the psyche-up procedure. The audio stimulation actually amplifies psyche-up efforts and wearing headphones makes it impossible to be interrupted or distracted. I use music to seize control of the audio element and prevent outside intrusions.

9. Don't overplay your hand. There is nothing holy or sacred about this exercise and don't load it down with extemporaneous, superfluous philosophic or religious baggage. No visions, hallucinations, gods or demons will appear. This is a mind exercise, pure **Brain Train**; a no bullshit approach, refreshingly free of touchy feely New Age-ism or Hitlerian exhortations.

10. A smart man can perform his Shikantaza procedure and follow up with a few rounds of auto-visualization without a single other person being aware of the incredible internal transformation taking place. Please don't use this profoundly personal method egotistically.

Save the Shikantaza/auto-visualization procedure for the big sets of the day. Give the procedure a test drive on a set using the top poundage in a given exercise. The body has a limited amount of adrenaline and done correctly, every time you get seriously fired-up using our one-two, Brain Train procedure, the body will dump precious adrenaline reserves into the bloodstream. With a finite amount of adrenaline available, don't fire your hormonal guns off on meaningless warm-ups sets. Practice makes perfect. Give our two stage, brain train tactic an extensive test run; to be fair about it, make a commitment to use the procedure for at least two or three weeks on the top set of all the core exercises. Any less and you're really not giving the system a fair chance. The more you practice the quicker you'll be able to rid yourself of clinging thoughts and the more vivid your visualizations will become. When that happens poundage soars, reps increase and muscles will, as if by magic, begin to burst and expand—all strictly through brain power!

Suggested Reading

- *Zen Training: Methods & Philosophy* - Katsuki Sekida
- *The Marathon Monks of Mt. Hiei* - John Stevens
- *Zen Meditation and Psychotherapy* - Tomio Hirai, M.D.
- *Zen in Motion* - Neil Claremon
- *Yoga for Every Athlete* - Aladar Kogler PH.D
- *The Zen Way to the Martial Arts* - Taisen Desimura
- *Zen and the Art of Archery* - Eugen Herrigel
- *Nirvana Tao: Techniques of Taoist Masters* - Daniel Odier
- *Secrets of Chinese Meditation* - Lu K'uan Yu
- *Zen Mind, Beginners Mind* - Shunryu Suzuki
- *The Awakening of Intelligence* - Krishnamurti
- *On Zen Practice* - Hakuyu Taizan Maezumi

A 10 Step Program Based on the Kogler Brain Train Approach

1. *The Power of Self-Awareness*

   All athletes need to keep a training log. Tracking progress through the use of a training log allows the bodybuilder to identify trends, both good and bad. Doctor Kogler wants us to take the log one step further. In addition to writing down physical and training statistics he requires we also record our psychological status. Our training diary should include detailed notes on our ongoing and ever-shifting psychological status. Body sensations, feelings, thoughts; all are considered pertinent data and all are logged. His system rests on the athlete's ability to accurately and objectively assess (and then modify) his mind-set.

2. *Autogenic Training for Sports*

   Autogenic Training is a highly systemized method of self-suggestion. Champion powerlifters intuitively practice a form of Autogenic Training. Watch any great champion prior to lifting a weight. They don't just pick up a weight and start repping; they go through a mental checklist, a procedure. Dr. Kogler shows how we can develop this championship mental attribute—positive self-suggestion. Sport modified Autogenic Training is a reworking of our psychological hardwiring into a configuration more conducive to athletic success.

3. *Individually Tailored Autogenic Training*

   Dr. Kogler's Autogenic Training approach is further refined to help the athlete meet individualized goals. The athlete creates a series of meaningful self-suggestive phrases which are used to reinforce a desired response. Phrases are developed that increase workout intensity, encourage self-confidence and deal with specific performance problems. These phrases are practiced on a regular basis (daily) and always in conjunction with the basic heightened autogenic state. These individualized phrases are utilized in practice and competition.

4. *Examining Athletic Experience*

Dr. Kogler encourages the athlete to discover and develop their own "positive self-talk", an individualized internal dialogue. Through "concentrative analysis" the athlete relives peak performances of the past. Self-talk is converted into clear and precise autogenic phrases. These phrases are applied in different athletic situations. Past experience assists future performance.

5. *Self Confidence*

A key factor in athletic success is redesigning the athlete's self image. Self confidence is reinforced in Kogler's system with several techniques. Two tried and proven Aladar Kogler tools are modeling and self-video. In the former, the athlete emulates a role model. In the latter the athlete produces a video tape of his/her best performances.

6. *Autogenic Training and Self-Hypnosis*

Kogler introduces the athlete to self-hypnosis. The subject is discussed and a rudimentary method of self-hypnosis is described. All aspects of this subject are discussed and reservations are dispelled through Kogler's clinical descriptions.

7. *Ideomotor Training and Vivid Imagery*

The vividness of the mental movie is critical: beginners have fuzzy visualizations lacking in clarity, detail and focus. Elite Iron Curtain athletes, through repeated use, were able to generate amazingly detailed movies of themselves, succeeding in the athletic event about to happen, a clean and jerk, a bobsled pilot taking himself through the course, a high jumper, long jumper or shot putter—the better the IT image the better the results. Practice increases the amount of detail and clarity that the athlete can create.

8. *Preparing for Competition*

Dr. Kogler believes that each athlete needs to develop a detailed mental game plan for the day of the competition. The elite also know what to do when plans go awry. Kogler's system incorporates specific steps for refocusing when things go wrong. Kogler insists that the athlete regularly rehearse the "game plan" prior to competition. His athletes use autogenic phrases during competition to help keep focused on the positive and simultaneously diffuse stress and anxiety.

9. *Putting Together a Complete Mental Training Program*

Knowledge is a wonderful thing, but results are what counts. The goal of any psychological training should be improved performance. In the gym that should trans late into more poundage handled, more reps, and quicker recovery. All of which will translate into bigger stronger muscles; which is the reason why we lift weights. Any psychological training should show real results in concrete terms. Otherwise the whole thing degenerates into a touchy-feely love fest that is delusional and ineffectual. The nice thing about the Kogler approach is that it has been battle-tested by international level Olympic athletes for over thirty years. Dr. Kogler offers up a basic template for designing a mental training program. The athlete then tailors this basic blueprint into a highly individualized game plan.

10. *The Utilization of Yoga for Improving Self Control*

For years top athletes have incorporated stretching into their training. Done prior to and after a training session, stretching helps prevent injury by elasticizing muscles and speeds-up recovery by forcibly circulating toxins rather than allowing them to settle. Yoga is a 5,000 year old system of stretching and Dr. Kogler uses a stripped-down, modified version of Yoga to center and focus the athlete. The athlete develops a high degree of control over their mental and physical functions. The ability to stay calm and centered in the heat of competition can be developed systematically through the use of Yoga stretching.

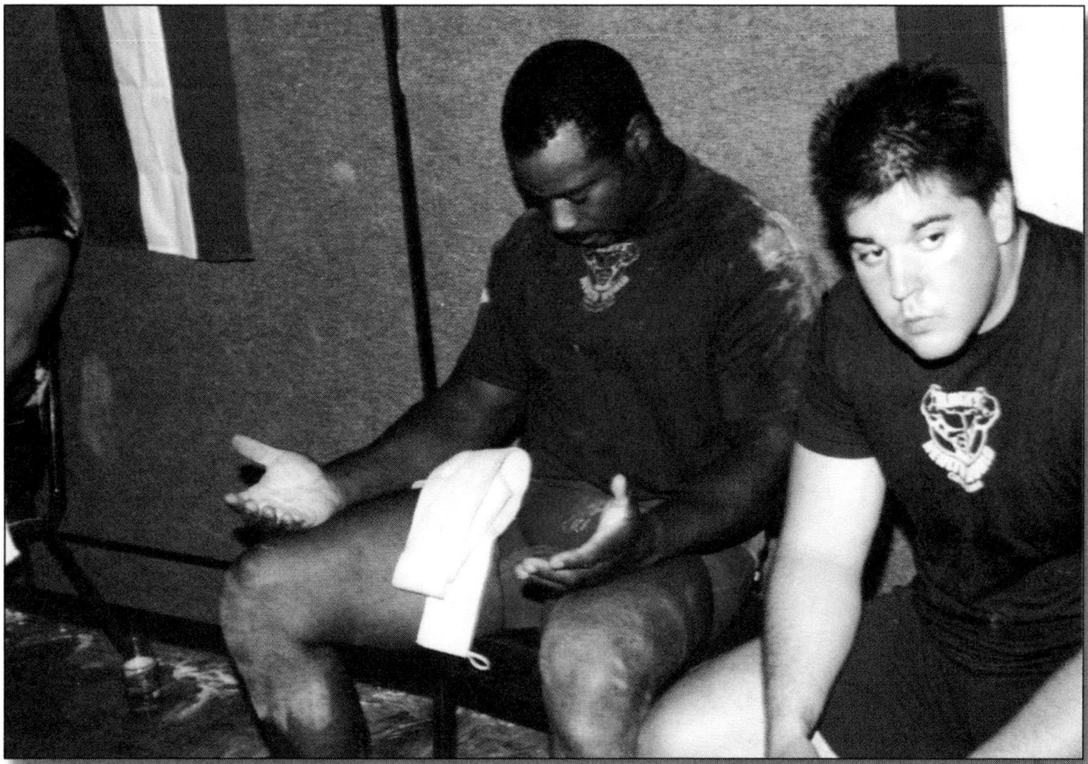

Witnessing mental recalibration in real time: National and World Powerlifting Champion, Willie "The Hammer" Bell, sits backstage and "psyches up" at the National Championships. He is mentally preparing for an 832 pound deadlift in the 242 pound class. Willie is using ideomotor/visualization techniques to "zone in" for the final attempt. He is running a movie of himself performing the lift. Over and over, with an ever increasing degree of realism, Bell is mentally picturing himself doing the about-to-happen lift. He is not concerned about thoughts of winning or victory or celebration, rather he is grooving in his technique; using mental imagery to reinforce that the lift will be done with absolute technical perfection.

He also is reinforcing the idea the weight will feel light—this is important. He lifts the poundage before it actually takes place. When his name is called he stands, strides to the platform and turns mental movies into championship reality. He made the lift and was crowned National Champion.

Mind Essays

During the white hot intensity of high level competition, the athletic elite have discovered how to effortlessly reside in the immediate present. Without distracting thoughts, without thoughts that project or reflect, free from preoccupation and extraneous internal chatter, they attain a thought-free concentrated mindset. This intense, laser-like focus allows them to enter into a state of heightened perception and awareness that leads to improved athletic performance. The "thinker" the "observer" has disappeared. The athlete has entered "The Zone." They are "One" with their athletic activity.

PURPOSEFULLY PRIMITIVE PSYCHOLOGY

Purposefully 'Mindless' Pursuits

Cleaning up cow manure, making love to the exquisite courtesan—all the same!

—Ling Po, 17th century Zen master

There is real value to being able to immerse yourself in an activity to the point that you lose all sense of time and self. You will do what it is you are doing far better, and with much greater concentration and focus. There is a tremendous psychological benefit to periodically practicing purposeful mindlessness.

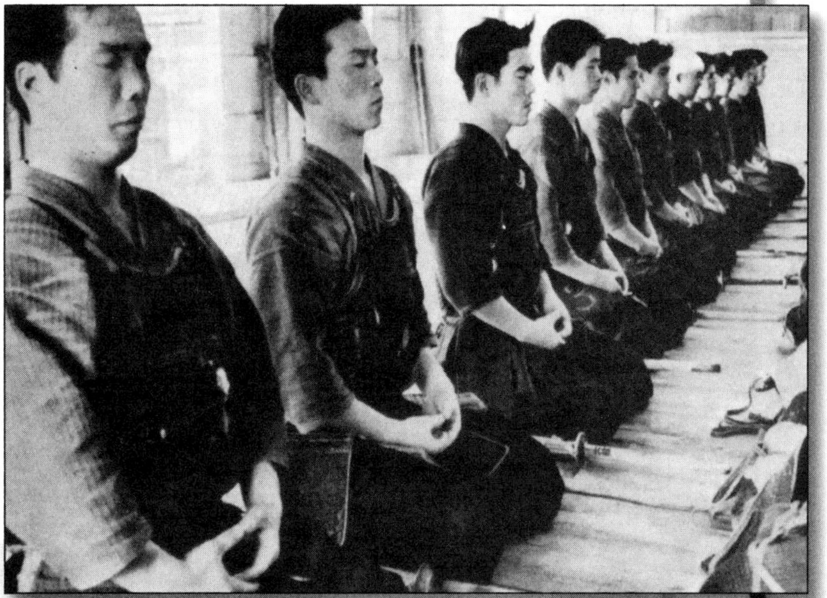

Moku-san is formalized Zen meditation used before engaging in sport. It has been used in Japan for centuries. Here a gang of Purposefully Primitive Hard Men clear their minds of extemporaneous thought before bashing the hell out of each other with wooden boken swords. These men seek to achieve a mental alertness called "sword of the non-abiding mind" prior to Kendo practice. We rip a page from the book of Budo for our own Westernized purposes. Mushin no shin, the 'mind of no mind' seeks "the establishment of something that transcends mere technique; explainable as a spontaneous mind that embraces a sixth sense."

Think of the human mind as a muscle. Like any muscle, if it is overworked it becomes over-trained and overtraining, as is the case with any muscle, leads to fatigue and performance degradation. The over-trained, over-worked, over-thinking brain becomes metaphorically overheated. The remedial solution is purposeful quietude; give the over-active mind some rest.

A mind that chatters ceaselessly eventually exhausts itself and an exhausted brain does not function nearly as well as a rested brain. Thought is self-perpetuating and by allowing internal dialogue to continue unabated 24-7-365, mental burnout lies just around the corner. Humans instinctively realize this and this is why drugs and alcohol are eternally popular: both allow the individual to dampen and suppress thought and reality. By stupefying the senses, by chemically altering the functioning of the brain, mental relief and euphoria are acquired. Anyone who has ever been drunk or high can attest to the fact that chemically altering the mind creates a pleasurable experience and pleasure is physically and psychologically addictive; especially if you can purchase pleasure in a bottle, pill or substance.

The desire to escape psychological reality and replace it with an altered reality is common and craved; always has been and always will be. Sufi Whirling Dervishes, Zen Monks, yoga aesthetics, sequestered Christian contemplative monks, Taoist priests, all seek to alter reality—though they would argue that they are amplifying reality not stupefying reality.

One common thread that ties the various holistic and natural contemplative methods together is that they all seek to silence the internal voice of conscious thought, one way or another. Thought creates a thin milky psychological layer that obscures reality. If thought is operating you are preoccupied.

When the internal voice grows silent, that thin continual sheen, the thought-chatter that obscures reality (and reality *always* unfolds in the instantaneous present) is scraped away. When the mind is silent and the senses engaged, you truly are able to *see*. Zen monks sit in formal meditation for upwards of twelve hours a day. In Zen meditation the idea is to quiet the mind without suppressing the mind and that presents a very tricky psychological dilemma. When thought finally falls silent the monks experience 'true original self.' The Zen brain, subjected to continual daily practice, eventually grows quiet and in that quietude an electric alertness emerges during which no thought arises. If thoughts do arise they are not 'clung to.' A thought might occur, but the reflective act of consciousness does not spring into action and examine or expand on the initial thought. And that is the end of it. No "thought chain" or "Nen sequence" occurs. The initial thought might arise, but the nen-chain does not take root. When a single thought arises, no amplification or expansion occurs and the electric alertness reemerges. Crisp clarity returns.

After a period of continual no-thought, a 'Samadhi' state occurs. Samadhi is inexplicable; words cannot describe a wordless state. If pressed it might best be described as an ecstatic state-of-being that happens when the brain becomes silent yet remains alert. A vibrant stillness envelopes the body as the "sense gates" become amplified. Hearing, seeing, tasting and feeling are heightened and remain heightened as long as conscious thought does not interfere with the delicate non-verbal state. Samadhi, heightened sense phenomena, rolls on unabated.

> ***"Moment after moment only the present comes and goes during the period of Samadhi, a continuous stream of the immediate present. Only in the precise instant of the immediate present can we be said to exist."***
>
> —Katsuki Sekida

If a single thought takes root and creates a nen-chain of subsequent thoughts, the gossamer strand that is the Samadhi state is shattered. Formal meditation practice eventually filters over into day to day existence and relates back to Ling Po's quote, wherein he references the idea that when the electric quietude becomes a regular part of normal existence, mundane chores like washing the dishes or cleaning up manure have no greater or lesser significance than peak experiences such as attending a Super Bowl or making love to a supermodel.

When the vibrant state of intense internal quietude is present, everything is experienced intensely and equally. One attribute of the Samadhi state is the total lack of mental *reflection or projection.* You cannot be in the immediate present if you are reflecting or projecting, Thought uses memory to conjure up "Remembrances of things past" or conversely thought projects ahead on things and events yet to happen. Not to say that there is not a time and place for memory and projection. Humans however, are continually and eternally preoccupied, an unceasing and continual blathering within the brain occurs during nearly every waking moment. No activity is done without the "thinker" engaging in internal dialogue. People find that only when engaged in some intense activity does the thinker fall silent: sex or sport, life or death experience, something so exotic or dramatic that full attention is demanded. We have even coined a pop psychology phrase, "peak experience" to describe those undertakings or events so captivating and enthralling that the internal thinker, the verbal diarrhea, fall silent; trumped by events so intense that the individual stays in the immediacy of the exact present with every ounce of their being.

Is all this talk about internal dialogue mere arcane abstraction with no real relevance to Americanized fitness or athletics? Hardly. Sport masters need to be in the absolute present when applying their tradecraft.

Dogen Zenji, Krishnamurti and Thomas Merton, all the mystics and seers, inform us that the inky film of thought prevents you from being in the exact present. Of course drugs and alcohol can obliterate thought and with it the web of personality, but like going to the circus, sooner or later you have to come home. Athletes and improvisational jazz musicians are aware of the thought-free bliss of the immediate present. An athlete in the white hot immediacy of a competitive event has no time for conscious thought. Actually, conscious thought can be detrimental for the athlete.

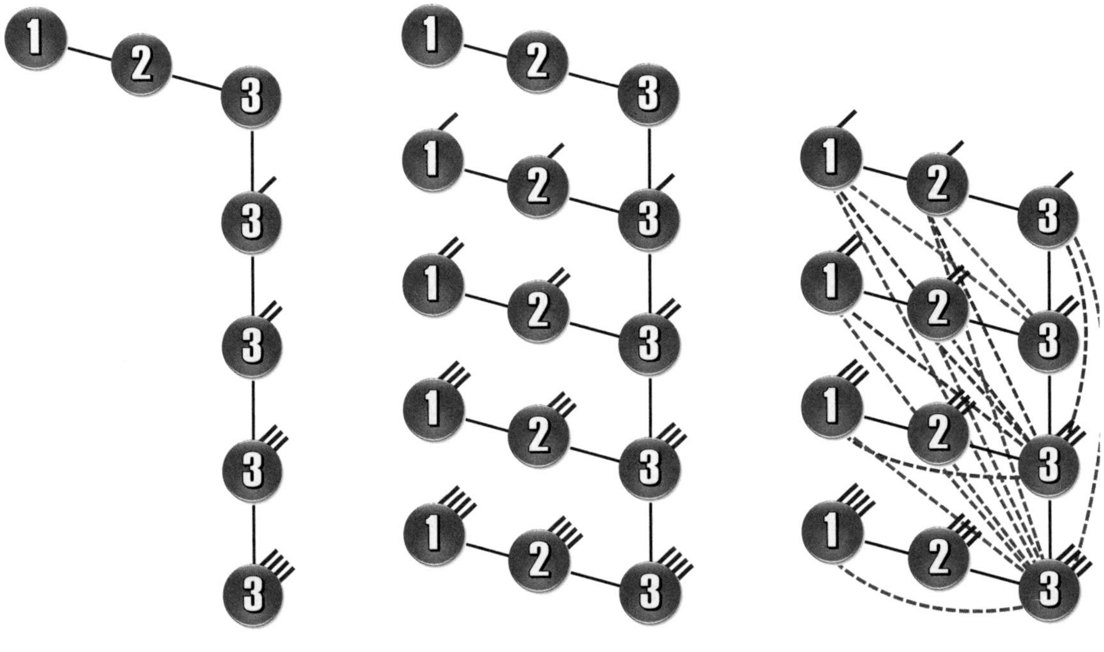

Sekida's Zen Nen Chain Diagram describes passing and clinging thoughts. #1 represents sensory input. #2 is the 'reflecting act of consciousness,' the little voice in our head. #3 represents 'clinging thoughts.' When a person, place or thing enters into our sensory radar screen, that is #1. When people, things or events pass 'into and then out of' our perception, without thought amplification, that is a 'passing thought,' #2. When we enter into internal mental discourse about the object of our mental focus, then we create 'clinging thoughts,' #3. There is a problem with allowing 3rd Nen clinging thoughts to take root. When 3rd Nens are active, perception of the ever-unfolding instantaneous immediate present is impossible. The best psychological positioning is mental quietude combined with mental alertness. A thought-free mind is vibrant, engaged and amplifies the five senses. The factual reality of the immediate present emerges out of mental silence.

If you are on the receiving end of a 125 mile per hour tennis serve, thinking will doom you. There is no way you can consciously think about how to react and still react in time. Try thinking about how you should move for service return, "here comes the ball; it's heading to the left forward quadrant." By the time the internal voice barks the order, "Move four paces left, use a backhand return to his left forecourt," the tennis ball has gone past you like a cannon shot.

The capable and competent elite athlete moves mindlessly and surrenders motion and movement to the wordless subconscious. The elite allow the intuitive mind to move the body in the correct fashion to the correct location and initiate the proper physical response. All this is done in a split-second, an eye-blink. If conscious thought intrudes, the athlete is lost.

Elite jazz musicians are improvisational masters. When it is their turn to solo in the middle of a torridly paced tune, they know that conscious thought cannot move fast enough to allow them to improvise the perfect solo at breakneck speed. The jazz improviser in full flight has no idea how or why his fingers respond to the audio input of the accompanists. He listens with perfect and relaxed concentration and surrenders to that same electric alertness the Zen Monk experiences when deep in Samadhi. This is a musical Samadhi state wherein the thinker within the brain falls silent. Any preoccupation, any reflection or projection will derail the solo. When unleashing a series of 64th note glissando arpeggios against a breakneck tempo, a single clinging thought will smash the flow like a brick thrown through a plate glass window. The jazz master's brain is perfectly still. The improvised solo unfolds and reveals itself to the wonderment of not only the audience, but also to the musician who spontaneously creates it.

Krishnamurti encapsulated these psychological phenomena in his master work, "The Awakening of Intelligence." He makes the case that when the unceasing internal voice finally becomes quiet, a whole new dimension of reality and existence is revealed: vibrant, exciting and wonderful. He states that the peak experiences of the Jazz musician, elite athlete or Zen Master can be experienced by all of us as we go about our day to day lives. We can improve our psychological well-being by consciously engaging in activities that cause the chatterbox to fall quiet. Pursuits that require intense concentration naturally cause the mind to fall silent. Art, music and sport can become activities that allow the mind to fall silent, but there are numerous activities that potentially allow you to "lose yourself." Some folks 'become selfless' working on their custom cars, doing carpentry, knitting or playing chess. Others achieve the electric alertness doing T'ai Chi or Qigong.

I personally seek to engage in a variety of activities in which I lose all sense of self. Intense physical training short-circuits and quiets the conscious chattering of the "observer" every single time. There is no way in hell the brain can be chit-chatting about "what's for dinner" or "how will the Redskins do this weekend" while underneath a 500-pound barbell per forming backbreaking squat reps. Ditto for an intense game of racquetball, tennis or basketball. The lightning pace, the sheer physical exertion, makes sure there are no superfluous mental projections or reflections.

Any competent musician will attest that, if preoccupied, their playing suffers from distraction. Focus and selflessness are the keys: classical piano virtuoso Glenn Gould spoke of "A state of wonder and ecstasy" that enveloped him when playing at his best. Even something as mundane as concentrated reading requires a degree of concentration and focus that preclude the observer from making inane comments. Intense competition, be it chess or target shooting, shuts the internal talker down and requires total and complete attention and concentration. The participant must stay in the immediacy of the mindless present in order to perform optimally.

Do you engage in some sort of activity that requires that you "reside lightly in the immediate present?" Does your reflecting or projecting internal voice mindlessly blather ceaselessly and endlessly? Does the thin inky film of continuous chatter prevent you from experiencing the electric alertness of the immediate present? Are you able to become 'lost' in an activity? For your own mental health you should seek activities that demand total and complete attention. If you want to renovate your physique, you will need to learn how to immerse yourself in hard training.

If you are able to carry on a conversation with yourself while training, you lack intensity. Mental silence is an indicator that you have taken your training performance to the next level. Learn how to immerse yourself so totally and completely in an activity that thought falls silent of its own accord. Chatter and preoccupation impedes performance, regardless the mode or activity. Champion athletes and elite performers know and understand this. So should you.

REPROGRAM THE CENTRAL PROCESSING UNIT OF THE SOFT MACHINE

Willpower is a Finite Mental Propellant

Successfully engineering a complete physical renovation is largely dependent on the trainee's ability to psychologically reprogram their current way of thinking. Optimally we seek to replace bad habits with good ones, exchanging detrimental behavior in favor of beneficial behavior. If you are able to derive pleasure from the process, transformation is just a matter of time. The Mind can be your biggest ally or worst enemy. It largely depends on your particular psychological makeup. Initially, beneficial changes are *legislated* through willpower. However, all acts of willpower must cease at some point. Eventually you want genuine enthusiasm to take over from willpower. When enthusiasm powers the psychological process, chances of success radically improve.

Willpower is a finite mental propellant. Once you burn through your quota, it takes a long time to restock. Enthusiasm is infinite. It replenishes itself. Human nature loves to repeat pleasurable experience and if hard, intense, endorphin-releasing training is perceived as pleasurable, the Mind will seek to repeat this pleasurable experience. The more you train the better the gains, the better the gains the more you train...round and round it goes.

Disciplined eating is a psychological horse of a different color. It is far more difficult to become enthused about legislated eating. No endorphin-releasing pleasures, no training partners, no mathematical sense of accomplishment...eating requires the modification of conditioning and overcoming habit force. In our approach, proper nutrition is arrived at through the principle of *creeping incrementalism.* Tiny steps are taken, nutritionally speaking, using a wide range of foods and the end result is that the individual morphs detrimental eating habits into beneficial habits—new habits replace old ones—some through sheer trickery.

In the world of eating Taste is King. To pretend taste doesn't matter or that it can be overcome through suppression or by some massive act of willpower is naïve, simplistic and doomed to failure.

Several easy to understand steps are taken to recalibrate our nutritional approach. Everyone has certain food preferences, foods that are totally acceptable. First off we identify foods that we like that are also acceptable and beneficial. It might be shellfish or carrots, turkey or garden salads—once we identify those foods, we "heavy up" on their consumption. Secondly, we come to grips with our own food preparation. That's the big one. We learn how to prepare tasty versions of the foods that we like and that are beneficial and acceptable. Then we make lots of these acceptable foods ahead of time. Which ties into our next incremental step: we never allow ourselves to become hungry, particularly at night…that's when the binging occurs. A person who is satiated is less likely to binge on sweets or junk food than someone who is ravenous.

Another step is the trickster fake out of dealing with a sweet tooth by having on hand "engineered foods" that are sweet taste treats, yet are nutritionally acceptable. Will a sport nutrition bar equal the taste of a pint of Ben and Jerry's ice cream? No way, but if the individual has on hand a sport nutrition bar when the sweet tooth urge hits, he/she can satiate the sweet tooth and avoid the ice cream binge. There are other tricks of the nutrition trade that will help a person morph from bad eating to good eating, but the greatest single motivator is success. Nothing fires a person up more than losing a substantial amount of body fat. Nothing fires a formerly overweight person up more then when people comment about their new lean look without being asked.

When tangible progress becomes readily apparent, disciplined eating and regimented training become effortless. Joyful experience begs the Mind to replicate it, over and over, again and again.

Habit-force is a bad thing when the habits are physically detrimental. Habit-force can be quite beneficial if the habits are positive. What does all this psycho-babble mean? Look for ways to make exercise fun. Certain physical activities are genuinely fun, but you need to make an effort to find them. Weight training can be quite enjoyable, particularly when planning is used. Half our brain is rational and logical and quite masculine while the other half of the brain is intuitive and spontaneous, artistic and feminine. A wonderful physical feeling descends and envelops the trainee after a properly aggressive progressive resistance workout. A state of physical well-being is brought on by the pure physical effort exerted.

Elite athletes are addicted to the endorphin rush that accompanies truly hardcore training.

Baby workouts, going through the motions, are insufficient to release endorphins and insufficient to trigger muscular hypertrophy. The Mind can be our most powerful ally in our effort to reconfigure our physiques. Have the rational side of the brain design a plan of attack and let the intuitive side take over during the actual workout. Try and make a mind/muscle connection during every set of every exercise. I like to listen to music as I train. I find I can develop a deeper level of concentration during a workout and music actually amplifies results derived from that workout. Plus it is damned near impossible to get roped into an energy-zapping conversation while wearing headphones. Deep concentration results in those extra growth producing reps or that additional poundage. More reps or more poundage (assuming there is no degradation in technique) means more muscle growth. Find cardio modes that you actually enjoy. They are out there, but you'll need to search a bit.

Too many people feel that unless cardio is done indoor on a treadmill, stair-stepper or in a step-aerobic class, the activity doesn't qualify as legitimate cardio. That is fallacious to the max and a good case could be made that prolonged cardio machine use can actually lead to repetitive motion injury. There is a lot to evidence that doing the same exercise on the same machine in the same way for days, weeks, months and years can literally wear out body parts. If you use exercise machines for cardio exercise, please be clever enough to vary machines and shift from one type to another on a periodic basis.

I prefer outdoor cardio: I run/power walk/jog on mountain trails. Every footfall is slightly different than its predecessor. Outdoor cardio, provides the body clean, highly oxygenated air. Compare that to the air breathed in the commercial gym. Have you ever thought about the toxic stew of stale, recycled gym air loaded with the carbon dioxide emissions from sick or hung-over individuals? It is far better to suck in fresh, clean, reinvigorating, unpolluted outdoor oxygen. Find a cardio mode you enjoy, or better yet develop a series of enjoyable aerobic modes that you enjoy and systematically rotate them. Find modes you enjoy and you will learn to love exercise instead of dreading exercise. Enjoyment breeds enthusiasm. Enthusiastic participation takes over where willpower leaves off. Beneficial physical activity is enthusiastically anticipated.

Let us make the training process enjoyable. Let us subtly reprogram the brain, the Central Processing Unit of the human body. William Boroughs dubbed the human body "The Soft Machine" and that description is incredibly apt. Open your closed mind. Try some new and different physical activities, activities intense enough to trigger the release of those blessed endorphins! Training intense enough to trigger endorphins is also intense enough to trigger hypertrophy!

Making the Mind/Muscle Connection

A Muscle Parable

James wasn't getting any training traction and couldn't figure out why. It was easy for me to see why. He trained at the same time I did at the local steel house and any old timer who casually observed his training could pin the tail on this donkey in five seconds flat.

His sloppy, bounced bench presses looked liked belly heaves. His butt came so far off the bench on each rep that you could have driven a mini-van between his glutes and the bench surface. He would load up the weight belt when he did parallel bar dips, but his rep stroke was all of about four inches; he neither went down in his dips nor did he lock out at the top. His squats were the nose bleed variety, so named because of how sky high they were. He would load up the squat bar with impossible poundage, wear powerlifting knee wraps cinched so tight they cut off leg circulation and put on a weight belt so gargantuan he needed help buckling it. I doubt he dipped more than six inches on any squat rep. Ditto for his ridiculous leg presses: same lame procedure…load about fifteen 45 pound plates on each side, wrap his knees, wear the gigantic belt and press the weight maybe six inches. He got a better *back workout* loading and unloading the leg press plates than his legs did pressing the weight. His cheat curls looked like reverse cleans and it is no exaggeration to say that his spinal erectors got more work then his sad little biceps. Triceps pushdowns required he use the whole stack, but the push traveled maybe three inches. Lateral raises were done with 60 pound dumbbells and he used more momentum to get the bells moving than an Olympic shot putter uses propelling the 16 pound steel ball 70 feet.

Plus the yelling; how could I possibly fail to mention his bloodcurdling screams that accompanied the final reps of each set? It sounded as if the boy was having his fingers mashed with a 20 pound sledge hammer. His screams were impossible to ignore—which was the intended purpose—this kid was not only misguided in his training, but obviously starved for attention. I thought of each scream as a pathetic cry for help. Eventually, it grew old and the management made him an offer he couldn't refuse: cease and desist with the blood curdling screams, the loud cursing, his lifting chalk strewn everywhere—or find a new place to train.

When Tim the night manager told him one night to shut up or he was going to kick him out on the spot, the boy stumbled backwards like he'd been shot in the gut with a rifle. The screams and cursing, he protested, were a natural expression of his incredible effort. Tim held tough and from that point forward the kid moped around like a castrated steer. Without his screams, without the profanity, James was Samson shorn of his locks.

I was shocked when later that week the boy approached *me* and asked if I had a spare moment. I was taken aback; I'd never spoken a word to him and was mystified as to what he wanted. To make a long story short, James was actually reexamining his training efforts and asked if he could train with me! Essentially he asked if I would I show him the training ropes. I was dubious, but he seemed sincere. I told him the only way I'd agree to this was if he trained exactly as I did. And no talking—the only talking would be by me. I neither wanted nor needed his input. He would play the part of the compliant deaf-mute training partner. I told him to show up the following Monday at the appointed time and we'd hit a chest and triceps workout. He agreed. I secretly decided to drive him into the ground; not purposefully or maliciously, but I would not compromise my own training efforts.

Normally when introducing a well-intentioned beginner to my style of training, I would be nice and ease them into the game. I would not ease this potty mouthed youth into my style of training: I would throw him into the deep end of the pool and see if he could swim. His problem (in a nutshell) was that he'd been so poundage crazy he'd shortened his rep strokes to next to nothing. His range-of-motion was nonexistent and his technique so sloppy that he wasn't coming within a country mile of working the targeted muscle.

When I spoke to him about "zeroing in on the muscle" or making "the mind-muscle connection" it was like trying to describe the Space Shuttle to a Brazilian rainforest tribe member. He scratched his head and scrunched up his face as I described proper bench press technique. Not only would he keep his ass on the bench for each and every rep, but he would also pause the poundage on his chest before firing it skyward. He started to protest when after a warm up set I loaded the bar to 185. He indicated that he was "easily" capable of 250 for reps. "Not anymore." I said.

He struggled with 185 for 5 reps using the proper pause technique. Ditto for incline dumbbell presses, which I insisted be done strict and with a pause. His dumbbell flyes, which used to be indistinguishable from dumbbell bench presses, were now done so wide and so deep that the bells touched the floor. I noted that his chest was actually trembling as we segued into dips. He looked around for the weight belt. "I can do 10 dips with 90 pounds strapped on." He proudly proclaimed. "Not anymore." I said.

I made him drop all the way down and pause before pushing upward to a complete lock-out. “Hold the lockout for a full second.” I demanded. He made two full reps using only his bodyweight before collapsing on number three. By the conclusion of our third set of bodyweight dips, he was unable to do a single rep. Lying nose-breakers and overhead dumbbell triceps extensions were done with a full rep stroke and pee-wee poundage—since that was all he could properly handle. Triceps pushdowns were done with full ROM. I stood behind him and pinioned his elbows to his side to prevent him from using his old trick of heaving at the start to get the weight moving.

At the conclusion of our 70 minute workout he was shaking like he had malaria. I made him drink a triple serving of protein/carb powder in shake form and sent him home. I wondered if I’d ever see him again, I doubted it. The next day was leg day and James wandered in dazed and confused. “My pecs and triceps are so sore I can’t lift my arms. I couldn’t shave or comb my hair this morning.” He moaned. “That’s really too bad,” I said, “Because yesterday’s chest and triceps workout is a happy-time picnic in the park with a gorgeous super model compared to what we’re going to be doing today.”

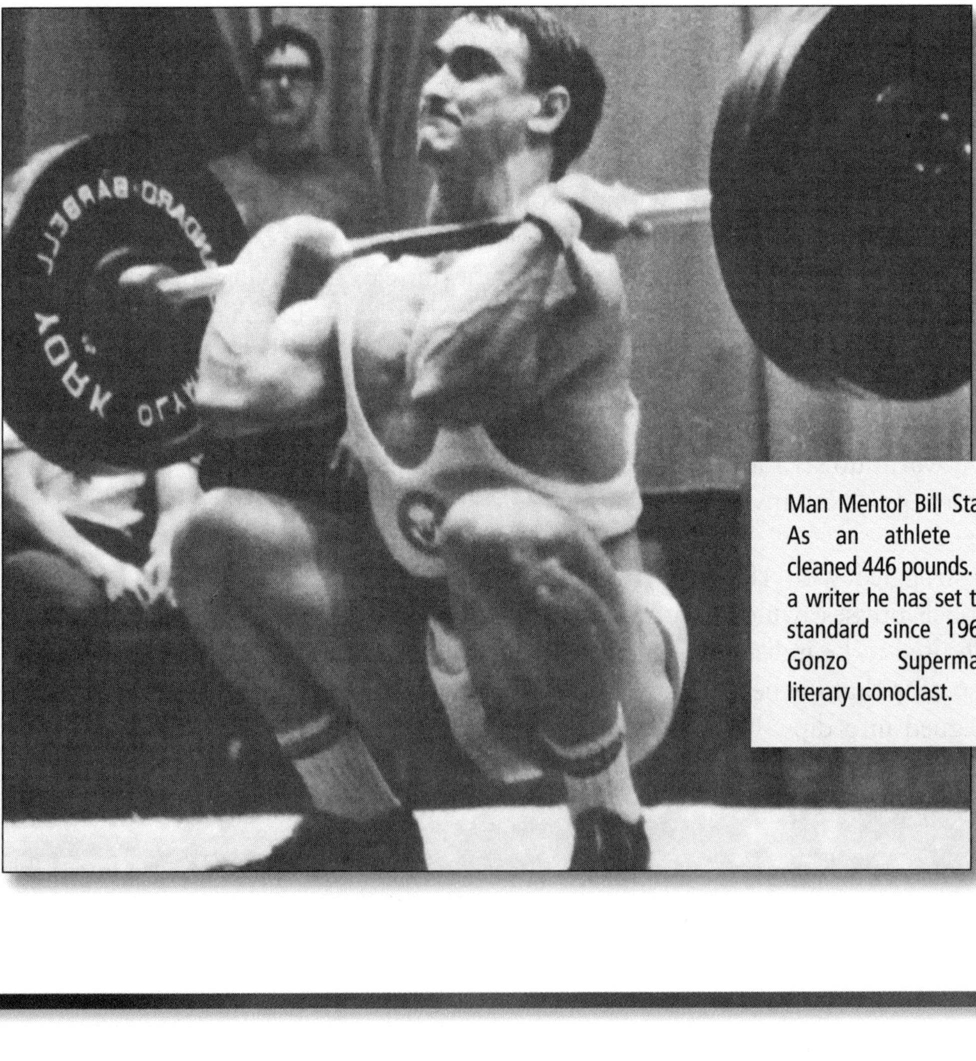

Man Mentor Bill Starr. As an athlete he cleaned 446 pounds. As a writer he has set the standard since 1964. Gonzo Superman, literary Iconoclast.

He looked positively frightened as we began full squats. Squats are hell. That's why they're so damn effective. I made the kid do something he'd never ever done before; go all the way down in the squat without any supportive gear. On his 1st set he reached for his knee wraps and lifting belt and I told him to stuff them right back into his gym bag. His 400 pound partial squats dropped faster than the stock market after the Enron collapse. He struggled with 185 and 205 was positively traumatic. I had to help him complete the 5th rep. "Oh my God, my legs are on fire!" He hissed. James was gulping air like he'd just run a marathon, but I made him do two more sets: 155x10 caused him to convulse so badly I thought he was going into a seizure.

Leg presses caused him to run to the bathroom and toss his breakfast. He wobbled out pale and shaking. I had made James take the sled down until his knees touched his chest. He locked out fully and two 45's per side were all he could handle. He looked white as a ghost. "Feel better?" I said. "No!" he moaned, clutching his gut. We finished off with calf raises super-setted with lying leg curls. I went on to standing calf raises and stiff-leg deadlifts. He sat in the corner curled up in a fetal position and called in sick to work the next day.

He surprised me. I thought it at best a 10% proposition that he'd ever return, but he showed up a few days later ready to train shoulders. He still walked funny three days later. "I got home that night after leg training and had to sit down halfway up the three flights of stairs leading up to my apartment. I still walk like I'm drunk."

On shoulder day the procedures were repeated and again the full-range-of-motion exercises sent him reeling.

We performed five sets of standing dumbbell presses followed by five sets of press behind the neck. His 60 pound lateral heaves turned into 10 pound super strict laterals. Now his screams were real and not for show. Back day finished the training week: let me just say that by the time we finished deadlifts, power cleans, rows, chins, shrugs and 9 sets of biceps spread over three different exercises, the boy was a ball of pain. "Be sure and eat a ton of protein this weekend." I said. Wordlessly he wobbled out the door.

The following Monday James showed up for the start of his second 'real' training week. "I am still reeling," he said, "My body is torn to shreds from my neck to my calves...I laid on the couch all weekend eating...every muscle still aches." I smiled. He seemed battered, but buoyant. "I have never felt the degree of fatigue and muscle soreness I am now experiencing."

To his everlasting credit, James stuck with it. In three months he underwent an amazing physical transformation. The winning combination was full range power training and making the mind muscle connection—along with ample eating—all of which caused his body to explode. He packed on twenty five pounds of muscle and looked like Bill Pearl winning Mr. America in 1955. I told him, "You'll never survive this style of training unless you eat like you've never eaten before; without copious calories your body will collapse." He was firing down 5,000 calories per day.

James packed on 25 pounds of muscle in 90 days and because he ate clean and kept up his early morning cardio, 95% of his gains were lean, fat-free muscle.

His training poundage increased rapidly after week one; this despite my insisting on technical perfection on every single rep of every single set. His recovery improved dramatically and eventually he was able to completely recover by the next training session. "I think the biggest single thing I learned," he said in a reflective moment many months later over dinner, "was to make a mind-muscle connection. I trained all sloppy and poundage crazy and never gave the mind-muscle connection any thought. Until I began training with you I never had been really sore—I'm talking deep muscle soreness exactly on the targeted muscle. There is a real art in performing an exercise in such an exact fashion that the muscle you are supposed to be training actually feels it." Well no kidding.

Take a tip from James and crank back on the training poundage and establish the critical mind-muscle connection. Are you able to pinpoint and target the exact muscle with the right exercise? Use an extended range-of-motion and a perfect technique to achieve muscle isolation. Unless you are able to do so, your foundation is built on sand. So take a tip from James: lose your ego and your preconceptions regarding how a person is supposed to look and act when they train. Establishing proper technical basics will be the smartest training move you can make. Trust me.

PHYSICAL AND PSYCHOLOGICAL WEAK POINTS

If arithmetic, measuring and weighing
Be taken away from any art,
That which remains will not be much
...for measure and proportion
Always pass into beauty and excellence."
—Plato, Philebus

What's the toughest lesson to learn in all of fitness-dom?

I would nominate prioritizing weaknesses and *not* continually playing to our strengths.

Let's loop back around to human nature: the reason we are strong in certain areas and weak in others relates directly to bias, preference and enjoyment. We all have our likes and dislikes and we seek to repeat experiences that we perceive as pleasurable. We avoid things and experiences we perceive as dreadful. In our fitness efforts we are inclined to repeat that part of the transformational process we perceive as pleasurable. Perhaps we love a particular cardio mode, like tennis. We get up at 5:00 am year round and go to the local tennis club and play for a solid hour with other tennis fanatics; all before the rest of the world is even awake. I know such a collection of tennis fanatics exists because I used to see them flailing away first thing in the morning as I passed the windows overlooking the indoors courts at the posh club where I used to train. I would be on my way to train with like-minded group of weight training fanatics.

That which we perceive as pleasurable causes us to make great sacrifice in order to squeeze the pleasurable activity into our hectic and harried life. Often our training preferences, taken to an extreme, will result in physical dis-proportionality. We train a certain muscle or group of muscles to such an extent that our physiques become physically unbalanced and asymmetric. If a person loves to do curls and does them often, after a number of years those biceps are going to become proportionally larger than other muscles neglected during that same time period.

Maybe you love a particular cardio activity and despise resistance training. You avoid any and all muscle strengthening—then hurt your back picking up a forty pound child. Perhaps you can bench press 400 for reps, but cannot walk up a flight of stairs without getting totally out of breath. Maybe you are diligent at weight training and love cardio, but have zero control over the knife and fork. You end up very strong, extremely fit (in a cardiovascular sense) and obese, all at the same time. The NFL is loaded with this type of athlete, 350 pound offensive tackles that can bench press a house, run a marathon (albeit not very fast) and still are clinically obese. The point being, we all have our fitness preferences and dislikes.

Likely the areas on your physique that need improvement are developed using modes, techniques or tactics you don't particularly like. Working on weak points is the absolute fastest way to make physical improvement. A weak point is likely to be at 50% (or less) of total genetic potential. When you mount a serious effort to bring up a weak point, the room for improvement is vast.

Factually, that hypothetical athlete who loves to curl would find that if suddenly he devoted as much time and effort to a bodily weak point (say his bird-thin legs) as he has on his over-developed arms, huge physical improvement would be realized and realized quickly. He could add two inches to his under-worked, underdeveloped legs in a matter of months. It would take *years* to bring his arms up that much because he is likely already at 90% of his arm growth potential.

Logic dictates a continual shift in the training emphasis: the wise man goes from one under-developed body part to the next, until every muscle and muscle group on the body is uniform and proportional. But that's logic and humans are not robots.

If you want to make progress at a neck-snapping, head-spinning rate, look at the Purposefully Primitive Training Triad and with a cold hard eye identify your particular weak points. Then draw up a four week battle plan that specializes on weak aspects of your game.

If you're strong as a gorilla, but fat as a pig, then eating is your weak point. Your food selections and quantities are undercutting the rest of your efforts, so focus your energy on disciplined nutrition.

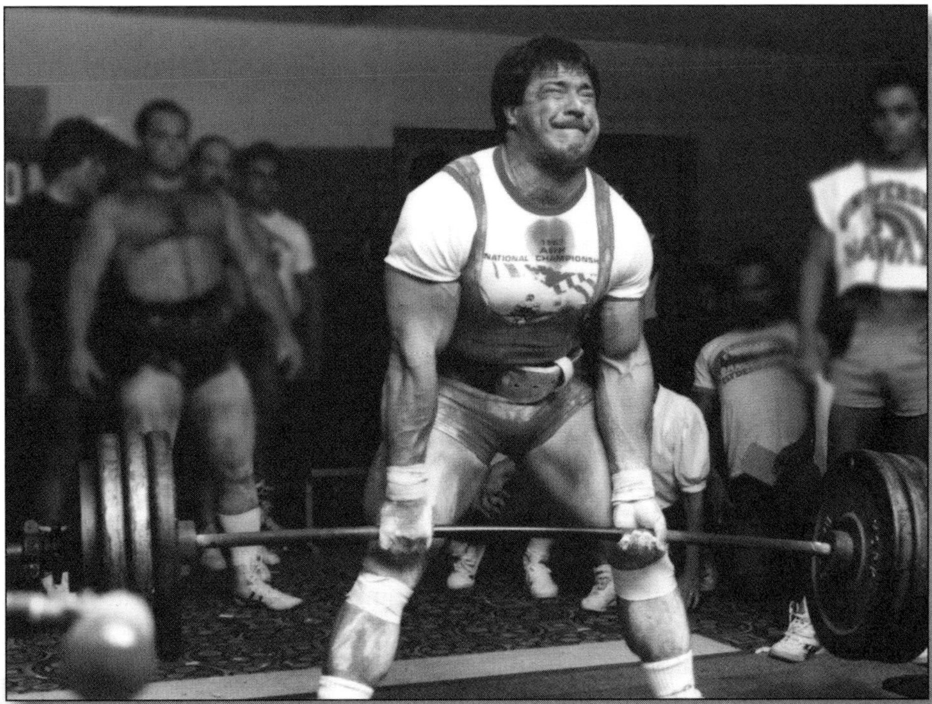

Work the weak points: Pat Brago's face captures the degree of pure physical effort required to trip the hypertrophy switch. He is 'willing' his body to exceed what he is actually capable of. Pat demonstrates the top pull position in this 750 pound Sumo deadlift. His weak side lags slightly. The deadlift was Pat's weak point. By prioritizing weaknesses and not continually playing to his strengths, he ultimately achieved physiologic balance The blood stain on his t-shirt occurred when he pushed so hard on his third attempt squat that the membranes inside his nose exploded and shot blood out in projectile fashion.

Do you have to train so hard your nose explodes? No, but Brago's facial expression alerts you to the degree of effort the top men exert on the final reps of a top set.

If you are doing way too much cardio and zero weight training, get down to some serious iron pumping. Habit-force is a bitch to overcome, but fighting against our basic preferential human nature is the way of a champion. If we always and forever do that which we love, ignoring things we don't, then we are digging a deep, deep trench that becomes nearly impossible to overcome or escape.

People who do the same thing for too long become fossilized and incapable of change. Progress and change are synonymous. Without change, without subjecting the body to new and different tests and stresses, nothing of any physical consequence will occur. The human body does not favorably reconfigure itself in response to sameness. Identify weak points and give them priority. This is the toughest of tasks, but the one with the most growth potential. Play to your weaknesses, not your strengths.

BRAIN TRAIN

Music Trumps Mechanical Sounds
Natural Silence Trumps Music...
The Poundage Is Constant Even If You Are Not...

People sometimes ask why I listen to music when I train. "The iPod seems out of character." One acquaintance said after training with me one afternoon. Actually, if he knew me better, he would have known that listening to music while training is very much *in* character for me. First off I always try to find a proper selection of music for that particular day. I am interested in 'mood elevation' as it pertains to the workout, so ballads and somber songs are usually out. Music elevates and amplifies my ability to concentrate and get totally zoned in on the athletic task at hand. And to such a degree that I believe my workout results improve if I hit the right tunes on the right day at the right time. It all relates to my individualized psyche-up procedure.

Top athletes get psychologically fired up immediately prior to undertaking a limit or near limit feat. Conversation interferes with psyching-up. Wearing an iPod is particularly important if you train at a commercial gym where potential distractions are just waiting to happen. I really don't want to get caught up in a conversation with a well-meaning gym member when I'm about to blast away at my top set in the deadlift. Talk is counterproductive. If you are a nice person and allow yourself to be interrupted in the House of Iron, then you have a problem. It is not psychologically possible to stop mid-sentence during an involved conversation, casually stroll up to a limit poundage barbell or dumbbell, and lift it with any hope of success. The poundage is constant even if you're not. Don't be thick-headed: In order to have a prayer lifting a weight that equals or exceeds current limits, you need to develop a personalized psyche-up routine.

What, prey tell, does that mean?

Psyche is a centering process. A proper psyche is tinged with aggression and purposeful machismo, even if you're distaff. Focus and ferocity are required to tackle something you've never done before. Anything less and you're toast.

Bring your "A" Game to the training session. Over time, learn how to fire yourself up like a berserker. The psyche doesn't have to be outwardly demonstrative. While psyche-up is still no absolute guarantee of success, this approach improves the odds considerably. Select mood arousal music and in about the time the java hits the bloodstream you'll be raring to tear up some weights. The deeper I get into the workout the better my concentration becomes. I mentally review the about-to-happen lift immediately prior to actually commencing.

I was first introduced to the concept of 'visualization' by Mac McCallum in a two-part 1965 Keys to Progress article called, "Concentration." Over the past forty years I've gotten to the point where I can routinely *will* my body to do more than it is capable of on that particular day.

I visualize myself in whatever physical setting I find myself in, I close my eyes and see myself sitting as I'm sitting...I tell myself, 'picture the room in detail. What color shirt do you have on? Are there stripes on your gym socks?' Detailed recall and focus requires complete concentration. My mental picture is rich and detailed. I see myself stand up and do whatever preliminary things I would need to do for this particular lift. I see myself step to the bar and as I grab it appropriately and take control, the weight always (in my mind) feels light. I handle the poundage for the appropriate number of reps in pristine style then replace the weight. In the gym I open my eyes and take a huge breath. I stand up and attempt to turn the visualization into reality.

Do I use psyche on every dink-ass itty-bitty exercise? No way! But on the big stuff, the important stuff, the limit stuff, I make myself use "the procedure." It is also a surefire way to reduce the chance of injury.

If you want to end up making a quick trip to the emergency room, attempt a limit lift half-heartedly or in a state of distraction.

Regardless of the rep range limit is limit, and poundage stays constant even if you aren't. The weight makes no allowances for your spaced-out inattention. The weights will hurt you if you disrespect the precise technical boundaries of a lift.

A walkman/iPod discourages conversation and aides in the seriousness and centering that needs to occur if you are going to safely stretch the envelope. When I do cardio I love the walkman/iPod because it helps me with pace, stride-step length, cadence and general awareness. I love to glide along, breaking a magnificent toxin-expelling sweat, while listening to some amazing piece of music that provides a dramatic and appropriate soundtrack to the natural beauty I am seeing and smelling. And to think, I'm burning off body fat, elevating my basal metabolic rate, improving my endurance while building a set of lungs like a Porsche turbocharger. Often my hour long daily nature run turns out to be the highlight of that particular day.

Early morning aerobics done on nature trails or in some wonderful public park listening to perfectly selected music can be a transcendental experience. My rule of thumb for outdoor iPod use is this: if I can hear any mechanical sounds or manmade hubbub I wear the iPod. In Marty World, music trumps mechanical sounds or voices every single time. If I'm lucky enough to catch a real natural silence…birds and wind, leaves rustling, branches creaking...natural silence trumps music every single time. Do yourself a favor: if you are serious about bumping progress upward a few notches try using music to develop an embryonic psyche-up routine. Try some outdoor cardio. Feel the wind at your back and the sun in your face as you tool along at 80% of age-related heart rate max while some subtle, sultry, siren seductress murmurs through your head phones. Outdoor cardio in a serene natural setting is psychologically addictive and has incredible physical benefit.

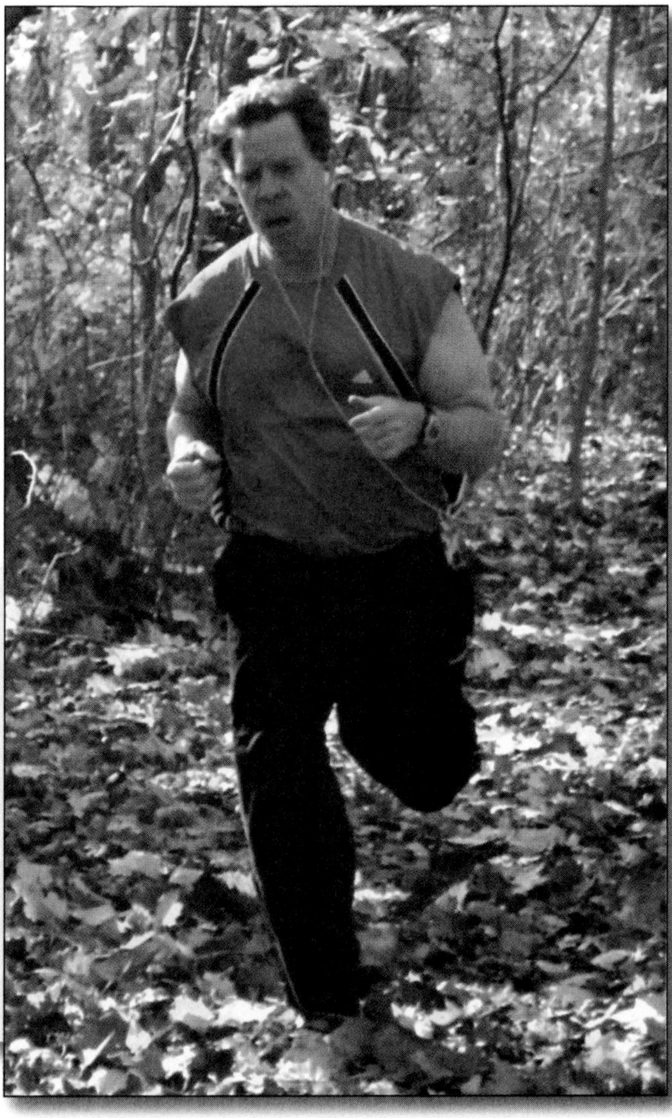

One Nation under a Groove: I wear my iPod when I hit the woods for cardio. With 1,000 songs of my own choosing, I can sync up any preexisting mood with a soundtrack. I usually use the shuffle function to surprise myself. I also wear the iPod in the gym. It's a perfectly acceptable way to discourage the enemy of progress: conversation. It's damned hard to make small talk to a guy wearing earphones.

THE PSYCHOLOGY OF A CHAMPION ATHLETE

The mind, the brain, the internal thought process, can become your biggest ally or worst enemy in the battle to transform your physique. Psychological repositioning is critical; optimally the athlete *must* be enthused, excited and fired up about the training session. They also need to be excited and enthused about the overall game plan.

Construct a 6-12 week fitness battle plan and do so with the care and intricacy of a ship-in-a-bottle builder. Once you hatch the plan, you should be so excited and so jacked up that you cannot wait to train and when you train you attack the workout. The "berserker" mindset in a training session results in amplified athletic performance. Think of individual workouts as pearls on a string that together form a necklace: each new cardio and weight workout represents a new pearl on the strand. String together an uninterrupted series of workouts and create genuine physical momentum.

Once physical momentum is achieved, results suddenly amplify past all realistic expectations. I've seen the phenomenon of momentum occur in myself and in others a hundred times over. The athletic elite understand how important the creation of momentum is and seek to generate it. A successful weight or cardio workout builds muscle tissue or oxidizes stored body fat. Intense physical training releases narcotic-tinged endorphins into the bloodstream and the workout becomes a physically and psychologically pleasing experience. Human nature seeks to repeat experiences it deems pleasurable. The enthusiasm quota is replenished and the whole process pushes forward one solid step.

String together a series of successful workouts and after 10-14 days tangible physical changes begin to manifest. Once tangible physical change occurs, the elusive physical *and* psychological momentum takes root. Establishing "Big Mo" is the immediate goal. Fourteen days of complete adherence will create momentum and can change a person's life. Obtain that critical toehold by stringing together successful workouts. Workout quality is elevated by total focus on the athletic task at hand.

Get fired up: log results and exult in the continual, numerical, tangible, undeniable physical progress: "I bench pressed 200x8 on Tuesday and bench pressed 205x8 on Friday."

That's certifiable, objective progress; the kind that translates into muscle and strength gains. Too often civilian trainees coast through their workouts and use training time as social inter-reaction time. How many times have I walked into a commercial gym and seen folks gabbing away to the person on the cardio machine next to them, or yakking it up with an acquaintance? The most unpardonable sin of all is when they talk to each other *during* a weight training set. Blasphemy

Innocent, but not harmless; I consider conversation in the gym the equivalent of an energy leak. You have a finite amount of energy when you walk through the door of the gym to train. Every conversation, every belly laugh, every engaged interplay, depletes the precious finite energy reserve to a slight or significant degree. Conversation prevents heightened awareness.

If you access "The Zone," you will be able to squeeze out extra reps and/or handle increased poundage—strictly by generating a particular mindset. Talking between or during sets may seem the amiable or sociable thing to do, but unless you maintain a silent, concentrated awareness between and particularly during the actual set, performance will suffer. The worst of all gym sins is when you allow muscle-head poseurs to engage you in intense conversations *about training* or training strategies or various athletic personalities, instead of focusing on the training that is actually taking place! In *A Moveable Feast* Ernest Hemmingway lamented that he had to stop frequenting the Parisian Café scene during the Lost Generation period of the 1920's because all the writers were wasting their precious creative writing "juice" *talking* about writing and instead of staying home in the their lofts and Left Bank apartments and *writing*.

Talking about training and training itself are two different things entirely. Another tale, a related tale, this one about *faux* awareness as opposed to true awareness...

> ***In May of 1954 Krishnamurti and four other religious leaders were traveling west from New Delhi in an open Mercedes en route to a religious retreat. The vehicle was chauffeured and allowed the gurus and mystics to discuss esoteric topics of great depth and complexity. The day was perfect as they tooled along dirt roads lined with 5,000 year old shrines and temples. The conversation amongst the exalted turned to the subject of awareness, 'We need be here in the present; we need be alert and aware and alive!' said the high priest. 'Alertness at every instant is the key to living life to its fullest!' The sage responded. The mystic chimed in, 'You must be here in the here and now!'***

The discussion became heated and intense as each religious leader (each practiced and quite at ease at persuasive pontification) fought hard to be heard in the rapid-fire word exchange. 'Suddenly,' remembered Krishnamurti, 'we ran over a full-sized goat. It impacted the car with a loud thud. No one noticed.' Krishnamurti related this while shaking his head. The seers and teachers were so engrossed with their animated conversation about awareness that they as a group became oblivious to actual awareness. "It was a delicious moment." said the only man who noticed the road-kill.

I often take people hiking in the woods. It is interesting to observe how different people react. Some silently soak in the scenery and truly absorb the beauty of wild nature. Others don't see it at all. They want to talk about bench pressing or the validity of body fat calipers. Meanwhile they miss the red tailed hawk circling lazily overhead on an invisible thermal current. They want to talk about theoretical periodization strategies of great complexity; they want to talk about cardio—despite the fact that they are missing out on the cardio we are actually doing. They want to talk about anything; they avoid immersing themselves in the silent immediacy of the actual moment. This repeated and predictable occurrence is the equivalent of running over a goat in a car and not noticing.

I've noticed that champion athletes have a common ability to zero in on the workout with a focused intensity that is positively frightening. They have an ability to literally will themselves to lift more or force out extra reps. The athletic elite effortlessly make themselves run faster or further, jump higher or longer. The top guys routinely add 10% to their training sessions, strictly through the use of extreme concentration. So what does all this have to do with running over goats or not seeing the circling hawk? People who are preoccupied, distracted or mentally scattered rarely have the single-minded ability to focus on what is happening now. These self-same individuals also have a related problem of being unable to string together quality workouts and as a result, fail to establish real momentum.

There is a fierceness of concentration that the athletic elite effortlessly muster that allows them to do more than they are actually capable of. This is a learned skill and improves with time. Learn to focus in on the individual training session. Become hyper-aware of your surroundings, be it in the gym or outside. Concentration increases in direct proportion to the decease of internal chatter. This inky film of continual, *unceasing* thought prevents clear perception of what is actually occurring in the immediate present. An elite athlete has taught himself to focus totally and completely on the immediate athletic task at hand. So should you. Don't be talking to your neighbor while lifting weights or doing cardio. Please try and get psyched up prior to the heaviest set of a particular exercise. Learn how to conjure up alert concentration.

Mental chatter needs to be minimal and external chatter nonexistent. Please, no talking while working out. How are you going to get fired up for the top set of dumbbell bench presses if you're over at the water cooler yapping about how Tom got screwed on American Idol? Beware the seductive lure of *talking* about fitness and training instead of actually doing it—talking about training in a heated and engaged way is an energy leak of epic proportion. It is great to be liked and be social, but performance suffers in direct proportion to how much you engage in gab during your precious time in the gym. Take energy leakage seriously.

Can you take athletic efforts seriously enough to make changes in how you conduct yourself during the workout? Once you are able to develop real focus and concentration, performance skyrockets. Improved results equate to more muscle mass and less body fat. When you are out and about, try and pay attention to your surroundings. Henri Troyat said of Leo Tolstoy "He went through life with his eyes wide open, his nostrils flared and his ears pricked." So should we all. Tolstoy wasn't preoccupied. He would have seen the goat *before* they ran it over and he damn sure would have seen the hawk circling overhead.

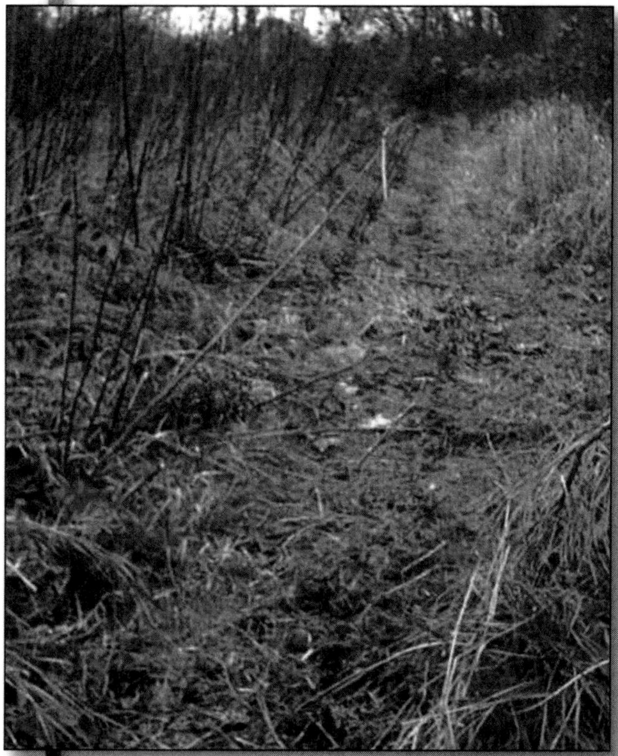

Where is Waldo? I have taken to placing a red fishing bobber somewhere along the mountain pathways I most frequent. When clients come up, part of our Fitness Day Camp is an intense hike on the steep trails that crisscross the Catoctin Mountains.

At the start of our power-walk I inform them that there is 'no talking' and further, anyone who finds the red bobber while we are on our hour long, lung-searing hike will win a prize. I will forgo my fee and the entire day is free. They all light up at that and off we go. Their visual searching for the bobber initially keeps them in exactly the right concentrated mindset: outwardly silent, inwardly silent, searching intently. Since the bobber is "hidden in plain sight" towards the end of the hike, their communal concentration has long since evaporated by the time we pass over it. Real concentration is quite draining.

Needless to say, no one yet has found the red fishing bobber. As soon as we pass it, I stop them and point it out to them. It lies big as life right in the middle of the trail. As soon as I point it out they all go, 'How could I have possibly missed that?!' I sincerely hope that someone finds the red bobber. I suspect the person that does will already be a physical and psychological adept.

PURPOSEFUL LAYOFFS

He came, He saw, He capitulated

—Winston Churchill

People often ask me how they should train while away on vacation. That presupposes that I would insist they should train while on vacation. My counterintuitive advice surprises them: why not synchronize a *purposeful layoff* from training while on vacation?

If you are due for a vacation, if you are going on an extended business trip, or coming up on a period where for whatever reason physical training will be difficult, cumbersome, inappropriate or impossible—why not plan ahead and plan to *not* train! Planning not to train sounds like a contradiction in terms, but it is not.

Elite athletes routinely 'cycle' periods of complete rest as a regular part of their periodized training regimen. Why not purposefully redouble the training effort leading up to the vacation and while on vacation avoid training altogether? Rest and heal the body fully and completely and then jump back in the mix (physically and psychologically rested and reinvigorated, ready for action) after the vacation?

One strategy I use repeatedly is to push hard, heavy and often in the Steel House during the month leading up to the vacation. Peak out, perhaps get a little burned out, err towards too much training then forget all about *resistance* training while vacationing. This approach is hardly heretical stuff rooted in laziness, sloth or lack of dedication. Competitive athletes always lay off after a major competition in order to allow the body to recover from the pounding they have subjected it to leading up to the event. Every elite athlete and coach knows that the human body cannot be trained all-out year round. Periodically there need to be purposeful layoffs. The post-competition layoff creates a necessary contrast to the intense physical and psychological preparation leading up to the event. A layoff 'detunes' the body; purposefully relaxing it physiologically and psychologically inducing a heightened state of readiness.

This is a good thing.

Progress is never an unbroken graph line pointed ever upward. Psychologically the mind also needs a chance to heal. Competitive preparation is stressful and intense; in the weeks and days leading up to a competition, an athlete thinks of little else and this mental single-pointed focus takes a terrific psychological toll. Like any other over-trained muscle, the brain loses its freshness and alertness in the post-competition let down. Regardless if the athlete has exceeded expectations, or tanked and done terribly, psychologically he/she is a mess. Trying to maintain anywhere near the training intensity built up for the event after the event is a surefire recipe for injury.

Better to rest the body, rest the brain and once recovered, jump back into the mix—but jump back in using lower overall training volume and lower overall training intensity. After a healing layoff it is time to start the purposefully slow and deliberate ramp-up procedure for the next event.

Rookies and novices find all this counterintuitive. "Won't I lose everything I've worked so hard to achieve? Won't all my gains disappear?" The obsessive-compulsive types that cannot stand to vary the training volume and intensity invariably hit the "sameness wall." The sameness wall is an insurmountable barrier. The sameness wall occurs when the trainee insists on training when a layoff is in order.

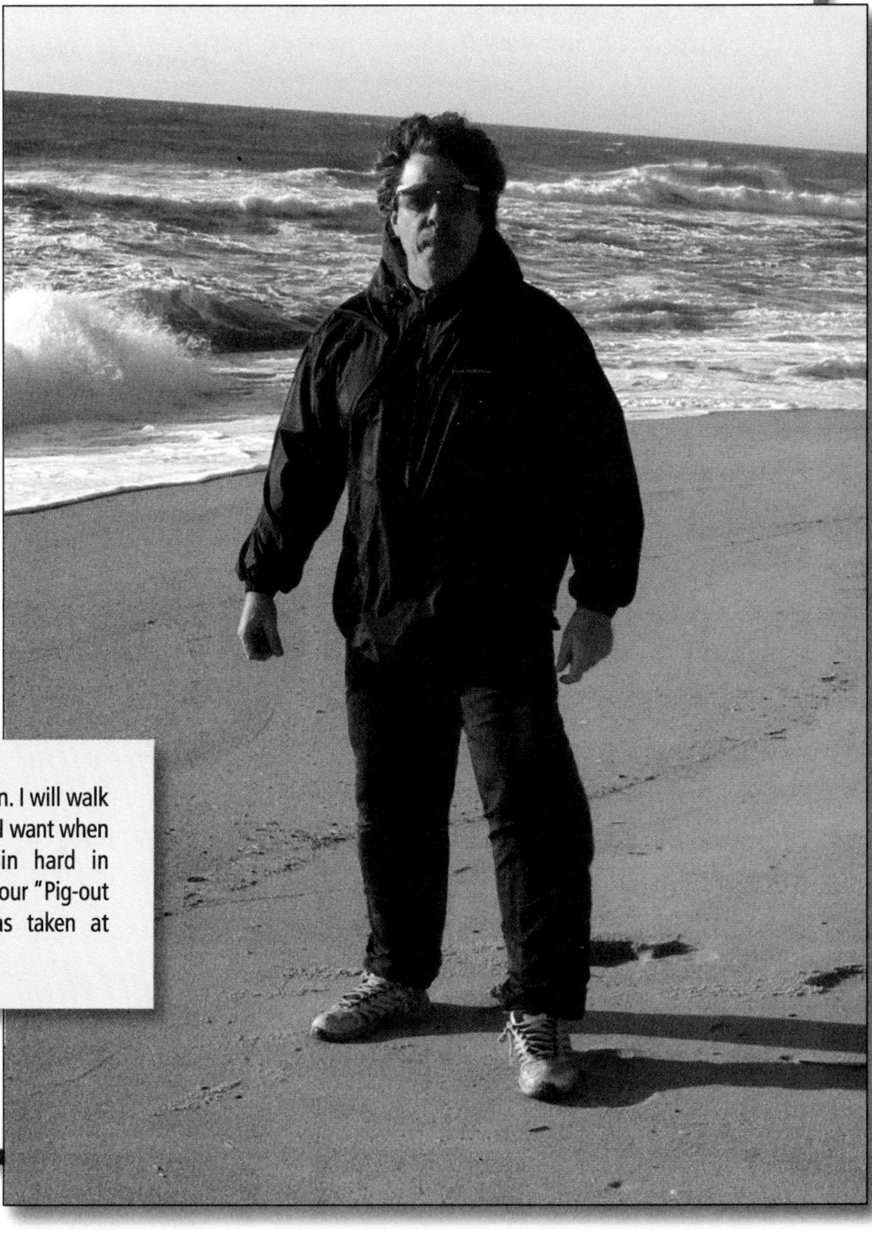

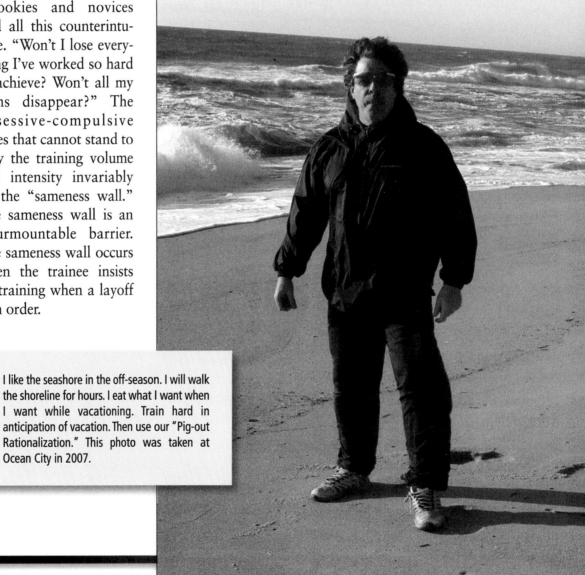

I like the seashore in the off-season. I will walk the shoreline for hours. I eat what I want when I want while vacationing. Train hard in anticipation of vacation. Then use our "Pig-out Rationalization." This photo was taken at Ocean City in 2007.

Unwilling or unable to stop, the compulsive athlete continues to train all year and ignores the fact that all measurable and quantifiable progress has totally ceased. This type usually incurs some sort of injury attributable to a combination of overwork and fatigue. Burnout and inertia are the constant companions of the obsessive-compulsive fitness devotee: too much of a good thing is never a good thing.

Elite competitors want the body to get slightly 'out of shape' so that when they begin anew, the renewed training program will produce "the training effect." In the olden days, my first mentor, John McCallum, referred to this as "softening up for gains." It was, and is, a deliberate strategy.

Once you are peaked out, the best thing you can do is cease and desist training for a proscribed period of time. Again, this is all predicated on the foregone conclusion that after the purposeful layoff you will get back on the training bandwagon.

If you are peaked-out, burned-out and over-trained, you need to take some time off. If you've gone in a particular training direction as far as you can go and gains have ceased, then a planned layoff is appropriate and actually stimulates progress in the long run. Obviously if you are lollygagging along, engaging in half-ass, halfway pretend training, you can use the "softening up for gains" approach as an excuse to become even more slothful. You are a fool fooling yourself.

Taking a layoff after a peak period of intense physical training has a liberating effect on the body and the mind. Better yet, if the planned training sabbatical is synchronized with a wonderful vacation at some remote location, it can be a fun and exciting experience. Enjoy friends and family without the compulsive-obsessive behavior that mars interaction with others. "I'd loved to go to the boardwalk with you guys, but I have to find a gym and train legs for two hours." Besides for most people vacations usually become one long extended cardio session. I always seem to end up walking my legs off going hither and yon, running or romping, being super active with some sort of water-related or nature-related vacation activity. While on vacation I love seeing, doing, enjoying, partying and moving about. Who sits in their hotel room while on vacation? I love eating more and trying different foods. I worry less and I forget all about barbells, dumbbells, progress and my "quest."

Oddly, towards the end of any vacation, my thoughts invariably turn towards training since I really enjoy it. By forcing myself to not train, other than vacation-related cardio activities, I build up a real desire to get back into weight training. By the time I get back to the real world, I am positively itching to commence some serious iron slinging once again. Now I am rested and ready and psychologically hungry: I'm fired up. I always make fantastic gains in that post-vacation period. My biggest concern is jumping back into the training mix too hard, too heavy, and too often and then crippling myself because of my over-the-top enthusiasm.

So when I get these questions relating to how best to train while on vacation, my first thought is, "Don't train!" If you have been hitting it hard and intense, why not blow it off altogether? Now let's loop back around to our original premise: Lazy or smart choice? It all depends on how you spend that last month leading up to that vacation.

BRAIN TRAIN FEATS AND TACTICS

I once wrote an article on psyche-up tactics for weight training in *Muscle & Fitness* Magazine and in response Jeff Everson wrote that you "don't have to read Plato before a set of triceps kickbacks." I'm pretty sure this barb was aimed at me. In my book on the incredible Ed Coan, I wrote that while getting your mind right was not all that important on the little stuff, like a set of triceps kickbacks, on the top set of a really heavy exercise using limit poundage, being centered and in the moment, undeniably helped performance. This is what Arnold called "the heightened arousal mode"

Every single top athlete I've ever had the pleasure of working with has some method of getting themselves psyched-up for a big gym effort. The top guys are the top guys because they have an ability to mentally force their body to perform beyond its awesome actual capacity. There is no handbook or single mental technique that is universally used and each of the iron elite has developed their own individualized psyche-up tactic. One of the best athletes I ever saw in action was the great John Kuc, a multi-time World Powerlifting Champion and a guy built all wrong for the sport. To be a really great powerlifter requires you have thick muscle density in relation to your height. Top powerlifters are heavy and thick, squat and stocky. The best powerlifters are short in relation to their bodyweight. Thickness and bulk provide incredible leverage. In a time when a top 242 pound lifter stood maybe 5'7" Kuc stood a basketball player-like 6'1". He looked positively skinny. With his thinning hair and lean look he seemed more like a college professor than a power dominator. Much of his dominance could be traced to his ability to put himself into a trance state that bordered on psycho.

I remember in the late 70's watching Kuc come out for a World Record deadlift of 852 pounds. With bugged-out eyes and an odd stutter-step gait, he looked like a zombie in Dawn of the Dead. He looked menacing and possessed. The barbell was loaded and he was making his way to the platform to attack the weight when some goofy official stepped in front of him and asked some asinine question. I doubt Kuc even saw the guy. He was so deep into his psyche space that his mad eyes drilled holes through him. Kuc's crazed eyes made Charles Manson's famous killer stare look like a high school yearbook photo of a sci-
-

ence club nerd by comparison. He said not a word and refused to acknowledge the man's existence because taking an instant to say, "Get the hell out of my way, little clown man, before I rip off your head and piss down your neck!" would have shattered his carefully constructed psyche as surely as throwing a glass figurine against a concrete wall.

Pompous and imperious (as some officials are) the blazer-clad butterball took offense and asked once again, this time in more insistent voice. He was determined he would have a piece of Kuc's spotlight. He knew all eyes in the packed auditorium were on John and by default on the official who was inserting himself into Kuc's orbit with his frivolous inquiry. The second request was forceful and indignant; the official *would* have his answer and if that destroyed the delicate strands of Kuc's gossamer spider-web psyche, then so be it.

Another elite lifter, watching in awe from the immediate vicinity, caught the gist of what was happening and without a second thought unceremoniously and violently jerked the hapless glory hog in his blue blazer by

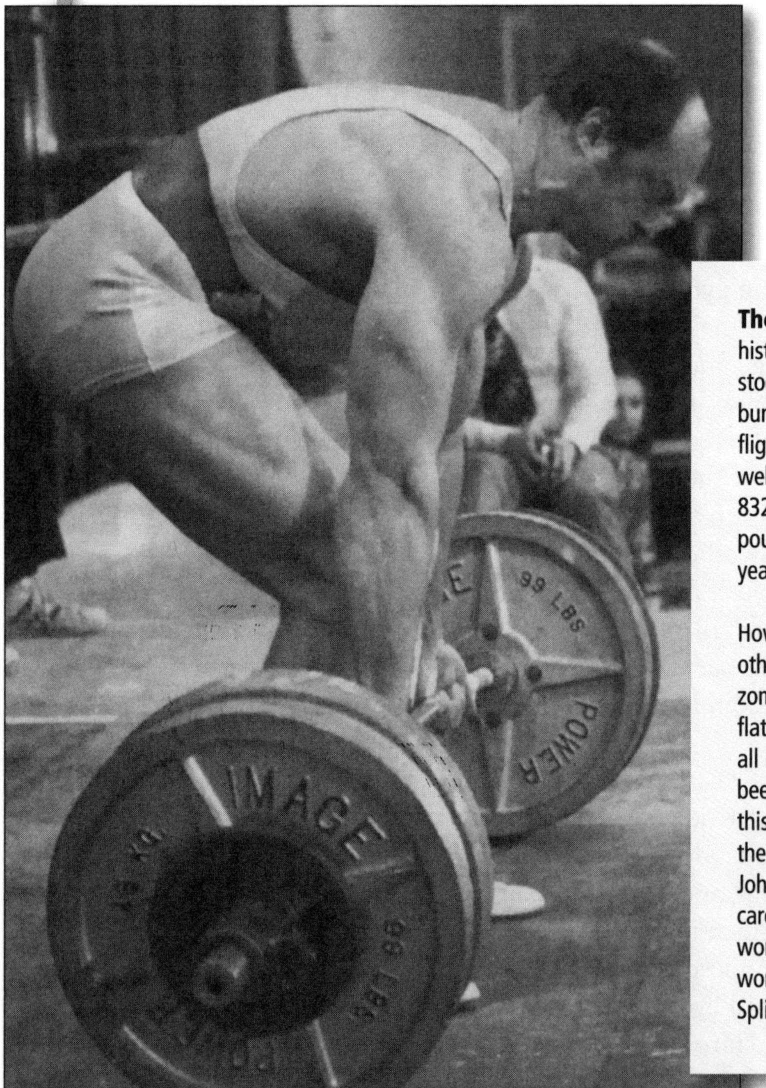

The Iron Bumblebee: Mind Master John Kuc launches his historic 871 pound deadlift weighing 239. This World Record stood for 19 years. Kuc was the lifting equivalent of the bumblebee: Physicists insist the bumblebee is incapable of flight—power experts would insist that there is no way a man well over 6 feet tall weighing a mere 240 pounds, could squat 832, bench 500 without a shirt and deadlift 871 for a 2204 pound World Record total. The total record also stood for 19 years.

How did Kuc's bumblebee achieve flight? I suggest it was his other-worldly psyche abilities. He could morph into a psycho-zombie capable of strolling through brick walls in two minutes flat. Ferocious, fearless, fanatical, frenzied, scary and awesome, all at the same time, John Kuc was an Iron Immortal and had I been able to contact him, I would have proudly included him in this book as a featured athlete. He was the training partner of the greatest bench presser of all time, Jim Williams. Big Jim and John trained at the Scranton YMCA. At the beginning of his career, young Kuc pushed his bodyweight up to 340 pounds. He won the World Title then reduced his weight down to 240 and won the world title again. Astonishing! "Walk on Guilded Splinters!"

the scruff of the neck, ripping him out of Kuc's zombie path. He shook the little man like a rag doll. Kuc, now unimpeded, walked on by, lost in his Private Idaho where the mind wills the body to do that which it is incapable of doing. He strode to the barbell while the audience screamed encouragement he did not hear. He pulled the barbell effortlessly to lock out.

It was a great example of athletic psyche. It also portrayed the reverence other lifters have for a psyche-up-in-progress. It is totally taboo amongst those in the know to walk up to a lifter prior to an all-out attempt and make small talk. More than once I've seen ignorant gym rats stroll up to an elite lifter readying prior to a set of, oh say, 705x5 in the deadlift, only to be roughed up by the lifter's training partners. When a man is getting prepared for an assault on gigantic poundage they need to be prepared mentally and this requires utter and complete internal focus, free of all distraction. Other top lifters know this and woe unto any civilian, gym mullet or ignorant passerby who wanders up to a psyching lifter and asks, "HEY! Are you using this 5 pound plate?" Or my favorite, "How much longer are you going to be? I need to use the squat rack for my pathetic curls." I've seen mullets swatted over benches. I've seen 'em backhanded and dropped on the spot. I've seen 'em so traumatized and terrified they pissed their pants. I've seen 'em so frightened they left the facility and never returned.

If you would like to realize a 10 to 15% across-the-board performance bump, strictly through some applied brain train, develop a good psyche-up regimen. It will enable you to routinely squeeze out more reps and/or extra poundage. If you are casual about your weight training you'll reap casual results. If you are intense, focused and dead serious than....well, you know the rest.

WANT TO CHANGE YOUR PHYSIQUE? START BY CHANGING THE WAY YOU THINK

Psyche Up to Improve Workout Performance

Kirk Karwoski was pacing back and forth at the National Powerlifting Championships getting mentally prepared to lift. He would be attempting 1003 pounds for a World Record squat in the 275 pound weight class. As he paced back and forth, like a caged animal at the zoo, tears streamed down his face.

To the casual observer, it might have appeared something tragic had befallen this muscle-laden giant; had he just been informed of some catastrophic event? What calamity could bring this iron giant to tears? To the contrary, Karwoski's tears were tears of white hot rage; his tears were the tears of a crazed lunatic. He'd twisted himself into such a psychological frenzy that the tears that ran down his face were the tears of a berserker about to throw himself into battle and kill someone or something.

I was Kirk's coach and one of my many jobs was to keep at arms length all the well-wishers, glad-handers and anyone else who might disturb Karwoski's well-constructed psyche. He had purposefully put himself into this state of aggravated agitation on purpose; he knew a proper psyche-up was worth an additional 10-15% in performance. He wore a Walkman and listened to his favorite rock group play his favorite tune—over and over and over and over. He listened to the music and used it to exclude outside influences. He was working himself into a bug-eyed frenzy worthy of a Kamikaze pilot prior to dive bombing a U.S. carrier during the Battle of Midway. His was a carefully constructed competition psyche-up routine, one honed to psychological perfection for over a decade. He was a seven-time National, six-time World Powerlifting Champion, and in order to tackle the giant weights he needed to have his head screwed on just so.

His procedure was extremely formalized: he would walk exactly ten paces in one direction, wheel and walk ten paces in the other direction. He kept his head down, his eyes purposefully unfocused. He listened to the music; it was all a soundtrack to a movie that was running in his head: a movie of him squatting 1000 pounds perfectly. Over and over he would run the movie; an intense visualization of him and the weight. Each time he ran the movie the visualization grew clearer, more realistic and detailed. He ran the visualization over a dozen times in his head in the interlude between his previous successful squat, 963, done a few minutes ago, and this final World Record attempt.

By the time I signaled him that it was time for him to lift, Karwoski had worked himself into a barely controlled emotional state of fury and rage. Having acquired his crazed state of mind, he now would unleash his psychological Tsunami on the unsuspecting barbell. Wordlessly, he removed his Walkman, threw it into his gym bag. He had his training partner Nacho Del Grande wrap his knees. I pulled his lifting belt tight. He chalked his hands and strode onstage. He effortlessly shattered his own World Record by 40 pounds. This particular record, 1003 pounds, still stands as this is being written, twelve years later.

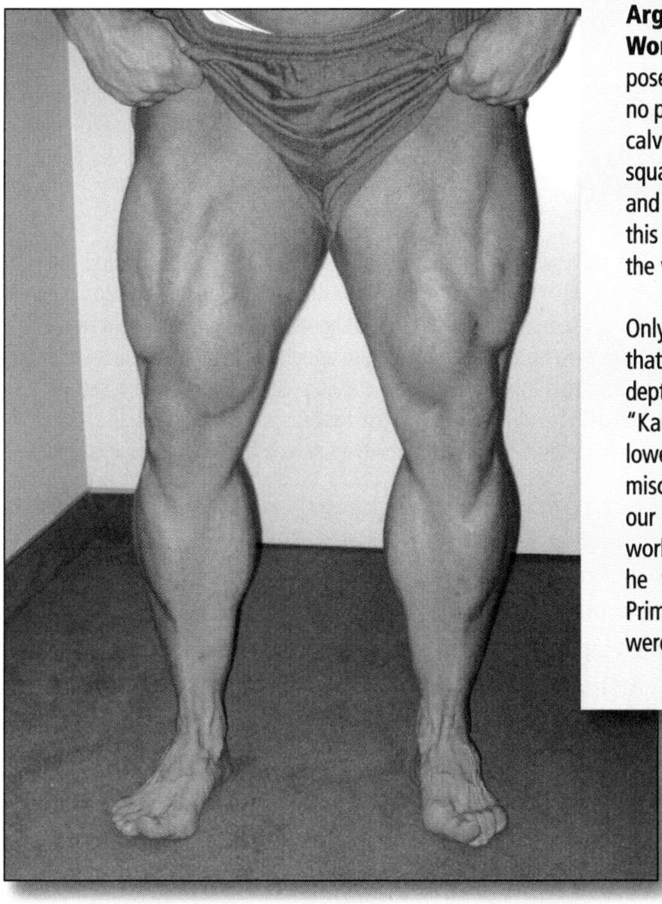

Arguably the Strongest Legs in the World: Kirk rolled out of bed and I made him pose for the photo on the left. Stone cold with no pump his thighs measured 33 inches and his calves 20.5 inches. A few hours later he squatted 826 pounds. He weighed 241 pounds and I think a strong case could be made that at this point in time he had the strongest legs in the world.

Only Ed Coan would be capable of handling that poundage taken to the extremely low depth at that bodyweight. As I told the tale in "Karwoski Remerges," the 826 was actually lower poundage than we had planned on. A miscue on his previous 804 caused us to lower our 840 projected 3rd attempt. Kirk and I have worked together for almost twenty years and he was and is the penultimate Purposeful Primitive. His focus and psyche-up abilities were otherworldly.

Technical Perfection: Later that same day, here is how low Kirk rode 826. This photo tells you everything you need to know about the low position of a perfect squat. His hips are well below the tops of the knees. Also note how his left knee is directly atop the ankle of his left foot and his right knee is slightly out of position. As a result of this imbalance he experienced a quad tear in this leg on his ascent. Note the upright position of the torso and bar position in relation to the hips. Snapped at the exact instant descent becomes ascent, a fraction of a second later he would throw his head back in conjunction with his upward thigh thrust. His hips will stay beneath the torso and shoulders as he initiates leg drive. Pure push perfection. Kirk had an ability to psyche himself into rage states.

Do you have to work yourself into a state of bug-eyed frenzy with tears streaming down your face before attempting a new personal record with 150 for 10 repetitions in the bench press? Certainly not—however, employing some rudimentary mental tactics and having a real psyche-up procedure in your mental trick bag can add 5-10% to your efforts. Handling more poundage or squeezing out extra repetitions in training equates to a vastly improved physique. Take a tip from a psychological berserker and take lifting seriously: casually approaching a limit attempt makes no sense from a performance or safety standpoint: be serious and be respectful. Get psyched!

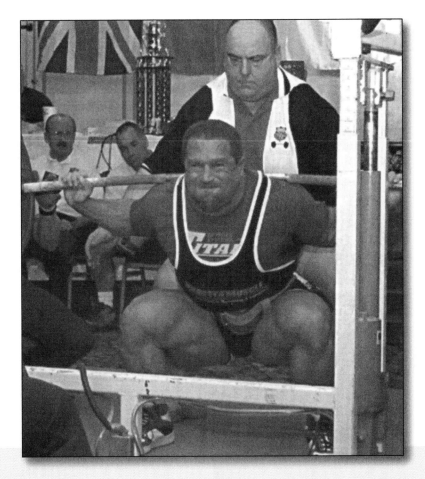

Cardio Masters

The human heart doesn't care <u>how</u> it gets elevated – just as long as it <u>gets</u> elevated.

—Iron Master Bill Pearl

Purposefully Primitive Cardiovascular Exercise

Like everything else in the world of fitness, aerobic exercise has been made way more complex than necessary. The human innards, our guts, our internal organs, need exercise as surely as our muscles. What's the best way to exercise, strengthen and build our internal mechanisms? Systematically increase the heart rate and hold it there for a specific and protracted period of time. That's pretty damned simple. Aerobic exercise done consistently strengthens the muscles involved in respiration and actually enlarges the heart muscle. That's a good thing.

A stronger, larger heart has a radically increased pumping ability and far greater stroke efficiency. The arterial pathways are cleared of plaque and sludge as the elevated heart rate forcibly pumps torrents of enriched blood through the arterial highways at an accelerated rate. The resting heart rate decreases; circulation improves and blood pressure is reduced. Consistent cardio increases the total number of red blood cells in the body which helps the body become more efficient at the transport of oxygen. Aerobics also improves the ability of muscles to mobilize body fat during exercise and builds endurance. Improved endurance means we are able to work harder, longer, more often and recover quicker.

Over time the storage capacity of energy molecules (fats and carbohydrates) within the muscles is increased. Over time when subjected to specific cardio training protocols, the muscles actually reconfigure their composition, increasing mitochondrial density. More mitochondria (cellular blast furnaces) means improved energy processing ability: nutritents are utilized with far greater efficiency. After a torrid aerobic session, the basal metabolism is dramatically stimulated and remains elevated for hours afterward. Incredible physiological benefits are bestowed on the conscientious trainee if cardiovascular exercise is performed on a regularly reoccurring basis.

Mr. Analogous Strikes Again

My wife calls me "Mr. Analogous" and in keeping with that title I describe the body's cardiovascular component parts as analogous to engine parts: imagine that the human body is a supercharged racing engine…perhaps a 426 Chrysler Hemi with two four barrel 650 cm Holley carburetors set atop a 6-71 GMC supercharger. The carburetors are the equivalent of the lungs and take in oxygen from the atmosphere. The oxygen is mixed with fuel in the carburetors and sent to the supercharger that serves the same purpose as the human heart: both supercharger and heart muscle are *pumps* that push fuel/nutrients to the engine/muscles. The supercharger/heart muscle pumps oxygenated fuel, oxygenated, nutrient-laden blood, to the cylinders that are analogous to muscles.

The cylinders/muscle cells are where the actual work is done. In both cases energy fusion occurs and waste products are created as a result of violent acts of combustion. Within the cylinders in the engine and within the mitochondrial cells of the muscles, energy is produced and waste products must be efficiently eliminated through an exhaust procedure. Optimally the lungs, heart and muscles work in close synchronization during cardiovascular exercise. If the balance is thrown off the body shuts down. Often during cardiovascular exercise we *purposefully* seek to put the body off balance by zeroing in on the heart, lungs or muscles exclusively. We seek to impose cardio stress using different methods in order to elicit differing cardio responses. The purposeful creation of cardio imbalance creates differing cardio effects.

- *Steady-state* cardio is when heart, lungs and muscles operate in synchronous balance.
- *Interval* cardio purposefully disturbs the balance in order to spike the heart rate.
- *Hybrid* cardio adds an element of muscular intensity to aerobics and creates new mitochondria.

Many Roads Lead to Cardio Rome

The Purposefully Primitive cardio adherent utilizes a periodized cardio game plan that lasts for 4 to 12 weeks. During the designated time period the individual stair-steps their way upward into ever-improving degrees of cardio condition. Using creeping incrementalism we start off slightly below capacity and over the 4 to 12 week timeframe ease our way into ever better physical condition. We are able to go longer, faster and more often; we reduce body fat as our endurance and vitality improves weekly.

Close coordination of cardio exercise with a solid diet plan creates continual "windows of opportunity" that result in stored body fat being mobilized and preferentially burned as energy. We create these windows through the expert use of exercise and dietary timing. Over time the cardio exercise effort gains more and more traction. The more cardio you perform the better your endurance becomes, the better an individual's endurance the longer, faster and more we can train. More training equates to more progress. All these factors combine to create momentum.

There are three separate and distinct cardio types and periodic rotation of the three types within the training template is required. Variety keeps cardio fresh, vital and fun. Human nature seeks to repeat pleasurable experiences and avoid unpleasant ones; so we make cardio both effective and enjoyable. Cardiovascular creativity enables us to develop a deep love for aerobic activity. As pointed out earlier, you can see a lot further and a lot clearer standing on the shoulders of a true giant. You can see over the vision-obscuring fog of conventional thinking that rolls along at ground level. While standing atop the shoulders of a giant you are able to see over the product pushing pygmies, the charlatans, hucksters and hordes of fitness frauds frantically waving their puny arms to attract your attention. Fitness frauds continually obscure clear viewing at ground level.

Let's get straight on our cardio facts. We start by absorbing some unvarnished truths spoken by a true cardio giant. Cardio is not an option and the key to conquering cardio is learning to love it.

Getting Our Cardio Facts Straight

Fitness product makers compete for market share in the never-ending quest to persuade consumers to purchase their particular product. "Hey look at me! I've got a revolutionary new device that will melt fat off you faster than you can say abracadabra! You'll lose ten inches off your waistline in two weeks!" This type of outright fraud is commonplace in fitness. Product makers continually make outrageous claims for products that can't possibly deliver 1/10 of what they promise. Their claims are physiological impossibilities. The product pushers feel the only way they can attract attention or differentiate their mode, device or method from other vendors is to make ludicrous claims. Adolf Hitler defined this sales strategy in *Mein Kampf* "A big lie is easier to get the public to believe than a little lie." Fraud merchants promise quick and easy physical transformation using whatever it is they are selling.

Meanwhile I have the unenviable task of convincing you that you need to get back to the cardio ultra basics that you likely never learned to begin with.

Aerobic activity is indispensable for health and wellbeing. Cardiovascular results are the quickest to appear and the quickest to disappear. Whereas resistance training gains are slow to appear, they are slow to disappear. Strength gains stay with the trainee long after he ceases training. Aerobic activity bestows its numerous benefits almost immediately, yet the downside is that benefits flee as quickly as they appeared once the trainee stops training. We use this phenomenon to our advantage. We generate immediate momentum and infuse enthusiasm into the process by performing cardio every day. Quick cardio progress jump-starts the transformational process; we feel great, both physically and psychologically, in a matter of days.

In order to engage in a sensible and result producing cardiovascular program you need to purchase a heart rate monitor. This is the lone hi-tech device we Purposeful Primitives endorse wholeheartedly. We will show you how to use this incredible tool in a manner even the makers didn't envision.

The heart rate monitor allows us to assess cardiovascular intensity and cross-compare exercise modes. We use the monitor to determine which modes are effective and those modes that are a complete waste of training time. The systematic rotation of modes and methods is mandatory. The body will neutralize the beneficial effects of *any* exercise protocol to which it is continually subjected. By varying the kind and type of cardio exercise we engage in, we keep the body off balance and that is a good thing when the name of the game is steady physical progress.

Integrate aerobics with resistance training and underpin the training with a rock solid nutrition program. Our goal is to ignite physical synergy: a unique physiological state that elite athletes are intimately familiar with. How do we start? First establish and identify realistic goals. Then set these goals into a timeframe. Break the goal into weekly performance benchmarks. Systematically set about achieving the weekly goals. It is a relatively easy task to design a customized cardiovascular plan, one that melds with your lifestyle and available training time.

- Establish a realistic goal
- Set the goal within a specific timeframe
- Reverse engineer results: work backwards establishing weekly performance benchmarks

Weekly goals are established. Weekly goals are achieved in three cardio benchmarks: frequency, duration and intensity. Other sub-categories can also be periodized.

Each week we inch ahead, using the theory of creeping incrementalism. Log results and continually refer back to predetermined goals: where *are you* in relation to *where should you be*? How is ever-unfolding reality comparing to the predetermined game plan? If a systematic cardiovascular regimen is sensibly coordinated with precision nutrition, body fat is mobilized and oxidized. We expropriate elite bodybuilder nutritional tactics and meld them with specific cardio protocols; the goal is to systematically "trick" the body into mobilizing and melting stored body fat.

Unfortunately most fitness experts have a collective cardio blindspot: they are ignorant of, or refuse to acknowledge altogether, one critical aspect of cardiovascular exercise: *aerobic intensity*, i.e. how fast does the heart beat in relation to exercise-induced physical stress. Fitness experts and personal trainers have become needlessly entangled in a spider web of cardio confusion wherein exercise *mode* is confused with cardio *goal*. Most experts champion a particular mode or device and lose sight of the goal: as mentor Bill Pearl once said, "The human heart doesn't care *how* it gets elevated, just as long as it *gets* elevated." That is a profound and liberating aerobic insight. Does the mode selected successfully elevate the heart rate to the predetermined target? If the answer is yes than that mode is deemed effective. This all presupposes you actually have a predetermined target heart rate and the ability to monitor it.

While anal-retentive personal trainers make nuanced distinctions about miniscule aspects of resistance training and split infinitesimal hairs over the science of nutrient selection—most remain stridently, defiantly, belligerently ignorant or downright dismissive about a critical element of the cardio report card: the trainee's heart rate during the actual exercise. An obese trainee forced to jog could be operating way past the safety redline, perhaps at 110% of their age-related heart rate maximum. Blind-spot personal trainers ignorant of this critical piece of data exhort the obese to, "Go faster! Pick up those knees!" and put at-risk clients in real danger. Most personal trainers do not monitor the heart rate during cardiovascular exercise.

Would you lift weights without knowing the poundage?

Of course not! So why would you perform cardio exercise without knowing the impact the exercise was having on the heart rate in real time? It's a classical example of arrogance cubed with wilful ignorance.

LEONARD SCHWARTZ, M.D.

Aerobic Avatar

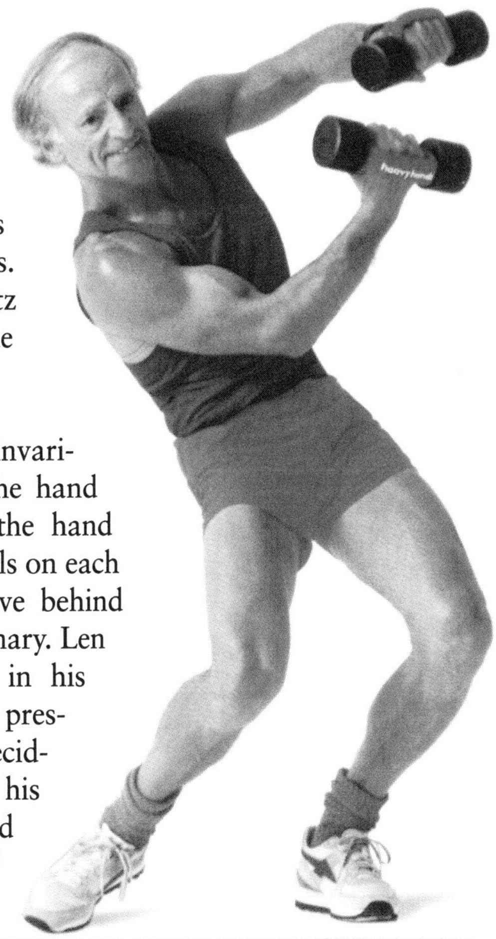

Leonard Schwartz is a medical doctor, psychiatrist, exercise researcher and inventor of *Heavyhands*. We have all seen joggers running along carrying little red hand weights. Those are Heavyhands and Len Schwartz invented these devices as adjuncts to his unique cardiovascular exercise system.

If you were to watch the Heavyhand jogger, invariably they use the hand weights incorrectly. The hand weights weren't meant to be *Carry Hands*, the hand weights were meant to be raised to different levels on each and every stride-stroke. The hand weights have behind them a system that is both radical and revolutionary. Len became interested in cardiovascular exercise in his fifties. An overweight smoker with high blood pressure and chronic back problems, Dr. Len was decidedly unfit and decided to do something about his own health and fitness. He became a jogger and found that wanting. He then immersed himself

"How much muscle do you want? Physiologists speak of 'excess' muscle, probably meaning the amount {of muscle} that encroaches on the efficiency of oxygen transport. Weight training is the best manufacturer of muscle. If you aspire to hulkish proportions, big weights lifted for low reps are the answer. There are few occupations, outside of competitive sport, that make good use of gargantuan strength...The best body, when it comes to good work, is the strongest, smallest body you can finesse through life. I'll lay odds that no single system can produce that as well as Heavyhands."

in the various fitness theories and strategies of the day and came away decidedly unimpressed. Being a medical doctor, he began accessing available research.

One day the proverbial light bulb went off over his head as he was investigating athletic VO_2 maximums. The highest VO_2 maximums ever recorded by a group of athletes were not registered by endurance runners, which is what he had logically presupposed before his investigations, but rather by Russian and Norwegian cross-country skiers. Why was this? He wondered. It didn't take long for him to come up with the answer: the skiers generated propulsion using all four limbs. The runners used only their legs.

The cross-country skiers were registering Maximal Oxygen Consumption rates, per kilogram of bodyweight per minute, of 94. The long distance runners were topping out at 85. Rowers came in a 75, bicyclists 70 and speed skaters 65. Everyone registered substantially below the skiers. The skiers propelled their bodies across the landscape using the legs and the arms on every single stride. While the majority of the aerobic world used two limbs, the legs, in their respective modes, the skiers were using *four limbs* to power locomotion. A cursory examination of the other sports and cardio activities revealed that most disciplines required only two limbs to generate propulsive movement.

Len wondered how he could recreate the quad-limb exercise form and reap the amazing cardiovascular benefits and endurance capacity of a cross-country skier. He began experimenting, imitating cross-country skiers "double pole action" by pumping small dumbbells while walking. The aerobic apple fell on the cardio Newton's head: Len was amazed at the aerobic effect of double-ski poling with dumbbells and soon envisioned a whole series of moves and patterns where he lifted light dumbbells to varying heights while walking, jogging, duck-walking, hopping or squatting.

The key was to force four limbs to "share" the aerobic workload. When legs alone were used to elevate the heart rate, the legs had to work considerably harder to attain, retain and sustain the target heart rate. How much easier it was to hit the same target heart rate when legs *and* arms were used in conjunction with one another. The athlete could generate an elevated heart rate quicker and maintain it longer when the workload was spread among four limbs. The work didn't seem as hard. While it might take considerable physical effort to reach a heart rate of 150 beats per minute running, it took far less effort to achieve the same heart rate jogging while simultaneously pumping light hand weights.

Len took his suspicions and suppositions to the University of Pittsburg sport laboratory where he was able to confirm scientifically everything he had suspected intellectually. He then went into the woodshed and developed a system—using hand weights in a series of freestyle movement patterns—that would replicate the huge VO_2 maximums that cross-country skiers were attaining. He codified and birthed an entirely new exercise system. This system would be efficient and deliver a multiplicity of results. It would teach Heavyhanders how to use varied movement patterns; these patterns done with certain poundage would have radically different results using increased or decreased poundage. Results would also be impacted by the session duration and frequency. The freestyle movement pattern possibilities were limitless. The poundage possibilities were limitless. A person moving a pair of 20 pound dumbbells short distances for 10 minutes would net far different results than a jogger throwing 2 pound hand weights head high for 60 minutes. Old and young, beginner and elite, fit and unfit, all could tailor custom routines that suited their needs, goals, capacity and degree of fitness. The possible combinations were limitless and the advanced user, once they understood the fundamentals of the system, would be able to devise their own workouts.

Heavyhands required no machine or device that locked the user into a specific motor pathway. The type of motion used could be altered in every single workout. Sessions could be conducted indoors standing in place, outdoors traveling over sidewalks or trails. You might use a short session with heavy weights, long sessions with light weights, short motions, exaggerated motions...the endless variety would eliminate boredom and the chance for repetitive motion injury. Heavyhands could inject a psychological aspect into exercise: Fun! After all, Leonard Schwartz was not only a medical doctor, but also a clinical psychiatrist.

Birth And Death Of An Exercise Craze

In 1982 Len published the best book on aerobic exercise ever written: *Heavyhands, The Ultimate Exercise*. He began selling customized Heavyhand weights. These were clever and needed: the handles kept the hand weights from slipping out of the user's grip, the padding kept sweat from messing up the grip and the adjustable weights allowed the user to start off using 1 pound weights and work upward.

For a while Heavyhands was a bona fide exercise craze and swept the country. The problem was subtle: though lots of people bought the hand weights, few read the book. In order to make the Heavyhand system work, the user needed to raise their arms to varying heights in order to elicit the desired cardio result. Len devised three height levels and the trainee was instructed to achieve a target height with every step. What happened was that people would buy the Heavyhands and carry them around. While Heavyhands was an extremely effective exercise system, Carry Hands was lame and ineffectual. People claimed that they weren't getting results and the craze petered out—which was too bad because a lot of people really needed what Heavyhands offered. It was a classical case of a very effective system dying because people refused to adhere to the ground rules.

Len's own transformation was mind-blowing and pointed out how effective the studied use of quad-limbed cardio exercise could be...

Age	50	57
Weight	147	132
Bodyfat%	15%	4%
Resting pulse	80	38
VO2 max Using legs	33 ml/kilo/min	60 ml/kilo/min
VO2 max Using arms	23 ml/kilo/min	70 ml/kilo/min
VO2 max Combining legs/arms	70 ml/kilo/min	90 ml/kilo/min

No cardio weakling, at age 71 I saw Len do 36 pull ups while holding his legs in the V position!

Len Sets Me Straight

I began conversing regularly with Len in the mid-nineties after I had interviewed him for several magazines. His medical background, the fact that he was a psychiatrist and exercise research scientist, gave us much to talk about. And talk we did, for years, several times a week, sometimes for hours. He was fascinated by my "short strength," my weightlifting and powerlifting prowess. He was genuinely interested in how my type of power was developed. In turn I quizzed him like a CIA interrogator working on a Guantanamo Detainee. I had cardio questions galore. He spun my head around. He took me to school and I was the willing student.

My motivation was to determine if athletes who did supplemental cardio training would benefit by substituting Heavyhands for classical aerobic modes. He taught me about oxygen pulse and how pulse accurately represents the effectiveness of heart and skeletal muscle working together in consort. METs (an abbreviation for metabolism) would tell us how much work was being done compared to resting. Oxygen pulse would tell us how efficiently oxygen was being transported at a variety of workloads. Cardiac output was one aspect of oxygen pulse—the other aspect was the rate at which muscles were able to consume oxygen.

> ***"The artery that feeds the muscle contains blood richer in oxygen than the vein that leads the same blood away from that muscle. If you measured arterial and venous blood for their respective oxygen content, you arrive at what is called the A-V Oxygen difference. Pump output and the A-VO2 difference determine oxygen pulse."***

He clued me into Heart-Skeletal Muscle Duets: what, he would ask, limits an individual's oxygen consumption ability, i.e., is the limiting factor the ability of the heart to deliver oxygen? Or is it the ability of the muscles to receive the oxygen? The answer varies person to person: with some individuals the "senders"—the lungs, heart, blood vessel and blood that feed the muscles—might be inadequate. While for other individuals the "receivers" might be deficient and the capacity of the senders would exceed the capacity of the receivers.

> ***"The elite marathoner runs at approximately 75% of his maximum workload capacity. A Heavyhand user can generate 50% of leg capacity, 50% of arm capacity and <u>exceed</u> the marathon runner's 75% of maximum capacity using legs only. This is why Heavyhands feels easier. Lots of units, each doing <u>less</u>, add up to more."***

Len pointed out that "First and foremost, Heavyhands is a heart conditioner." He drew attention to heart rate contractions and the effectiveness of those contractions at pumping oxygen-laden blood throughout the body. He also noted that by placing the arms under stress, measured as per unit of muscle weight and volume, arms can "out do" legs. Arms "have greater training potential; while leg endurance might be upped 10 to 25%, arm endurance can be increased by 100% or more through the use of Heavyhands. Arms are freer to move than legs and capable of swifter, more complex and less 'grooved' motion."

Being a psychiatrist he felt Heavyhand training could even improve intelligence. "The hands enjoy a denser network of connections with our brains than do the feet or legs. Hand work thus feeds into human intelligence more than less imaginative leg work." Len was the first to alert me that prolonged use of Heavyhands could literally reconfigure muscle tissue, morphing the actual composition of the working muscle by infusing it with additional mitochondria.

The trick to muscle fiber transformation was infusing the cardiovascular activity with an element of *resistance*. What if there was a type of strength, *long strength*, (he called it) that could develop significant power output and sustain this strength output for an extended period? Would this not, over time, result in the creation of muscle fiber that would have the anaerobic capability of a weightlifter *and* the aerobic capacity of a long distance runner? Heavyhands could split the difference. Training in this way would reconfigure existing muscle fiber, creating a new type of muscle fiber. Len Schwartz is a cardiovascular exercise genius by any yardstick or measurement you care to apply. Len devised a positively revolutionary system. It died an undeserved death bought on by misuse and misunderstanding.

Len Schwartz at age 75: Note the muscularity of the shoulders and arms. He was so lean, light and fit that his heart rate never elevated to any significant degree. He could engage in amazingly intense cardiovascular activity and his fit heart and small body would handle whatever stress he inflicted on it without any problem. He later experimented with free hand isotonometrics – pushing and pulling on his hands while exercising. I found this tactic particularly well suited for keeping a spiked heart rate elevated during high intensity power walking.

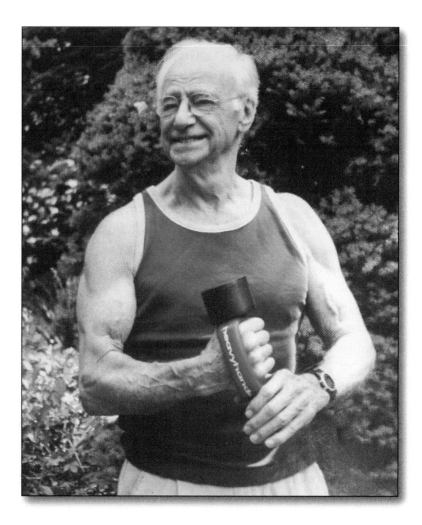

Cardio Methods

Muscle tissue is muscle tissue. A few minutes daily redirected towards cardio activity would quickly convert their {bodybuilders/powerlifters} muscle enzyme capabilities from 'one shot' to sustained performance. And give their hearts a steadied-out ride in the bargain.

—Dr. Len Schwartz

The Three Types of Cardio

The 1st Way: Steady-State

Pro

The Purposefully Primitive 1st Way of cardiovascular exercise is known as *steady-state,* or sustained cardiovascular exercise. The goal in steady-state is to attain, maintain and sustain an increased heart rate while moving along at a steady pace. Jog, swim, run, power walk—the mode is *less important* than the primary goal: elevate the heart rate to a predetermined level and keep it elevated in a sustained fashion for the duration of the session.

Regardless the selected cardio mode, be clear that the goal *is not* to become an expert jogger, runner or swimmer—those are spin off side benefits that naturally occur as a result of performing certain exercise modes on a consistent basis. The cardio goal is to *elevate the heart to a predetermined target level.* Steady-state, as the name implies, consciously seeks to attain a smooth and constant pace for the duration of the aerobic activity. Physiologically, the athlete motors along without triggering *oxygen debt.* The successful 1st Way practitioner operates just below the point where oxygen demand exceeds oxygen intake, thereby resulting in oxygen debt. The oxygen pulse should be balanced: "senders" (heart and lungs) need to be in perfect synchronization with "receivers" (muscles) as fresh, oxygen-laden blood is smoothly exchanged with toxic-laden blood full of waste products and lactic acid. The Soft Machine propels itself along smoothly and effortlessly, maintaining a delicate balance between senders and receivers.

1st Way cardio seeks to establish aerobic *efficiency.* Muscle contractions require oxygen and by staying relaxed the body achieves maximum oxygen efficiency. If the athlete tenses or flexes muscles as they propel themselves, oxygen demand is doubled. 1st Way cardio is exemplified by Kenyan long distance runners. These men glide as they run. Striding with complete relaxation, they skim along the surface of the earth; their footfalls barely leave a footprint or make a sound. They are able to glide along at 70% of their awesome maximum lung capacity all day long.

Con

Steady-state cardio, the 1st Way, is a valid arrow in the cardio quiver; another great tool in the exercise toolbox. Too many aerobic adherents use steady-state exclusively, to the complete exclusion of 2nd and 3rd Way aerobic practice. This is a major mistake.

1st Way cardio can become too efficient for its own good. Have you ever rode, strode or ran on a cardiovascular device or machine so ball-bearing efficient, so smooth that it was impossible to break a sweat or elevate the heart rate? Many aerobic machines and modes are too high-tech and too easy for their own good. Super efficient modes and machines used in steady-state style make it harder for the trainee to elevate their heart rate to the appropriate level; if they are even aware of the heart rate benchmark.

People that become exceedingly adept at 1st Way steady-state cardio exercise can, over time, learn how to run, walk, swim or bike in such a relaxed and technically efficient fashion, that as a heart rate elevator, as a calorie burner and metabolic elevator, steady-state becomes ineffectual. A steady diet of steady-state is not optimal. Beware the seductive honey trap of performing 1st Way steady-state cardio exclusively. We need some *inefficiency* in our cardio. Effortless steady-state, particularly on effortless cardio machines, results in negligible results. The body learns how to become efficient at cardio exercise and that needs to be recognized and avoided.

1st Way steady-state is ideal for a beginner. For advanced trainees, 1st Way needs to be in continual rotation with 2nd and 3rd Way cardio. Steady-state is the basis upon which all future aerobic efforts are built. Just don't make a religion out of it and don't use one particular mode to the exclusion of all others!

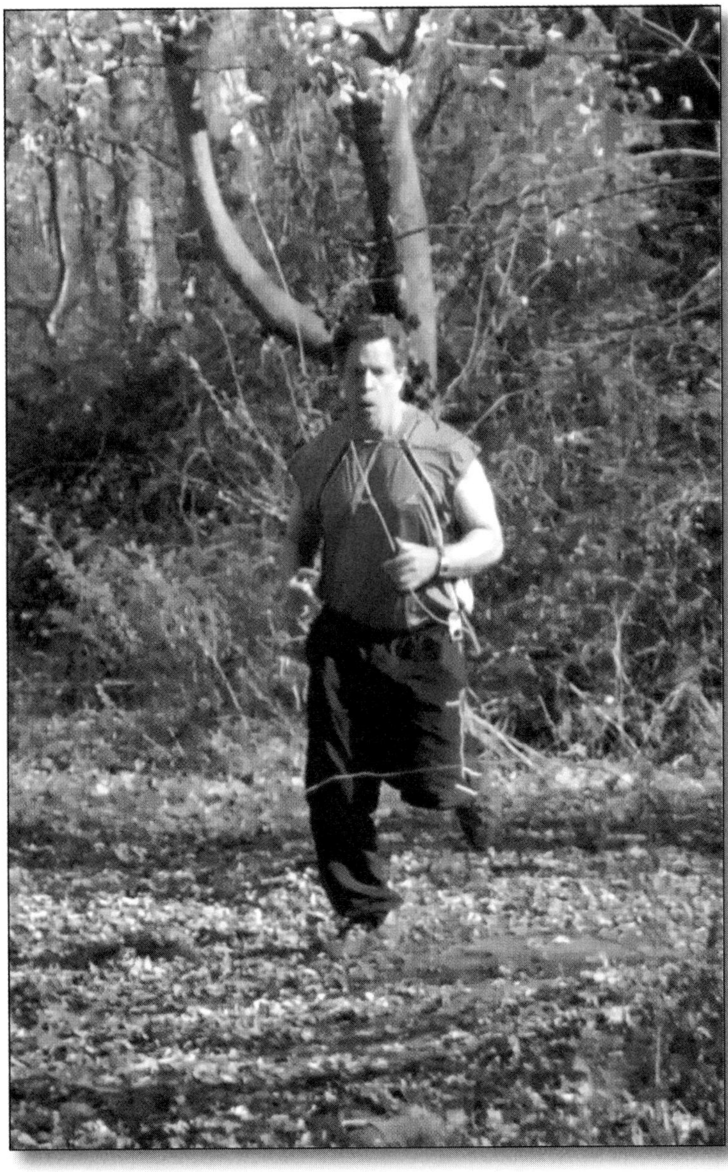

Steady-State propulsion through the woods: I seek to maintain 80% of my age-related heart rate maximum. If I spike to 90% I stop and allow lactic acid pools to dissipate and heart and lungs to resynchronize. When my monitor indicates I've dropped to 80% (130 beats per minute) I hit it again. Optimally I cruise along at a perfect 80% for the entire 40-60 minutes. I love two hi-tech devices: the heart rate monitor and my iPod; the latter provides a cardio soundtrack…transcendental altered-state surrealism.

The 2nd Way: Burst or Interval

Pro

Burst or interval cardio purposefully injects an element of *muscular effort* into cardiovascular activity. Classical Burst Cardio occurs when the trainee purposefully speeds up during an aerobic activity. Short bursts of intense effort are used to spike the heart rate upward quickly and dramatically. The 2nd Way cardio session is a series of bursts interspersed with rest periods or radical reductions in cardio effort. You could, for example, sprint for X number of yards, then walk or jog until breathing normalizes before sprinting again. Sprint, recover, sprint, recover...alternating intense effort and periods of recovery for the duration of the session.

2nd Way burst cardio possibilities are limitless: sprint, swim, shadow box, run or hike up steep grades, wrestle, grapple, play a torrid game of basketball, racquetball or football, jump, leap, climb...any imaginable activity that spikes the heart rate dramatically is Burst Cardio. You allow the heart rate to simmer back down then spike it again. Elite athletes use the heart rate monitor and spike the heart rate to 95/105% of age-related heart rate maximum before allowing the heart rate to drop back down to 70/80% before bursting again.

2nd Way aerobics always includes an element of muscular effort. The cardiovascular system is purposefully pushed passed capacity, then granted a short reprieve to regroup before another burst assault. This type of activity creates tremendous oxygen debt due to the incredible muscular effort. Muscles require oxygen to contract and we purposefully engage in activities that take us into oxygen debt. Rather than avoiding oxygen debt as in 1st Way, we force the body to cope and adapt. Burst cardio is powered by fast twitch muscle fiber and is particularly appropriate for athletes engaged in sports that require bursts of speed. Be sure core muscle temperature is raised before bursting. Tendons, ligaments and muscles are far less likely to pull, tear, rip or shear when warm then if forced to burst when muscles are cold.

Con

Another valid arrow in the cardio quiver. If the rest intervals between bursts are too long, the cardio effects are diluted. 2nd Way burst cardio is particularly effective if a heart rate monitor is used to determine rest periods. When the heart rate falls back to a certain predetermined level, hit it again. There is no better use for a heart rate monitor than in 2nd Way Burst cardio. Burst as fast as possible, perhaps you spike to 100% + of age-related heart rate max before "tying up." You glance at the monitor and allow the HR to "simmer back down" to 70 or 80%. That's your signal to hit it again. Heart rate monitors allow you to compare and contrast one exercise mode to another.

You may *think* your interval activity in tennis is effective until you strap on the heart rate monitor and realize that the periods of time that elapse between intense and sustained volleys are too long and render the whole effort ineffective. On the other hand you might discover that by allowing yourself another minute between 40 yard sprints, muscle recovery increases dramatically and as a result you are able to sprint 20% faster on each individual effort.

Burst Cardio users should neither lollygag nor go too quickly.

If you don't allow enough time for muscles to clear toxins and waste products, the quality of the next burst is diminished. There is an optimal time to rest between efforts: too long dilutes the overall effect and too quick diminishes performance. Done properly, 2nd Way Burst Cardio has tremendous benefits. Assuming the nutrition is in balance, burst cardio causes the mobilization and oxidation of stored body fat as the basal metabolic rate is skyrocketed and remains elevated for hours after the cessation of the session. Certain personality types need to beware of the tendency to rest too long between efforts. Other personality types need to beware of the tendency to go too quickly. Make sure 2nd Way burst cardio is in your regular rotation! Wear a monitor to check rest periods and to cross compare various exercise modes.

Bursting up a 45-degree incline: By definition interval aerobics spike the heart rate. Burst cardio needs to include an element of muscular stress. Burst formats are limitless; swim, walk, sprint, leap, use weighted implements – mode is secondary to protocol – use exercise to purposefully, dramatically, radically elevate the heart rate. Allow the accelerated heart rate to "simmer down" to a predetermined "floor" then burst again. Here I am sprinting up a ¼ mile 45-degree mountain path. I spike to 180+ then stop and allow my HR to drop. I can drop 40 beats in a minute. Once I bottom out, I hit it again.

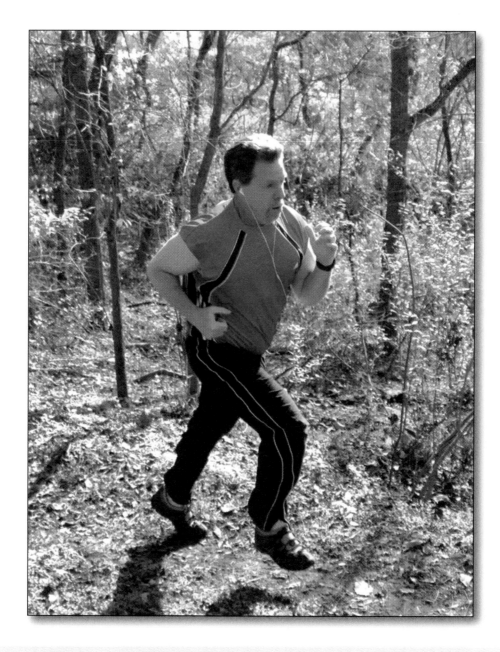

The 3rd Way: Hybrid

Pro

Hybrid cardio melds aerobics with strength training and in doing so reconfigures working muscles by adding mitochondrial density.

Len Schwartz, John Parrillo and Ori Hofmekler independently began advocating different exercise protocols, that each had the intended purpose of reconfiguring muscle composition.

I first sat up and took notice when in 1995 Dr. Len Schwartz began relating to me that he was working on a new type of exercise to develop "Long Strength." Among other positive attributes, the Long Strength exercise protocol would reconfigure the fiber composition of the working muscle. Over time the muscle would morph. By using Long Strength training tactics a muscle would acquire additional mitochondria, cellular blast furnaces. This I learned, was a good thing.

Quite on his own, John Parrillo began insisting that his fleet bodybuilders begin doing cardio with great intensity. He insisted that this would alter the composition of the muscle, causing the working muscles to add more mitochondria. He devised a resistance training program using a 100 rep extended set specifically designed to construct more muscle mitochondria. By building more cellular blast furnaces, "cardiovascular density" was increased and this resulted in the more efficient use of food/fuel. Nature's genetic growth limitations could be extended.

Ori Hofmekler spoke to me at length about his system of weight training, Controlled Fatigue Training, designed specifically to build a "hybrid muscle," a "super muscle" capable of generating sustained strength for long periods. CFT training would also, over time, reconfigure muscles by creating more mitochondria. Hofmekler was convinced that ancient warriors and early man had a preponderance of Hybrid Super Muscle. The ancients needed sustained strength *and* endurance for fighting, fleeing and rowing their massive boats for extended periods of time. When three of the smartest guys I know all feel the next frontier of modern fitness involves altering muscle composition, I pay attention.

How do you build 3rd Way hybrid muscle? Engage in aerobic sessions that have a strong element of resistance.

Con

3rd Way Hybrid Cardio requires a type of training that is both sustained and intense. Len, John and Ori all devised differing methods to arrive at the same destination: more muscle infused with more mitochondria. Technically we seek to create Type III Intermediate fast-twitch fibers; a cross between Type I and Type IIb. These hybrid fibers utilize both aerobic and anaerobic pathways for energy metabolism. To build mitochondria-infused super muscles requires the use of an extended, blended exercise protocol.

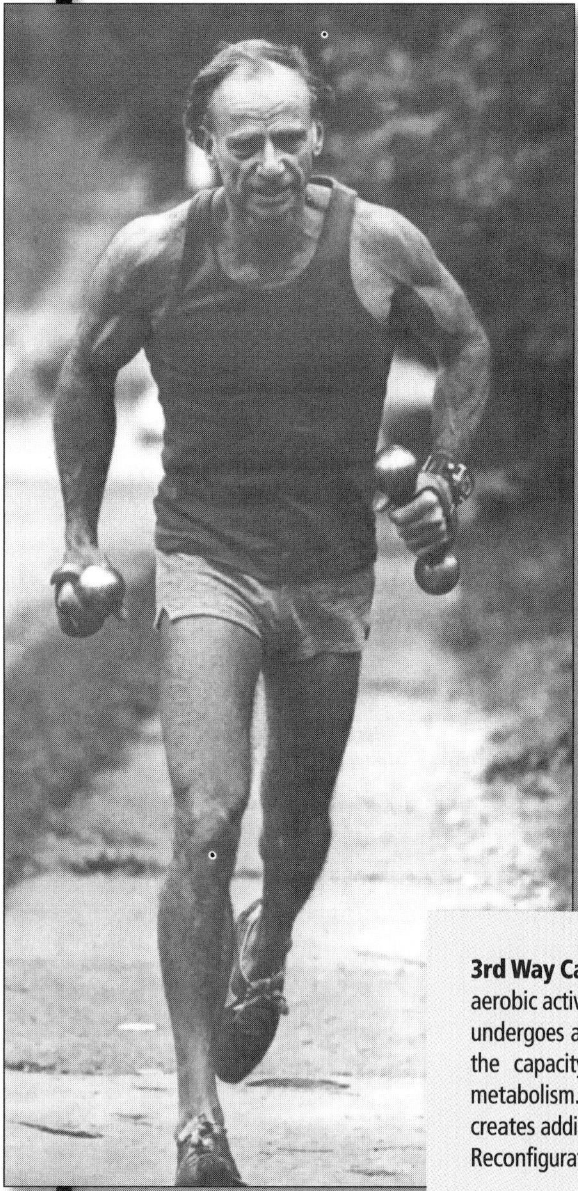

All three men devised training systems that required a muscle or group of muscles be worked for an extended time period with a maximum muscular effort. Len used his Heavyhand weights in combination with elaborate foot patterns to create quad-limbed stress. John used straight cardio done with maximum intensity or the 100 rep Giant Sets using standard weight training equipment. Ori's CFT utilizes pushing or pulling poundage or bodyweight for extended periods in an imaginative series of specific patterns. All three of these unorthodox exercise protocols force muscles to reconfigure.

The downside to the 3rd Way is that I find it incompatible with heavy weight training. By engaging in 3rd Way training I am unable to train for "absolute strength." I find recovery to be a problem and think that 3rd Way hybrid aerobic training needs to be practiced exclusively. I would suggest taking 4-6 weeks and practicing a 3rd Way routine to the exclusion of standardized resistance training. Mixed martial artists are converts to the

3rd Way Cardio Master in full flight: The goal of 3rd Way cardio is to blend aerobic activity with strength training. If properly executed existing muscle fiber undergoes a reconfiguration. A hybrid muscle fiber, Type III, is created that has the capacity to utilize both aerobic and anaerobic pathways for energy metabolism. Dr. Len calls this "long strength." A unique exercise protocol creates additional cellular mitochondria and improves cardiovascular "density." Reconfiguration requires aerobic activity include an element of muscular stress.

use of 3rd Way Hybrid cardio. To prevent "bonking" during fights they are infusing their cardio with a strength element: they flip tires, throw medicine balls, push weighted wheelbarrows and pound sledgehammers repeatedly to build sustained strength.

Muscle Fiber Nuts and Bolts

Type I

Type I muscle fibers are slow-oxidative fibers that primarily use cellular respiration. As a result, Type I fibers have (relatively) high endurance. To support their high-oxidative metabolism, these muscle fibers typically have lots of mitochondria and myoglobin. They appear red. In poultry Type I Fibers are the dark meat. Type I muscle fibers are found in muscles of animals that require endurance: chicken leg muscles, the wing-muscles of migrating birds. Long distance runners have leg muscles loaded with Type I fiber.

Type II

Type II muscle fibers primarily use anaerobic metabolism and have (relatively) low endurance. These muscle fibers are typically used during tasks requiring short bursts of strength, such as sprinting or weightlifting. Type II fibers cannot sustain contractions for a significant length of time. In poultry, Type II fibers are white breast meat.

There are three sub-classes of type II muscle fiber…

Type IIa: Fast-Oxidative

Type IIa are fast-oxidative fibers and appear red due to their high content of myoglobin and mitochondria.

Type IIb: Fast-Glycolytic

Type IIb are fast-glycolytic and fire quickly. They are powerful and can twitch upwards of 120 times per second. These are the fiber type of choice for a power lifter. They also tire the fastest. These fibers appear white due to their low oxidative demand, manifested by the lack of myoglobulin and mitochondria, relative to Type I and Type IIa fibers.

Type IIc

Type IIc fibers are created from a fusion of satellite cells to the corrupted Type IIb - so long as the cortisone hormone is inhibited. Type IIc possess the attributes of Type IIa and Type IIb.

Type III

Type III or "Intermediate fast-twitch fibers" are a cross between Type I and Type IIb. They can utilize both aerobic and anaerobic pathways for energy metabolism. This is the "hybrid" muscle fiber. To build mitochondria-infused hybrid Type III super muscle, use a blended protocol.

Muscle Fiber Reference Guide

Skeletal muscle fibers can be divided into two basic types: type I slow-twitch fibers and type II fast-twitch fibers. Type II is further divided, as follows:

Category	Type I	Type IIa	Type IIb
Myoglobin	High	Medium	Low
Mitochondria	Many	Moderate	Few
Fatigues	Slowly	Moderate speed	Fast
Color	Red "dark meat"	Red	White "white meat"
Diameter	Narrow	Medium	Wide

Mitochondria are cellular power plants. They generate most of the cell's supply of ATP (Adenosine Triphosphate.) ATP is used as a source of chemical energy. The number of mitochondria in a cell varies widely by organism and tissue type. Many cells possess only a single mitochondrion, while others can contain several million mitochondria. Resistance training *combined* with cardiovascular training, causes the composition of muscles to transform from predominately Type II (or Type IIb) into Type III. In doing so we extend growth limits Nature has imposed upon those muscles. By adding mitochondria genetic limits can be reset. More nutrients can be processed and mito-infused muscles possess the ability to work harder and longer. Mito-dense muscles are thus able to grow larger and resist fatigue for a far longer time.

The 1st, 2nd and 3rd Way Cardio Modes

1st Way **Steady State**

1. walk
2. power walk
3. jog
4. swim
5. cardio machines

2nd Way **Interval or Burst style**

1. power walking with a weighted pack
2. intense games such a basketball, handball, racquetball
3. sprint running, swimming, kayaking and biking
4. hoisting weighted implements: kettlebells, clubbells, medicine balls

3rd Way **Hybrid Super-Muscle Fiber Reconfiguration**

1. Heavy Hands
2. Parrillo 100 repetition Giant Set Training
3. Hofmekler Controlled Fatigue Training
4. Kenneth Jay's Cardiovascular Kettlebell Concepts

EVERY SELF-RESPECTING PURPOSEFUL PRIMITIVE NEEDS THIS HIGH-TECH GADGET

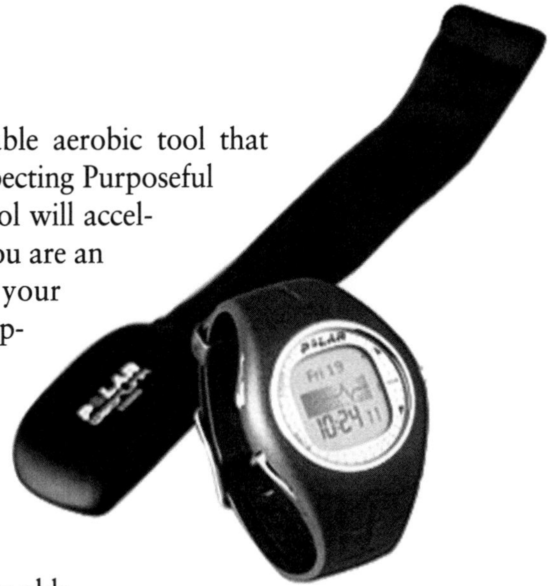

The heart rate monitor is an indispensable aerobic tool that belongs in the gym bag of every self-respecting Purposeful Primitive. The intelligent use of this hi-tech tool will accelerate results past your wildest imaginings. If you are an average individual looking to improve your physique, this device is a critical piece of equipment. If you are an intermediate or advanced trainee, you need it even more. This invaluable fitness tool allows the user to create, understand and make effective use of critical cardio data.

Once you've obtained an HR monitor you are able to monitor aerobic *intensity*, a critical piece of data otherwise unavailable to the exerciser. Newer versions of monitors have the ability to guesstimate calories oxidized during a session to an amazingly accurate degree. This piece of information can make for yet another interesting bit of aerobic data. Our approach is to devise a basic aerobic workout template then tinker with the component parts. The system promoted can be used regardless the exercise mode selected. It is advised that an individual eases into the aerobic mix gradually.

The Purposefully Primitive periodization principle of *creeping incrementalism* allows you to stair step your way toward ever improving physical condition. Each week you take mini steps towards the ultimate goal. Applying a periodization cycle to cardio is a new twist. In our hypothetical example the trainee starts off easy and by the end of the designated timeframe, the trainee is in undeniably better physical condition. The glide path is gradual, purposefully making it user friendly. In the 6 week periodization cycle the initial cardio pace is below capacity and training is done on an infrequent basis. This allows the trainee's body to acclimatize to the work and recover from one session to the next. As the weeks pass, the athlete systematically increases session frequency, session duration and session intensity.

I will assume the trainee has a monitor with a calorie counter. Over the six week time-frame, an ever increasing number of calories are oxidized during each session. If a disciplined approach to eating is used, stored body fat can be mobilized to fuel the session. Bodybuilders use a particular trick-of-the-trade that dramatically increases fat burning results: they perform cardio exercise in the early morning on an empty stomach. Due to a lack of food-fuel (glycogen) coming off the sleep-fast, the body is forced to mobilize stored body fat to power the cardio session. In the absence of glycogen, the body burns its second favorite fuel source: body fat. Combining an intense morning cardio session with a glycogen-free metabolic state creates yet another "window of opportunity," one similar to the post work-out window.

Poor eating habits can undo the entire exercise effort. You could burn 450 calories in a torrid 30 minute aerobic session, stop at the fast food joint on the way home, order an egg and cheese sandwich, hash browns and a soda and consume 1,000 calories. Congratulations, you just negated your cardio effort. Is it really necessary to eat after cardio training? I would advise to simply not eat. If you must eat, don't overwhelm the body with foods easily converted into fat.

The Three Benchmarks of Aerobic Activity

Duration: How long is the session?
Frequency: How often are the weekly sessions performed?
Intensity: How hard does the heart work during the session?

Duration and frequency are aerobic aspects easy to identify and quantify. Intensity is virtually impossible to access without a heart rate monitor. Intensity is how hard the heart must work to accomplish the work. Below is a rudimentary cardiovascular periodization game plan. The trainee uses steady-state 1st Way cardio. Modes could include walking, jogging, swimming or the use of a cardio machine. Preferably modes are alternated. The heart rate monitor enables us to cross compare exercises, an invaluable feature for determining how different modes affect you.

Six Week 1st Way Periodization Cycle

Week	Frequency	Duration *(minutes)	Intenstiy** (%ARHR)	Cals/ Min.***	Cals/ Session
1	3	15	60%	10	150
2	3	20	62.5%	10	200
3	4	25	65%	11	275
4	4	30	67.5%	11	330
5	5	35	70%	12	425
6	5	40	72.5%	12	480

** # of sessions done weekly. Initially allow a day or two between sessions.*

*** Intensity is measured as a percentage of age-related heart rate maximum.*

**** The rate at which calories are burned per minute.*

At the end of our hypothetical six week cardio periodization cycle, a multitude of goals are realized and copious benefits are achieved on a variety of levels. Initial cardio benchmarks are established and performance goals within each benchmark are ever so slightly increased each succeeding week. Weekly tweaking takes many subtle forms and momentum is generated by manipulating these different elements. Weekly benchmarks are gradually, subtly, imperceptibly increased over a protracted period. This skeletal framework can be used to devise a custom cardio periodization cycle that best suits the reality of your particular situation and circumstance.

I would highly recommend a heart rate monitor that has a 'blended session average heart beat' function and a calorie counter. The blended session average feature allows you to push a button at the beginning of the exercise session and again at the end of the session. The monitor calculates how many times your heart beats during the session. The microprocessor divides the total number of heart beats by the number of minutes. Advanced heart rate models guesstimate calories burned during the session. While it is never 100% accurate, it is accurate unto itself. I recommend paying a few extra bucks for this feature.

The intelligent use of a heart rate monitor allows you to identify the three cardio benchmarks and systematically plot progress. Below is a sound hypothetical cardiovascular training program for someone brand new to aerobic training. This expands on the six week cycle on the previous page. We use 1st Way steady-state and walking as the exercise mode.

The use of periodization tactics for the totally untrained individual is ideal: start off light and easy and below capacity. As the individual becomes acclimatized to the stress, we gradually increase the workload using the Purposefully Primitive theory of Creeping Incrementalism. Small incremental steps compound quickly!

Nine Week 1st Way Periodization Cycle

Week	Frequency	Duration *(minutes)	Intenstiy** (%ARHR)	Cals/ Min.***	Cals/ Session
1	3	20	60%	10	200
2	4	22	62.5%	10	220
3	4	25	65%	11	270
4	5	27.5	67.5%	11	280
5	5	30	70%	11	330
6	6	32.5	72.5%	12	400
7	6	35	75%	12	430
8	7	37.5	77.5%	13	500
9	7	40	80%	13	530

* *# of sessions done weekly. Initially allow a day or two between sessions.*

** *Intensity is measured as a percentage of age-related heart rate maximum.*

*** *The rate at which calories are burned per minute.*

This example is strictly hypothetical, but provides a terrific template for designing your own customized periodization aerobic routine: seek to gradually improve capacity, ability and endurance.

Frequency is easy to determine. Duration is easy to determine. Intensity requires the use of a heart rate monitor. If you have an overweight out-of-shape friend or relative, you might want to share this information with them before they fall into the clutches of a jogging obsessed Personal Trainer. Nearly every personal trainer will insist the unfit jog and that can lead to catastrophic injury. If a person can generate 80% or more of their age-related heart rate maximum simply by *walking* briskly, why would you insist that person engage in high impact jogging? The answer?

Bone-headed personal trainers have no earthly idea what sort of heart rate their clients are generating during the exercise. This can prove disastrous if the unfit are forced to run or engage in high-impact cardio exercise. The jogger-biased mentality turns off more obese beginners than any other single aspect of fitness training. The heavy person dreads the idea of being forced to run, they know that not only is it incredibly taxing, they also are aware they look awkward while jogging and the embarrassment factor is a very real psychological detriment. They are wisely unwilling to fall into the mongoloid clutches of a "No pain—no gain!" Sergeant Fury-style Knucklehead. Heavy people need to rebel against mindless jogger orthodoxy.

The Heart Rate Monitor Allows Aerobic Mode Cross Comparisons

My favored form of cardio exercise is traversing steep mountain trails. I use the blended session average feature of the HR monitor to cross-compare different cardio modes. If I'm feeling tired or off, I might power-walk. If I feel energetic, I might jog and sprint up and down the steep switchbacks. Other times my football knees might be aching so I'll load up a back pack with a 25-45 pound plate and power hike. Carrying a weighted backpack kicks my heart rate up 10 to 20 beats over weightless walking on the flat surfaces and 35 beats when walking up inclined grades.

At the end of the session I'll punch the magic button and the watch will issue my report card. It might tell me that for 62 minutes I averaged 132 beats per minute. I know that 130 BPM is 80% of my age-related heart rate maximum. I have quantified the session and can compare today's session to yesterday or tomorrow. I log the date, the duration and blended session heart rate average; this makes for a very telling and informative cardio log entries. Some days I will forget all that and simply refer to the watch continually: the face of the watch relates where the heart rate is the instant you glance at it.

Often I will take a (relatively) leisurely walk in the late afternoon. Not a formal, early morning kick-ass session, just a nice walk after dinner. On those occasions I will check the watch just to make sure I maintain 70% of my age-related heart rate maximum. Since I am so freaking old, this is a paltry 114 beats per minute. I really see no sense walking anywhere for any reason at a pace that doesn't generate at least 115! I am doubtful (in my particular situation) that any aerobic benefit whatsoever can be derived from anything less. By the way, my resting heart rate—early morning just waking up—is 41 BPM.

On other occasions I purposefully forget all about session duration, age-related heart rate max, blended session averages and all the rest and simply tell myself, I am going out and will burn 500 calories in this session come hell or high water. I use the calorie counter feature to gauge how I'm doing. If I kick it at a 15 calorie per minute pace, I can burn 500 in

33 minutes. If I lollygag along at a 10 calorie per minute rate it takes 50 minutes. Split the difference and use a 12 calorie per minute and I'm done in 42 minutes. I have "best times" for burning off 300, 500, 750 and 1000 calories per session. The heavier I am in bodyweight, the more calories I burn doing the same amount of work. The lighter I am, the faster I need to move in order to spike the heart.

The grade of the terrain is a huge factor: motoring up steep hills causes the heart rate to spike dramatically. Heart rate monitors allow us to compare one session to another and just as importantly cross-compare various exercise modes. How many calories did I burn playing three racquetball games in 45 minutes? How does this compare to 45 minutes of kayaking on my pristine mountain lake? What kind of blended average, age-related heart maximum can I generate jog trotting for 45 minutes on level terrain compared to 45 minutes of power-walking up and down steep trails wearing a weighted backpack? What's the HR difference between a 25 pound pack and a 55 pound backpack? I use the monitor to access cardio intensity and continually cross-compare modes. I use the monitor to create an aerobic periodization game plan.

I have found some athletic activities generate a surprisingly high heart rate—like throwing an aero-frisbie with a partner in an open field and sprinting to chase it down. I have found other cardio activities to be surprisingly disappointing—like playing tennis. If I didn't have the monitor, there would be no way of knowing that, for me, tennis is a complete waste of time, at least in terms of exercise. In the hands of experts, tennis is torrid and effective. In my hands it's a pathetic and wasteful athletic undertaking.

Cardio Essays

Man is the only animal who refuses to be what he is.

—Albert Camus

Aerobic Exercise Is Irreplaceable

The human circulatory system needs to be exercised as surely as the muscular system. Think of the circulatory system (Mr. Analogous again) as the body's internal plumbing. If the plumbing is rusted and corroded; if the pumps that flush the nutrients and remove waste products are overworked; if they are weak or clogged, a blowup or breakdown lies just around the corner. On the other hand, if the tubes and pipes that carry nutrients to the muscles and remove waste products are smooth as chromium stainless steel, if the heart and lungs are powerful pumps and super efficient exchange units, then the Soft Machine operates at peak capacity.

Aerobic activity by itself will never result in a complete physical transformation. It will, however, help the body better utilize quality nutrients for muscle recovery and growth. Consistent cardio increases the heart's stroke volume. Increased stroke volume allows the body to become more efficient at delivering nutrients to the cells and removing waste products. By performing all three legs of the Purposefully Primitive Training Triad (aerobics, nutrition, weight training) in a balanced, intelligent, ferocious fashion for a protracted period, the mysterious, mythical, ethereal *physical synergy* is triggered—when synergy takes root, results exceed all realistic expectations. Synergy only occurs in response to balanced application of the three interrelated elements: synergy only occurs when the diligent application of effective exercise is underpinned by performance-enhancing nutrition.

I hear stifled snickers and muffled laughs every time I tell hardcore iron pumpers that not only do I perform cardio, but they should too. "Aerobics is for girls!" is the predictable retort from far too many of my no-necked brethren. An unacceptable percentage of big strong men get gassed walking up three flights of stairs. A disproportionate number of ex-lifting champions drop over dead from heart attacks and circulatory health issues way before their time. Big guys should not be so dismissive of cardio-related activities, particularly after they retire.

The powerlifter purposefully adds muscle mass in order to increase the all-important ratio of muscle density per height in inches. A trained lifter standing 5'6" weighing 220 pounds, carrying a lot of muscle, is going to be one-hell-of-a-lot stronger than a trained lifter standing 5'6" and weighing 160lbs. The problem occurs after the 5'6" 220 pound lifter retires and balloons up to 260 after they stop training.

Often powerlifters quit training yet hang onto the massive eating habits they developed as young men trying to add muscle and size. One all-to-common scenario is that an elite lifter quits lifting, continues eating lots of refined carbs, sugar, beer and salted foods and adds 50 to 100 pounds of excess bodyweight. A high intake of artery-clogging food and zero cardio exercise makes for a deadly combination. An unacceptably high percentage of champion lifters are dying early and I think dietary restraint and some manly cardio would do wonders for big guys. Still, these bruisers would rather be caught with a transvestite hooker on an episode of "Cops" than be seen riding a stationary bike.

I myself hate cardio machines. I am disdainful of these boring gerbil wheels. When I use them the minutes tick by like hours. I hate doing cardio in a commercial gym, sucking in the rancid breath of the two guys riding bikes sitting two feet to my left and right. God have mercy on those in my cardio vicinity breathing in my rancid Sunday morning exhalations. The stale, recycled gym air is a toxic brew of expelled germs. Big Men, let's get outside and walk! Heavy guys are able to generate a 70 to 80% heart rate simply walking around the block. Hell, they won't even know you're doing cardio. Jettison junk food and massive booze intake. Manly Cardio doesn't suck! Dying decades before your time sucks!

Step Outside the Cardio Box

Obese people unable to exercise have a paucity of mitochondria. This partly explains why a 400 pound inactive individual can exist on 1000 calories a day and add body fat eating 1400 calories a day. After all that's a 40% caloric increase. Meanwhile the 240 pound competitive bodybuilder who hits early morning cardio sessions and weight trains ten or more hours weekly can consume 6,000 calories a day and not gain an ounce of body fat.

The obese individual has a sluggish metabolism and far fewer cellular furnaces than the bodybuilder. Over time the champion bodybuilder elevates their metabolism to a point where "only" eating 3500 calories a day causes him to *lose* body fat. Imagine! Meanwhile the obese dude eats a pint of Ben & Jerry's ice cream and gains three pounds of fat! Cardio exercise needs to be done for a variety of reasons, reasons that we've gone into tremendous detail on already.

Use a heart rate monitor to access with pinpoint accuracy the impact of your efforts. How might a typical steady-state, burst or hybrid session shake out using the HR monitor? This depends on your inclinations, preferences and psychological make up. Steady-state heart rate usage is pretty self explanatory. Perhaps the most fundamental form of burst cardio is sprinting. No need to run 100 yard sprints; 20, 30 or 40 yard dashes are more than sufficient to spike a heart rate through the ceiling and promote mitochondria growth in thighs hamstrings, calves and glutes. The procedure is primitive and effective: sprint one direction, cross the imaginary finish line and as soon as breathing returns to semi-normal, say 75% of age-related HR max for a fit person, sprint back the other direction. Obviously with each subsequent sprint the rest duration will increase. Keep this up for 30-45 minutes. You can use weighted implements such as weighted backpacks, kettlebells, clubbells, dumbbells with grip handles or medicine balls to create hybrid 3rd Way cardio katas. Use your imagination to create your own 3rd Way cardio protocols. I once tried doing the clean and jerk with 135 for 30 straight minutes...a truly painful memory.

Jump Start the Heart

I love outdoor power walking and will often wear a weighted pack while walking. Using free hand calisthenics to initially spike the heart rate, I will start my outdoor power walk with 2-4 minutes of free hand full squats, jumping jacks and push-ups to initially elevate the heart. I normally have a 75 beat per minute (BPM) heart rate after a few cups of coffee. Obviously I have on my heart rate monitor and will do my circuit of calisthenics for as many tri-sets as it takes to jump up from 75 to 130 BPM which is 80% of my age-related heart rate maximum.

I have found that repeatedly speed running up a flight of stairs is another great way to spike my initially sluggish heart up to the target zone. I use an 80% base, but that doesn't mean you should. Out of shape folks should initially work in the 50-65% ARHR max range. Once I spike my heart to my target baseline of 80%, I try and maintain that for the duration of the session. Be aware that there are periods where I will exceed the baseline and there are periods where I will fall short. The goal is at sessions end to have a *blended session average* that achieves the predetermined session target heart rate goal.

By way of example, I currently shoot for 82.5% of my ARHR max for 60 minutes. This works out to 134 beats per minute for 60 minutes. I have established a consistent base of 80% for 60 minutes and my new goal is to ratchet the intensity upward to a consistent 82.5%, 134 beats, for 60 minutes. I am keeping the duration intact, 60 minutes; keeping the frequency intact, 5-6 days a week and looking to increase the intensity. I continually manipulate one or more of the various cardio benchmarks in order to provoke progress. On other occasions I might seek to extend the session duration while maintaining intensity and frequency. Other times I tinker with frequency.

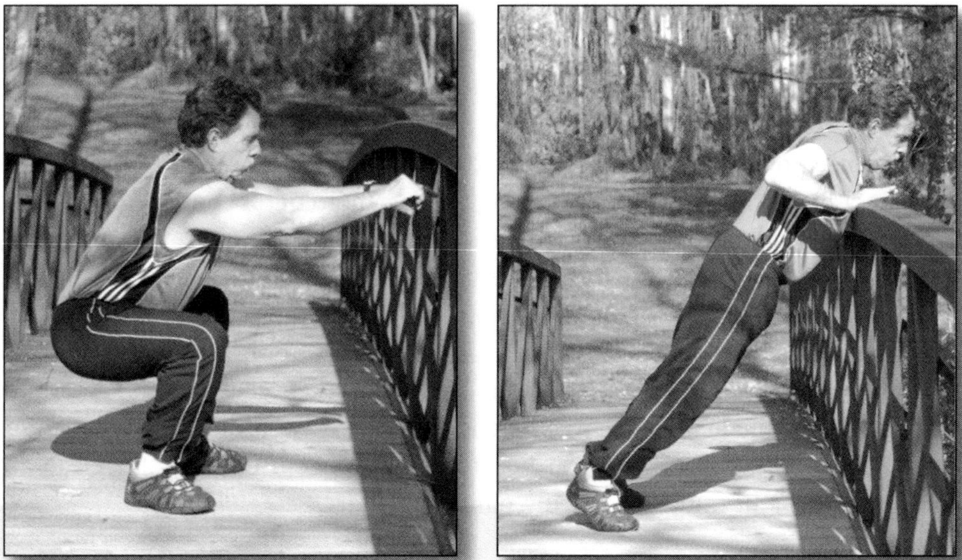

Punch up the volume: Physiologically speaking, the more fit the individual, the harder it is to elevate the normal heart rate. One trick of trade used to spike the heart rate is to start the cardio session with a series of rapid-fire free-hand exercises: squats, jumping jacks, pushups, etc. I have found sprinting up and down stairs is also a terrific way to "jump up" the heart rate. Once elevated to 70-80% (for fit individuals) it is relatively easy to keep the HR elevated.

Tricks of the Walking Trade

Some individuals will be able to maintain the target baseline heart rate simply by walking as fast as possible; others might need to wear a weighted backpack. In my case, I hike local mountain trails often wearing a backpack stuffed with a 35 pound plate wrapped in a blanket. After my free hand exercise warm-up (without the pack), I'll start walking as fast as possible or break into my jog-trot for ten minutes on the flat level terrain. My goal is to maintain my now established 80% heart rate.

Another method I use for amping-up the intensity of power walking is to throw my hands, clenched into fists, head height on each stride step. I have found that by conscientiously throwing each fist to head height on steep grades I can create a 20 beat per minute increase over "normal" walking. I recommend the clenched fist because it adds an element of muscle tension that spikes the heart rate. It feels like Len Schwartz's Heavyhands without using the hand weights.

In Cheng Tzu's *Thirteen Treatises on T'ai Chi Chuan* he references that when a T'ai Chi Master achieves the highest state of the art, "He feels as if he is swimming through air while performing T'ai Chi." I replicate that feeling using this procedure. The air feels thick and I feel as if I am swimming through air. At times of maximum stress, it feels as if I'm swimming through mud or concrete. Performing walking cardio provides a low impact form of exercise so the chances of incurring an exercise-related injury are radically reduced. If you are able to acquire and maintain the predetermined cardio intensity target strictly by walking, then that is enough, but if you want to take your intensity to the next level try these proven methods.

Stop and Smell the Roses

Walking at top speed up steep grades while throwing clenched fists to head height causes thigh muscles to burn and lungs to ache. Power walking can recreate Master Cheng Tzu's "swimming through air" phenomenon. On a steep 45 degree hill I am able to jack my heart rate from 115 to 170 using concentrated walking with fists thrown head high.

After a burst of this type, I stand still and allow my heart to simmer back down to my 80% "floor." The heart rate monitor gives me permission to take a complete post-burst break and not lose one single minute of cardio benefit. One of the biggest revelations I had using the heart rate monitor was the realization that I could stop completely after an intense heart rate spike. There is a heart rate lag time that enables me to get my wind back. While standing still and recovering I suck in crisp, outdoor, super-oxygenated air and receive a cornucopia of cardio benefits: working muscles are clearing lactic acid; and heart/lung/muscles are reestablishing their gyroscopic balance while oxygen debt is being normalized. The visual wonders of nature heighten my zoned-out, altered consciousness state-of-being and I receive the benefits of a still accelerated heart, pounding away at 170, now 158, 149, 141, 136, 130 now 128 and time to hit it again.

Now down to 80% of ARHR, completely recovered, I burst yet again. I hit it hard with rested muscles cleared of toxins and out of oxygen debt. Reenergized and revitalized, I repeat the procedure again and again for 60 solid minutes, or longer. I have no problem maintaining a blended session heart rate average of 80% using this procedure. Please don't run out and start blasting up to 100% of ARHR max or cruise along at 80% just because I do. That could be dangerous. Try alternating burst style cardio with steady-state during cardio training sessions. If you have never tried outdoor cardio, alternating steady with burst, it is exhilarating, intense and effective.

The human body craves sameness and for that reason we avoid sameness.

Get outside to a public park, put on the iPod and get lost in this transcendental form of cardio exercise. Why mindlessly submit to the tender mercies of some Hitlerian Personal Trainer who insists you jog or ride the bike without pause, all the while completely ignorant of the critical heart rate portion of the cardio equation? Liberate yourself; discover the unbridled joy of lung-searing cardio done outdoors in a visually exciting setting.

Isotonometrics to the Rescue

The Achilles Heel of power walking, even with a weighted back pack, is the precipitous and unavoidable drop in heart rate when the outdoor walker goes downhill. It seems that for every transcendental grade that spikes the heart rate as much as I want, over the crest of the ridge lie the downhill section that deflates the elevated heart rate, no matter how fast you walk or jog on the decline.

Enter Len Schwartz's *isotonometrics*.

By clasping the two hands together as you walk (or jog) and simultaneously pushing and pulling the hands, one against the other, I find that I am able to spike the heart rate an additional 20-25 beats per minute. Plus it's easy. Using Len's push-pull strategy I have been able to devise some basic isotonometric exercises that dramatically elevate the heart rate while walking down steep hills. These can also be done standing still; the key is to really push and tug on the hands.

Curl/Pushdown (see photos on next page)

Curl one arm upward while pushing downward with the other arm. The biceps muscles win. At the turnaround reverse the procedure, do a triceps pushdown while resisting with a negative curl. The push muscles win. Then shift to the other arm. Do this for 10 reps.

Static Chest Push

Push both arms together at the center of the chest, hands touch chest. Press the arms together equally and allow the hand clasp to drift as far forward as possible from the chest. Then pull the hands back to the chest maintaining the tension. Do this for 10 reps.

Hand Clasp Side-to-Side Push

Clasp hands and push to the right, resisting. After pushing rightward as far as possible, push leftward, resisting mightily. Do this for 10 reps.

Axe Mimic

Mimic swinging an axe with one arm and resist with the palm of the other arm. "Push" the axe back to the start. This represents one rep. Then switch arms. Do this for 10 reps.

Bench Press

Use the right arm, palm up in bench press position. Extend the arm, resisting. At full extension, push the right arm back to bench press start position. Switch arms and repeat bench press. Do this for 10 reps.

By continually referring to the monitor, I access the effectiveness of the push-pull movement and determine what impact it is having on the heart rate in real time. Here are five rudimentary isotonometric exercises I have devised: again, as long as the heart rate elevates, the type of pattern you select is of secondary importance. Create your own procedures. As long as the push pull pattern you invent spikes the heart it is valid. In most isotonometric push/pulls, one hand must "win." If you pushed or pulled with absolutely equal force the arms would remain static in a deadlocked isometric.

Allow one muscle to ever so slightly overpower the opposing muscle. Then, at the turnaround, reverse roles: allow the opposing muscle to ever so slightly win the push or pull back.

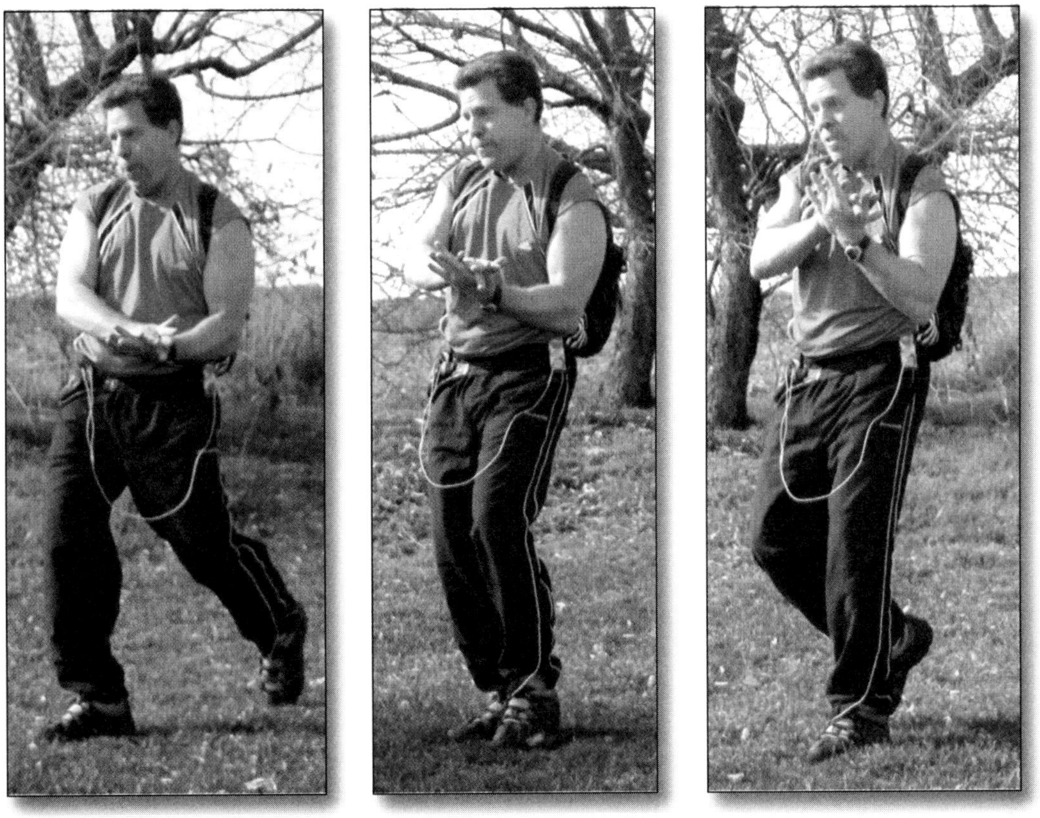

The possibilities are endless. Continually refer to the heart rate monitor to see which point/counterpoint isotonometrics are working and which ones are ineffectual. On one familiar down hill stretch I would have to walk or jog dangerously fast to maintain a paltry 115 heart rate. By using isotonometrics I was able to actually slow my walk pace yet generate a 135 heart rate! Isotonometrics rectifies the Achilles Heel of walking. I then turned and power walked back up the same hill and generated a 175 heart rate using the clenched fist thrown head high, swimming-through-air tactic. This was without a weighted back pack. Isotonometrics are another valid arrow for the cardio quiver.

Indoor Aerobics

I use kettlebells and assorted tools and weighted implements to generate 3rd Way cardio effect. 3rd Way cardio modes are perfect for training indoors when the weather is uncooperative. Try swinging, lifting, hoisting or flinging weighted objects for 30 to 40 minutes. I refer to the heart rate monitor to achieve the requisite intensity and pace my weighted implement session. If the implements are too heavy you will be unable to last for the predetermined session length.

I usually shift between implements. I might start with 50 reps in the big kettlebell sumo deadlift. This spikes me to 170. I simmer down to 130 (80% of ARHR max for me) then pick up the little kettlebells and power them around extended at full arms length until I spike back up to 150 or thereabouts. I might then pick up regular dumbbells and perform high rep snap clean and presses. I could follow this with "around the world" lateral raises. Then front squats holding a plate. After a few minutes of dumbbell use, I might jump on my Schwin Aerodyne bike (with the push/pull handles) for a torrid two minute sprint. I might swing the light clubbells creating a variety of different motor-pathways and grooves to end the session.

Sometimes I *power* the implements, moving the bells or clubs with purposeful slowness for maximum muscle tension. Sometimes I use a *natural and relaxed momentum* and swing the weighted objects. I might alternate loose-and-free momentum swings with slow-mo power grind moves, all within the same indoor workout. The heart-elevating effect of using kettlebells and clubbells is awesome. 30-45 minutes can go by quickly if you are clever. I can go through an entire 3rd Way Hybrid session and never once use the same tools or exercise as I rotate through a never ending series of cardio/strength moves. It's nothing to blast through a 45 minute session generating 80% of age-related heart rate.

Too many trainees use steady-state cardio exclusively and are unaware that their body has long since ceased deriving any significant training benefit from this mode. Do the same thing in the same way over and over and the ever-clever body eventually figures out how to neutralize the training effect. By alternating these three distinctly different approaches to aerobic exercise, we keep the body off balance and guessing, unable to figure out what is going on. This allows us to extract gains on a continual basis.

Outdoors I can perform steady-state jogging and flat out sprinting on flat grades, power walking in hilly territory, indoors I can play racquetball or other vigorous sports for burst cardio. I can perform 3rd way hybrid cardio using weighted implements. Again, as long as I have my heart rate monitor and as long as I have in mind my predetermined duration and intensity goal, I can guide any session to successful completion. Variety is the spice of life and we need variety to keep exercise exciting. If we have an entire menu of exercise modes and exercise tools to select from, enthusiasm can be kept at a fevered pitch. By playing vigorous sports, often with pals, instead of dreading aerobic exercise, we actually look forward to aerobic activity. We are able to inject fun into the fitness equation.

Once cardio exercise becomes a joy, the aerobic portion of the fitness equation is all but won.

WALKING FOR EXERCISE IS DIFFERENT THAN NORMAL WALKING

Most people who use walking as exercise cannot or will not walk properly. In order to derive maximum aerobic benefit from walking we need to learn how to walk *inefficiently*.

Walking inefficiently, using lots of arm swing, an exaggerated stride length and hip swivel, combined with a dramatically accelerated pace, burns far more calories and elevates the heart rate to a far greater degree than walking "normally".

Normal walking is *efficient* walking. Everyone walks and as a result we develop walking habits that are subconsciously efficient. To derive maximum benefit from *exercise walking*, the efficiency we've learned over the years needs to be exorcised. Being a self-regulating machine, the human body wants to do day to day repetitive activities in the most efficient way possible. Why does the body instinctively seek groove and repetition in life's continually reoccurring activities? It subconsciously seeks to preserve energy.

There are hundreds of subconscious activities carried out by the brain, organs and central nervous system, all of which occur just below the radar of consciousness. You do not think through the taking of every single step, you do not have to tell yourself how to maneuver the right hand in such a way so as to successfully pick a pencil up off a desk top—yet we are able to perform these complex bio-mechanical feats involving dozens of muscles without conscious thought. We subconsciously develop habitual patterns for complex bio-mechanical movements. Genetic hardwiring is encoded with directives to save energy (calories) at all cost. When the body is faced with a particular biomechanical mission, left to its own devices the body seeks to do what it needs to do in a way that expends the least number of precious energy-calories.

When it comes to cardio exercise, we want to expend the *maximum* number of calories and that requires concentrated inefficiency.

As a species we walk upright using our legs. A species subconscious consensus has been reached: walk with a minimum of torso movement for this is the most calorically efficient way to move. Look around and watch as people walk. The legs move while the upper torso stays limp and the arms hang at their sides. The best cardio exercise is not efficient, it is inefficient. We want to be inefficient, fuel-wise, when we exercise. We want to burn calories and we want to systematically flush the bodily plumbing. We want to force blood through the veins, arteries and organs. We want to send nutrient-enriched blood to muscles and remove toxic waste at an accelerated rate.

The upper body needs to be activated in a major way in order to turn lowly walking into an elevated exercise format. Embrace inefficiency: pump the elbows over their full and complete range-of-motion with each stride-step. Rotate the hips with each stride-step and attempt to extend the length of the stride. Turn the legs over as fast as possible. By purposefully pumping the elbows in synchronization with leg drive, by purposefully opening the stride and rotating the hips as we walk, the heart rate can be accelerated by as much as 30%.

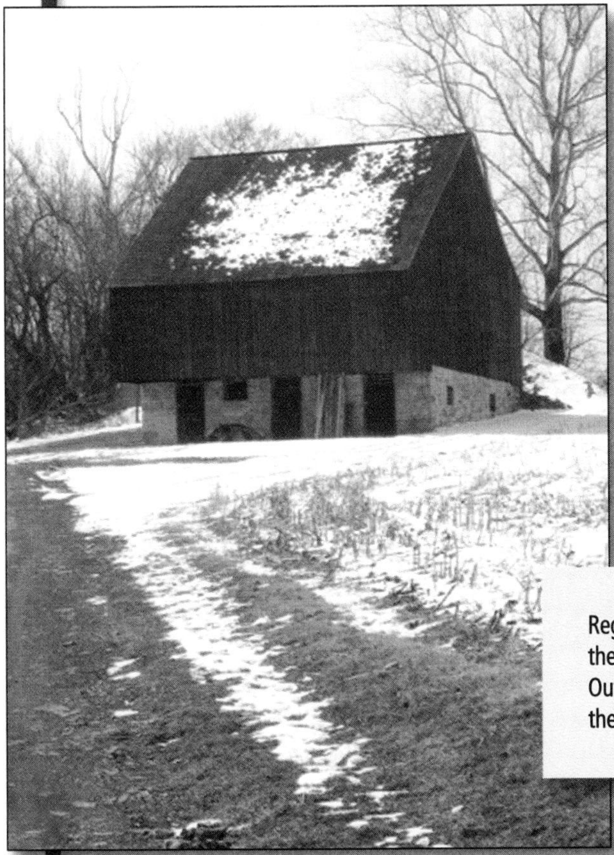

Exaggerated walking burns way more calories than "normal" walking. Purposefully pump those elbows high, hard and fast. Think of every stride-step as a rep and think about moving as fast as humanly possible without breaking into a trot. Try this test: walk as fast as you can without pumping your arms, without opening the stride or rotating the hips. Now walk as fast as you can while pumping the arms and adding extra movement and motion. This is akin to flipping the afterburner switch on a Jet. There is no way a person can walk as fast without pumping the arms as they can when pumping their arms.

Regardless of the weather I prefer outdoor cardio. All you need is the proper clothing. I took this photo during a morning run. Outdoor cardio is light-years superior to riding a gerbil machine in the stuffy confines of a gym.

Often a walker starts off using the "pump and swivel" exaggerated motion, but at some point they lose concentration and focus. The arms stop pumping, the hips cease swiveling and the torso goes limp, suddenly and without warning. It's a surefire tip-off the walker has morphed from concentrated and connected walking into distracted daydreaming. The breakdown of walking technique is an indicator that the walker is no longer focused and engaged.

There are a myriad of reasons we love outdoor walking as exercise....

Walk Outside When Possible

Almost every urban and suburban municipality has a public park. Get up early, go walk in the park. Trust me, in the early morning, public facilities are always deserted. Why stand on a cardio machine in a dank fitness facility breathing in the beer-laced carbon monoxide fumes of the guy next to you who drank 23 beers last night? Why breathe in the stale, recycled air and the germ-infused exhalations of other people? Instead suck in gobs of pure outdoor air. In the woods there is a richness and fragrance about the atmosphere. Clean pure air has a regenerating, supercharging effect on the body. Nature always changes and during an all-out, totally focused, outdoors nature walk, time seems to fly by. While the minutes seem endless riding a gerbil-wheeled cardio machine in a confined gym stuffed with people, walking outside in the sun, breathing fresh fragrant air, absorbing the visual kaleidoscope of natural colors compresses time. Suddenly 45 minutes have flown by and you don't want to stop. When cardio exercise becomes a joyful pastime, you make time for it and look forward to it. Over time the person who grows to love aerobic activity gains endurance, vitality, health and wellbeing. Coordinate consistent cardio with precision nutrition and burn off stored body fat.

Low Impact

Other than swimming, power walking is the least joint-stressful of all cardio activities—and you don't need a pool. High impact repetitive motion exercise can take a toll on the body of the trainee. The human body is a machine like any other, and repeated hard use of a particular body part in a particular way eventually wears out body parts. Knees, ankles, hip joints, elbows and shoulders are all quite intricate, delicate, and complex. Jogging on concrete is murder on the knees and ankles, particularly for the heavy out-of-shape person. Mix cardio modes. Find low impact modes that spike the heart rate sufficiently, modes you enjoy and rotate them continually.

Aerobic Machine Drawbacks

The tight, repetitive, (usually) circular motion of an aerobic machine is problematic. By forcing the human body to do thousands of repetitions (cumulatively it could be tens of thousands) using an identical motion or pattern, by using the same body parts in the identical same way over and over, body parts wear down over time. Factory workers that perform the same motion over and over for years on end often incur *repetitive motion injury.*

Those who religiously use a particular aerobic machine, one that locks you into an identical muscle pattern, (for months or years on end) run the risk of incurring repetitive motion injury. l. There are a significant number of fitness devotees who develop repetitive motion-related problems from using aerobic machines. Hip joints, knees, ankles and feet are particularly susceptible.

Uneven Footfall

One little discussed advantage of trail walking (or jogging) is that with every step the foot lands in a slightly different position.

This is a good thing.

The best way to avoid self-inflicted repetitive motion injury is to avoid doing the identical biomechanical motion over and over, ad infinitum. When walking or jogging on trails, each time the foot lands it lands on a different surface. The differing surfaces means the foot always is landing and pushing off from a slightly different angle. This is the exact opposite of walk/jogging on concrete. Sidewalk and street runners often complain of sore knees, ankles and hips joints. Shin-splints are a very real problem and usually traceable to pounding on hard surfaces. If you must run on concrete, learn to glide, not slam-step.

Kick Up the Cardio Walking Volume

Wearing a weighted backpack is a great way to jack-up the intensity of exercise walking. Place a 10, 25 or 35 pound plate wrapped in a blanket inside a school backpack. We've found that a sturdy kid's backpack—the kind the boys and girls wear to carry their books on their backs to and from school (available at any Wal-Mart for $15) are easily capable of carrying 10 to 35 pounds of weight. It is quite easy to spike walking heart rate upward 10-20 beats by packing poundage and taking a brisk hike. Don't go crazy and try to become a Sherpa all at once. Once you have the right pack and plate combo, this becomes a near effortless way to pump up the walking heart rate and still maintain the low-impact advantages of walking. Be progressive and smart: start light and work upwards slowly.

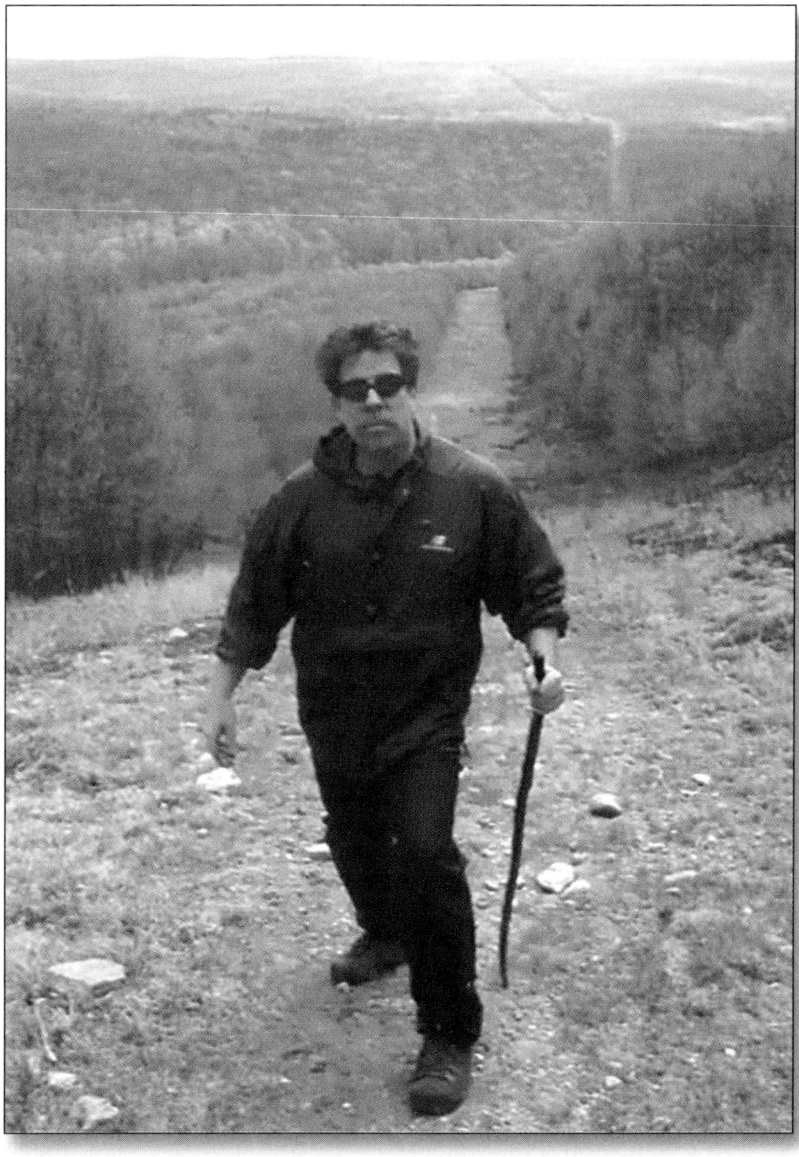

Exercise-induced Zen Samadhi: Three miles from my house are the "deep woods." Endless mountain trails crisscross endless mountains. I walk/jog for hours and routinely burn 2,000 calories in a session. No mechanical sounds of any kind: the wind in the trees, my own labored breathing, and the cry of an occasional bird of prey. Every step in this unforgiving terrain is uneven. I'd been going for two hours when we took this shot. This is my definition of "follow your bliss." I am deep in a mindless state of Cardiovascular Nirvana.

Zen and the Art of Walking– Dorian and Heart Rate Monitors

The Most Underrated of All Aerobic Activities is Perfect for Big, Muscle-Laden Men or Overweight Out-of-Shape Individuals

Walking is a great cardio exercise assuming it's done correctly. If you are a large man, if you are overweight or out of shape, if you are a woman over 150 pounds or a man over 200 pounds, walking should be your preferred cardio mode.

There are many acceptable cardio modes and types that can and should be rotated into the aerobic menu on a periodic basis; however *power* walking should be the default mode for big heavy people. The heavier you are the easier you'll find that you are able to spike the heart rate, dramatically, with simple speed walking. A heavy person doesn't need to do much, from an exercise standpoint, in order to spike the heart rate. It is a matter of mass times velocity.

While a 110 pound woman in good shape might have to jog intensely at a 13 calorie per minute burn rate to oxidize 400 calories, a 300 pound man can burn 400 calories in 20 minutes by simply walking fast. The walking rationale is a matter of basic thermodynamics, physics, payload (bodyweight) and propulsion. A truck loaded with 40,000 pounds of steel beams burns far more fuel traveling at 35 miles per hour for 60 miles than a 3,000 pound mini-van does traveling at 70 miles per hour for the same 60 miles. To haul around big payloads requires more fuel.

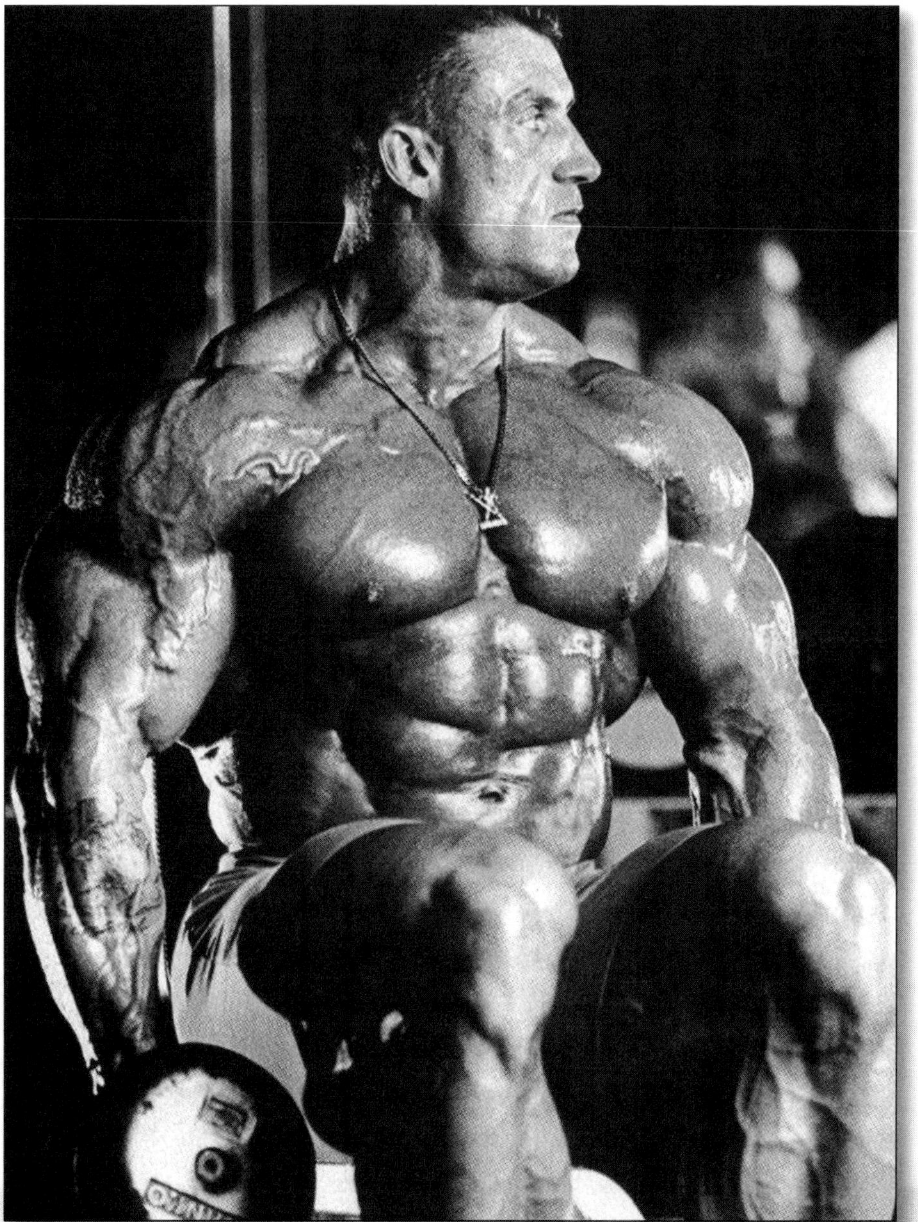

Dorian Yates in competition shape weighing 260 pounds. He would weigh 300 in the "off season" and in the 12 weeks leading up to a competition whittle down to the condition you see in this photo. Brisk walking would elevate his heart rate to the requisite 70-85% heart rate range. Please forget about the "fat burning zone" effete personal trainers mindlessly recommend. The amount of calories burned operating at a paltry 60% are insignificant and hardly worth the effort. Go hard and fast, burn off massive amounts of calories; build endurance and cardio density.

I never gave walking a lot of thought as serious cardiovascular exercise until I interviewed (then) Mr. Olympia, Dorian Yates, for an article in *Muscle & Fitness* magazine back in the nineties. Yates was a throwback Purposefully Primitive type of guy who reminded me of Bill Pearl, Reg Park, John Grimek or Sergio Oliva. He was the prototypical power bodybuilder and like the men that came up in the 50's and 60's, Dorain took great pride in being as strong as he looked. The old timers trained hard, ate big and recognized the undeniable correlation between growing stronger and growing larger. Yates seemed cut from that same cloth and had unusual ideas about training in general and aerobic training specifically.

Dorian "The Diesel" Yates seemed the antithesis of the Southern California, West Coast school of bodybuilding that emerged in the sixties, solidified in the 70's and still thrives today. The epicenter of the bodybuilding Universe is the LA/San Diego region. Serious bodybuilders relocate to these areas from all over the world to further their physique careers. They share information on training, eating and the black arts. Everyone basically uses the same methodology. I use to interview these men for training articles on a monthly basis. There was a dull uniformity to their training and eating methods. It taxed my skills as a writer to make sameness seem different.

Dorian Yates was iconic in every way: he lived in Birmingham, England and had a spectacularly unique approach towards resistance training, cardiovascular training and eating. His resistance training had more in common with power immortal Ed Coan than with his West Coast competitors. His nutrition was sane and sensible and his approach to cardio was astounding—at least compared to the accepted practices of the time. I quizzed him on his "off-season" approach to cardio training and he related a unique slant on cardio that changed my viewpoint.

He kept referring me back to the aerobic "goal." The goal, and I paraphrase, was to burn off fat and accelerate the metabolism. The danger, he repeated over and over, was doing too much cardio, thereby impeding the acquisition of new muscle or, horror of horrors, destroying the existing muscle he'd worked so hard to construct. Yes, he felt cardio was critical, but above all else he wanted to retain muscle mass. He never went overboard with cardio. On the West Coast, a lot of pro bodybuilders were spending more time performing cardio than they were lifting weights. One California bodybuilder spent three hours a day, seven days a week doing cardio. He was ripped, but emaciated, and never finished in the top five of the big shows.

Dorian, ever sensible, wanted to do enough cardio to stimulate the metabolic rate and oxidize body fat. He also drew my attention to the bodyweight variable. Dorian weighed 295 pounds in the off-season. He'd whittle that down to 255-260 on contest day. Being that heavy, it didn't take a lot to spike his heart rate—the goal of cardio exercise. He viewed aerobics as a necessary evil and never did one moment more of cardio than suited his purposes. He didn't want cardio "nicking" his muscle mass. To him, bodybuilding was all about building muscle and getting lean, not getting bloody good at riding an exercise bike.

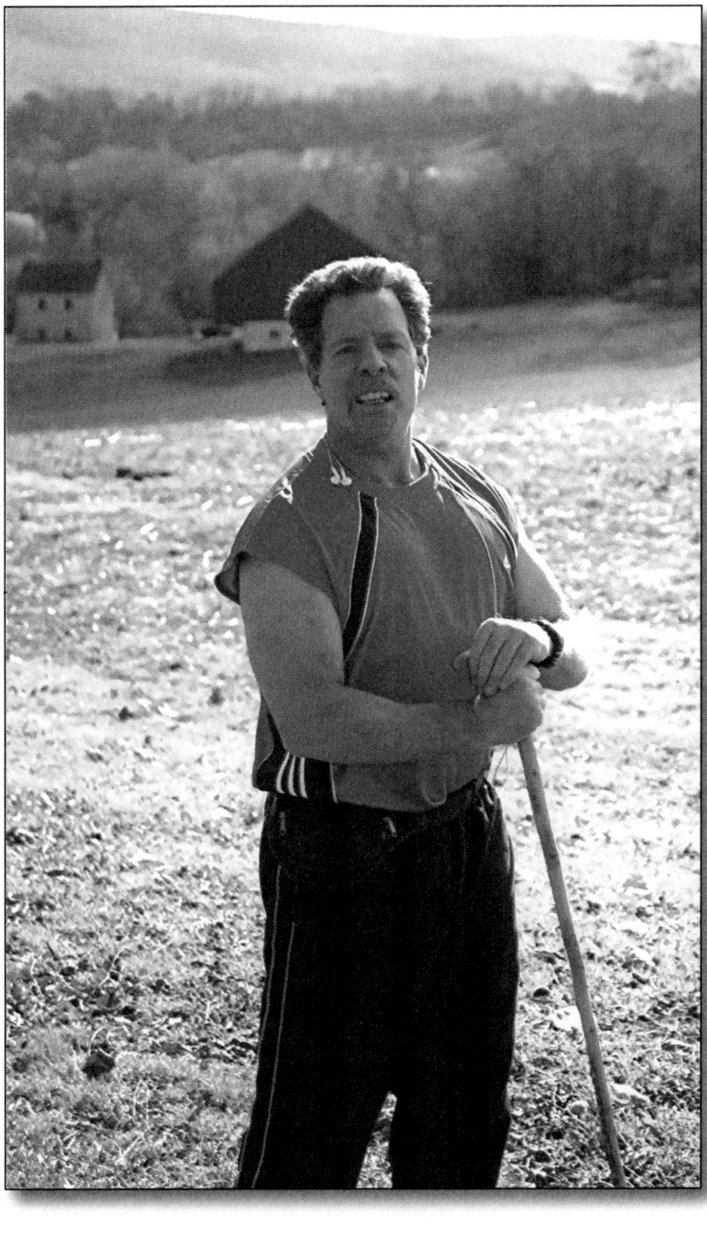

THE 1,000 CALORIE CARDIO BURN

Periodically I like to see how long it takes me to oxidize 1000 calories in a cardio session.

A lot of fitness experts point out that the calorie counting gauges on commercially available heart rate monitors are guesstimates at best and inaccurate compared to laboratory analysis of caloric expenditure during exercise. Point taken: on the other hand, the heart rate monitor is accurate unto itself. Once a caloric benchmark is created, using the same instrument will provide the user a valid frame of reference for future efforts. In addition, the truism that commercial heart rate monitors are inaccurate subliminally infers that they *overestimate* the amount of calories oxidized in relation to the amount of work performed—who is to say that they might actually *underestimate* the number of calories oxidized? Regardless if the instrument overestimates or underestimates the actual number, calorie burning provides a numerical frame of reference that I use often.

On this particular day I hit the farm at 8 am; it was Thursday, November 8, 2007 and I weighed 203 pounds. The temperature was 31 degrees. I started the session off with 50 jumping jacks to elevate my placid heart rate. Rolling out of the jeep and after two cups of coffee, I started off at 76 beats per minute (BPM.) I never eat food before my early morning cardio session as I want to operate in a low glycogen state and create a body fat oxidizing "window of opportunity." After the jumping jacks I performed 20 deep squats to loosen up my knees, hip joints and ankles. I glanced at my watch: 112 BPM. I fired up the 'shuttle function' of my iPod and began an easy run on the flat section of the farm. The trails were littered with autumn foliage and the scenery was surreally beautiful.

I was able to spike my heart up to 145 BPM within the first six minutes of my jog/sprint. I increased my speed as I felt my body coming awake. I run on a large circular path enclosed in forest canopy that takes three minutes to circumnavigate. By the end of two laps, six minutes, I am able to sprint at roughly 90% of my all out sprint speed maximum. I then hit what I call the "second leg" of the farm trek; a long stretch that runs along the trout stream I fish in from April to October. This section winds and twists yet remains level. By the time I finish this section my watch indicates I've been going for 30 minutes and was maintaining a consistent 130+ BPM.

These flat sections are ideal for interval sprinting and I would blast hard for 10-15 seconds, spike to 150+ BPM then ease off the accelerator. My body and heart, fully awake, sucked in the crisp cold super-oxygenated air. I felt alive and vibrant. I rolled into the third leg, a series of steep mountain trails that wind and twist upward. These Billy Goat trails require attention and care; one missed footfall and you will tumble down 100 feet into the trout stream. Normally I will run these steep trails, but today my goal was different. I wanted to extend the duration of the session as much as possible without dipping below 130 BPM.

In order to stretch the duration I power walked up these steep trails and had no problem keeping my heat rate at 140 +. The grade is so severe that simply walking as fast as possible, combined with high arm swings enables me to keep my heart rate effortlessly elevated. The work seemed "easier" than leg-intense sprinting on the level surfaces and my leg muscles actually recovered during this power walking phase. After walking as fast as possible up the mountain trail section, I emptied into a cornfield set on a high plateau.

I continue up yet another grade, skirting the perimeter of the field, reduced to corn stalks after the October harvest, Though not as steep as the previous Billy Goat section, the corn field circumnavigation was steady uphill for another half mile. By the time I crested out my heart rate is 150+ purely by power walking. I hit the 50 minute mark. In the past I have had problems keeping my heart rate elevated while traveling downhill. There is always a downside to traveling upward in the mountains. Heading up I might hit 170+ BPM but after cresting, heading down seemed a cardiovascular waste of time. I couldn't find a safe way to keep my heart rate from plummeting during the downhill phase.

I cured this problem by expropriating some tactics from Len Schwartz's *Whole Body* fitness approach. Len uses "isotonometrics" to elevate the heart. He discovered that by pushing and pulling on the hands while walking or jogging a significant bump in the heart rate occurred. I use a modified version of his system. While walking, or carefully jogging downhill, I push the two hands together or pull them apart, creating muscular tension. This procedure allows me to continue to keep my heart rate elevated. In downhill sections normally my heart rate nosedives from 140 to 105. I discovered that by using a series of "hand clasps that pit half the body against the other half," to quote Len, I could keep my heart elevated in the 125 to 135 zone.

I used to stop and do a series of jumping jacks, squats or pushups to spike the heart, but found these free hand exercises lacking. While the heart rate would spike in the immediate aftermath, the moment I stopped doing jumping jacks and started heading down hill my heart rate plummeted—as it does with all good athletes who are in good physical condition. On the other hand by pushing my two hands together, by curling one arm up as I pushed downward onto a triceps countermove, I created tension. By pitting one arm against the other, I could continually keep the heart rate jacked up as I walked or jogged. My heart rate would easily spike 10-25 beats over what it would be without the isotonometric push-pull protocol.

Coming off the extended downhill section and heading up and around the barn, I noted that I had burned 850 calories. I headed back to my jeep. I timed it so that as I popped out of the woods I had oxidized 990 calories. I flipped the watch to stop at exactly 1,000. My statistics were as follows: I had burned 1,000 calories in one hour seventeen minutes and 45 seconds. My blended session heart rate average was 134 beats per minute. I had achieved 82.25% of my age-related heart rate maximum for 77 straight minutes during which my heat beat 15,678 times. Far from fatigued, I felt invigorated and went straight to the unheated gym and worked my arms for another 30 minutes. By the way, I averaged 122 beats per minute for the lifting session and oxidized an additional 230 calories; all in all, a good day's work.

If you own a heart rate monitor with a calorie counting function, periodically see how long it takes you to burn 250 or 500 calories. Have caloric burn records. See how long it takes to burn X number of calories: establish burn benchmarks and seek to better these periodically. Those in better shape can go for the big numbers. Think of calorie oxidation records as another way to inject fun into the cardio equation. Sometimes it's nice to just forget about everything other than "How fast can I burn 500 calories?" It's a hell of a cool challenge.

Another mountain trail in my neighborhood. This one takes 40 minutes to crest. I repeatedly hit 200+ heart beats per minute scaling this near vertical grade. I take periodic breaks on the ascent to let my heart rate slow to my 130 BPM "floor," 80% of my age-related heart rate max. While standing still my heart and leg muscles recover and I still receive cardio benefit. I take in the breathtaking scenery and re-oxygenate my body. Time seems to compress when I engage in naturalistic aerobic exercise: at sessions end, instead of feeling exhausted, I feel invigorated.

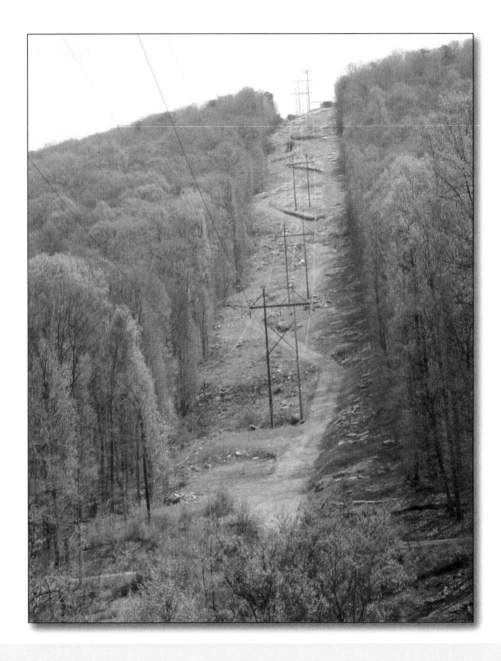

The Carefree Psychotic Peeks Inside Ali's "Near Room"

I had my first 100 degree workout of 2007 the other day in my garage gym out back of the Mountain Compound. It was a sauna. No fan either. I had the garage door open and a slight breeze kept the air moving. Now that I'm old, I actually like sauna-like training conditions. Heat seems to lube my joints. Warm muscle fiber fires far more explosively than cold, stiff muscle fiber and is far less susceptible to injury. Anyway, as I sat on the duct-tape covered incline bench between sets, my mind wandered back a few years to when Chuck Deluxe lived in the neighborhood.

We used to have some hellacious training sessions in the garage because he was freaking nuts and game to try any ridiculous physical activity I would suggest—and not just lifting. For example, for cardio we used to walk for miles and miles in the deep woods; hiking up and down the steep fire trails that bisect and trisect the mountains in my neighborhood. This was lung searing, leg burning Purposefully Primitive cardio: hiking up and down trails so steep one false step and you'd tumble hundreds of feet. It was exhilarating and exhausting and we always ended up drenched in sweat. I'm talking, take your t-shirt off, wring it out and have a stream of sweaty liquid fall to the ground. I would wear a back pack stuffed with water bottles and assorted junk. The pack was 30+ pounds and wearing it kicked my heart rate up 20 beats per minute, which is what I wanted. It was nothing to have my heart spike to over 200 climbing the near vertical grades.

The scenery was positively breathtaking and made these walks a transcendental experience. I loved the silence: you would hear your own labored breathing, the wind move through the trees, an occasional hawk or bird of prey might let out a shriek and other than that, no mechanical sound of any type. When was the last time you were outside and did not hear a mechanical sound?

He and I would carry walking sticks for viper protection. I had one coil up on me on another occasion. I came within three feet before I saw her, coiled, ready to strike and bite me. I call the snake "her" because I had a Special Forces buddy tell me the only reason the snake would stand and coil was if it were protecting eggs or her young. I was pleased with my own reaction: I froze and backed away, neither my heart beat nor pulse went up in the slightest. I know that for a fact because I was wearing a heart rate monitor at the time and I checked. I made like the late, great Steve Irwin and actually stood and studied the coiled snake from a safe distance. It was thick as my forearm and it relaxed as I backed off. It studied me as I studied it. I moved around to the right and was on my way.

On our jeep ride back home I came across a skateboarder. He was five miles out of town and just walking. It would have taken him hours to get to town at his pace. He was 18 or so with long hair and looked like Laird Hamilton the champion surfer. I stopped and yelled "Get in!" He let out a whoop. On the ride to town he talked to me passionately about the joys of meeting his buds at the town library and practicing their skate tricks all day long. Then he'd walk six miles back to the trailer where he lived with his widower dad. I dropped him off at the library and he generously and lovingly pulled a crinkled dollar bill from his pocket and handed it to me "for gas." I suspected it was his only dollar. I told him to keep it and drove off.

I thought "What a day! A creature of nature almost kills me and a beautiful kid restores my faith in humanity—all within a single hour." Chuck and I must have been one hell of a sight traveling over those mountain swells. Mountain cardio is the most exhilarating and effective way to perform aerobics that I know of. I would routinely burn 2,000+ calories on these endless enduros.

Our weight training sessions were also Purposefully Primitive to the max. I get bored easily and one summer we decided to try this crazed Russian ultra-high volume program that Pavel had translated and passed on to us.

We are admittedly mentally sick gluttons for self-induced punishment. We'd goad each other on like grammar school boys on the playground. We decided (well, actually *I decided*) that we would test ride this vicious squat program. The first week we did nine sets of 9 reps. Week two was eight sets of 8 reps, week three was 7x7 and week four 6x6. We were training in July and August and the gym thermometer routinely registered 95 to 105 degrees. Trust me, we glistened. I remember Deluxe weighing 205 hitting 440 for six sets of six, no suit, wraps, belt, no nothing. I was content with 405, six by six, weighing 195.

We were dying after the first set. The gym heat on that day was particularly vicious: 101 degrees with zero circulation. I even turned on the "air conditioning" which consisted of opening the garage door. No help today. Later Deluxe called our sessions, "The hardest workouts of my life." Nice compliment.

After training, as was our habit, we'd stagger to the deck adjoining my house and sit down, peel off our sweat soaked shirts and moan in ecstasy as the breeze would wash over our overheated torsos. I would head to the kitchen and mix us each a giant protein/carb Smart Bomb shake. I'd fire up the propane grill. Actually I would fire it up when we were on our final sets of squatting. When we walked to the deck we were ready to roll. We drink the shake and make some breakfast. Man Breakfast. Black Angus rib eye steaks sold to us by a local fundamentalist cult at their butcher shop. This was locally grown beef and not pumped full of steroids; this meat was restaurant grade. I'd leave the steaks out on the kitchen counter for a couple of hours before grilling to let the fat soften. Marty *knows* how to grill a perfect steak.

After drinking the smart bombs and allowing our leg tremors to subside, I'd sauté some local farm produce in a bit of olive oil using whatever veggies were in season. It might be asparagus spears, beautiful red and yellow peppers, succulent fresh broccoli, amazingly pungent onions, rich spinach...I could have a pan of sautéed fiber ready to eat inside ten minutes. While the fiber veggies were on the stovetop, I would walk to the blazing hot grill and lay the rib eyes, salted and peppered, atop the blazing hot grate. Sear on each side, turn the heat way down, shut the grill cover and let the steaks bake for a few short minutes. Internal temperature needed to hit 120 for me and 135 for Deluxe. I used a meat thermometer to make steaks consistently perfect every time. Chuck and I would be eating steaks and vegetables fifteen minutes after training.

"Mar-tee my man," Chuck would say with a drawl thicker than Fog Horn Leg Horn (incongruous for a guy with a law degree *and* a journalism degree) "This is 'bout what I'd imagine Heaven would be like for a powerlifter—assuming you believed in that sort of thing." I would laugh at his Jed Clampett inspired bon mots. He was an inexhaustible well of country wisdom and bunkhouse logic told with a Huckleberry Cornpone accent. Stuff like, "It's better to be a has-been than a never-was." And "Don't corner something meaner than you." Or "A bumble bee is faster than a John Deere tractor." That sort of stuff.

That boy could eat: I'd buy him two pounds of pure Black Angus and he'd gobble it down like a snack and be eyeing mine. "Are you going to finish that?" After that we would part company. I would take a shower and a power nap. Food never tasted as good as when we would eat that delicious, perfectly prepared organic food and those perfectly grilled steaks within a few minutes of a workout so torturous you'd think you might faint.

To follow the body crushing workout with a man meal, a hot shower and a power nap was heaven on earth. As my commando buddy Ori would say, "Life in paradise should be rugged." There was a physical intensity about those training sessions that caused me to access mental regions I hadn't visited in years. By the time we would get to the sixth or eighth set, by the time we'd be grinding out the 6th or 8th rep in that stifling garage, I was genuinely afraid of physical collapse. I would mildly hallucinate and have a detached sense that even though I was in my body, I was not really there. I was sort of an observer. It was intense and real.

It put me in mind of something related to the Ali-Forman fight. In the movie "*When We Were Kings*" Norman Mailer and George Plimpton retold tales related to the Rumble in the Jungle. Mailer in particular was great, morphing into a weird southern accent to tell Ali stories. Hunter Thompson was in attendance, but so bombed out of his mind he forgot what day it was and missed the fight altogether. But then again, he was the guy who had his ashes packed into a rocket, shot 1000 feet into the air and then exploded over a crowd in a fireworks explosion. Johnny Depp donated over a million bucks to fund the rocketman sendoff. They built a 50 foot tower on Thompson's Peacock Ranch in Woody Creek and constructed a rocket tower that had a gigantic double-thumbed gonzo fist. The rocket was shot off from behind the prop while below, revelers celebrated in fittingly hedonistic Gonzo fashion. Though, in view of Thompson's age and the age of his friends, it should have been called a gathering of the Tired Hedonists.

Who qualifies as a tired hedonist? I thought you would never ask. Cyril is addressing Vivian in Oscar Wilde's "The Decay of Lying." In my mind's eye I have always imagined Samuel L. Jackson as Cyril, while my role model, hero and literary idol, Camille Paglia, plays Vivian. We pick up the action...

> *CYRIL: Give me a cigarette. Thanks. By the way, in what magazine do you intend to publish your article, "The Decay of Lying: A Protest."*
>
> *VIVIAN: For the Retrospective Review; I think I told you the elect had revived it.*
>
> *CYRIL: Whom do you mean by "the elect"?*
>
> *VIVIAN: Oh, the Tired Hedonists, of course. It is a club to which I belong. I'm afraid you are not eligible. You are too fond of simple pleasures.*
>
> *CYRIL: Well, I should fancy you are all a good deal bored with each other.*
>
> *VIVIAN: We are. That is one of the objects of the club. Now if you promise not to interrupt too often I will read you my article....*

I think the party ethic exemplified by Hunter would naturally result in a tired hedonist at some point in time. I suspect he became a tired hedonist, recognized it and checked himself out when physical disability affected mobility. My wife thinks that I am far too lively to be classified a tired hedonist. She feels I more closely resemble Dorothy Parker's self-ascribed sobriquet, "The Carefree Psychotic." Stacy feels that the carefree psychotic moniker is far more apropos for me in my current state. And while I might logically be accused of being a hedonist, I am not yet tired. I label my wife "the upbeat cynic" so we make a good couple.

On to cheerier subjects: The movie, *When We Were Kings* and my viper encounter jarred my memory about a quote sport writer Peter Whitmer attributed to Ali in an post-fight interview after the Rumble in the Jungle.

> ***"In the 5th round during the rope-a-dope, when Ali was purposefully allowing Foreman to punch himself out, to hide from the firestorm Ali recounted a mental place he went to in his own mind. He would go to this mental hideout any time he was being pummeled for a prolonged period..."***
>
> ***Ali: "I went into the Near Room. The door was only half open. Inside, the room was neon orange with green blinking lights. There were bats blowing trumpets and alligators playing trombones. I could hear the screaming of snakes. On the walls were weird masks and actors' clothes."***

Ali would duck into the Near Room anytime he was in the ring in a fight and in trouble. To go inside the Near Room was to commit to self destruction. It was an interesting psychological insight into how one of the great athletes of our century dealt with the immediacy of severe athletic adversity. He would attempt to ride out the maelstrom and if still standing after the onslaught, he would be refreshed and revived enough to counterattack.

He had far, far more strategic successes than failures. I myself visited my own version of Ali's Near Room on the sixth set (all sets completed within 18 minutes) during the sixth of six reps. I went into my own version of The Near Room as I stalled badly attempting to push upward and lock out the 6th and final rep with 405. Time seemed suspended; in my detached state I saw the viper I'd run into on my hike, coiled and ready to strike me if I failed with the squat. I realized that if I missed this rep I would collapse so quickly and completely that the only help Chuck could provide was to call 911.

Metaphorically, if I missed the rep and collapsed the snake would strike me. As I ground upward with excruciating slowness I saw the snake clearly and distinctly...as I locked out the rep and as Deluxe helped me stagger back into the racks to replace the weight I could hear the snake scream. I missed the bats blowing trumpets and the alligators playing trombones.

Hammer Time!

Think Aerobics Are Sissy? Think Again Punk!

Mark "The Hammer" Coleman is without question one of the premier mixed martial arts fighters in the world. No one will accuse him of being sissified and live to brag about it. The Hammer has won the Ultimate Fighting Championship heavyweight title on three separate occasions and captured the prestigious Pride Tournament in 2000. I have interviewed Mark on numerous occasions about his overall training philosophy and specifically about his sport specific approach to cardio training. His approach exemplifies a hardcore cardio approach that is the polar opposite of the Richard Simmons School of sissy aerobics. He once told me, "Marty, if I don't puke at least once sprinting up hills, I don't feel as if I've really put out." Man Cardio.

Coleman makes the point that in addition to classical steady-state endurance, exemplified by roadwork or stationary bike, he also uses burst cardio and exotic 3rd Way cardio—though he wouldn't call it that. 3rd Way strength/endurance cardio is acquired through a specialized form of training that is becoming *de rigueur* in MMA circles. In "The Hammer's" world of mayhem he has to man-up and administer beat downs to monstrous opponents. To do so he needs to be able to put out incredible amounts of physical energy without "gassing." He needs to ground and pound, shoot and grapple, tug and kick, and do it minute after minute, round after round.

Riding an exercise bike will not give him the sustained strength that he needs to fight three brutal rounds with the likes of 6'5" 250 pound Brazilian jujitsu expert Antonio Noreiga. To build sustained strength he throws and tosses heavy implements; he pushes and pulls on training partners, he does all kinds and types of strength-infused cardio that requires intense, sustained muscular effort.

Mark purposefully injects an element of intense muscular effort into his cardiovascular training. He devises training situations that require extended effort. He might force himself to flurry punch when already tired; practice powering out of a submission; run up steep hills, sprinting all out or repeatedly throw a heavy medicine ball for protracted periods of time. He related one game he and his fearsome partner, Kevin "Monster Man" Randleman, use. It is an improvised game of 'fetch' that involves a heavy medicine ball. They throw the ball as far as possible to each other then scramble on all fours at top speed to retrieve it before heaving the ball yet again, over and over.

Another trick for building sustained strength is to grapple all out with an opponent and have a fresh opponent rotate in every few minutes. The Hammer is forced to deal with a completely fresh wrestler while he is exhausted, thereby pushing himself past his current strength and cardio limits to establish new and extended limits. He seeks extreme aerobic exercise modes that tax endurance and introduce muscle-stress elements into the cardio equation. Coleman makes a distinction between different types of cardio and recognizes each requires a different training approach. So should you. Don't make the mistake most modern aerobic practitioners make and practice steady-state exclusively.

The modern mixed martial artist needs absolute strength *and* sustained strength. They need sustained cardio capacity and burst cardio capacity; they need the ability to put out incredible amounts of power and strength over an extended period of time. This ability is not developed by simply sitting on a stationary bike pedaling along. Sustained strength is developed through sustained effort.

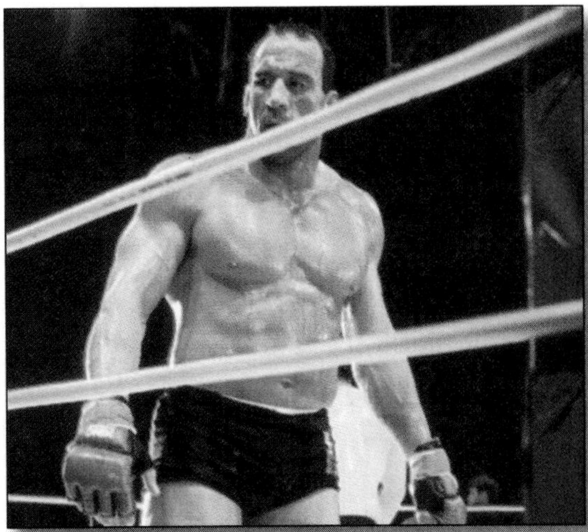

Hammer Time: Mark "The Hammer" Coleman is a mixed martial arts legend. The above photo was taken when he captured the Pride Tournament in 2000. Mark started his career as a world level wrestler and morphed his skill-set as he matured as a MMA fighter. He added knockout hand strikes to his pugilistic arsenal and his head-butts (pin the opponents arms down, butt him in the face with the forehead) were so effective and lethal that they were banned. His knees-to-the-head tactic was used to defeat Igor Volchainan and win the Pride Grand Prix. His physical training underwent as big a metamorphosis as his skill-set arsenal. Originally Mark trained in classic wrestler fashion. As the mixed martial arts game evolved, Coleman, a sophisticated and innovative trainer, morphed his training. "Bonking," precipitous drops in blood-sugar levels deep into fights, became a predictable problem. Mark and MMA giants like super-trainer John Hackleman determined that cardiovascular training needed to be melded with strength training in order to create sustained strength. Mark has gotten leaner over the past 15 years and now weighs 228.

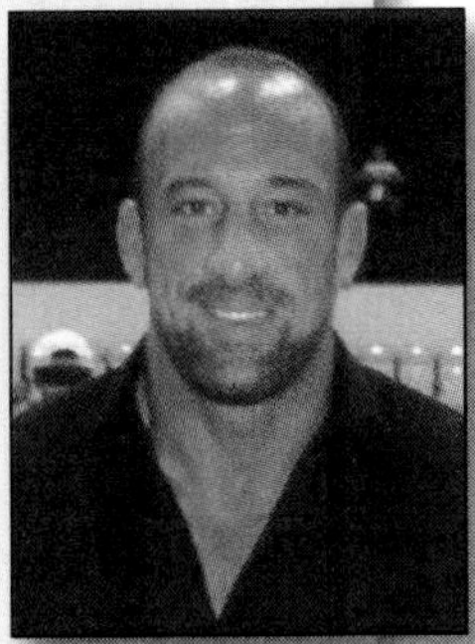

Martial Artists and 3rd Way Hybrid Cardio

In a recent TV show on and about Ultimate Fighters, the training methodology of mixed martial arts training Master John Hackleman was spotlighted. "The Hack" is the mentor of Chuck "The Ice Man" Liddell, the most dominant UFC fighter of the past five years. It was interesting to note that the training methods used nowadays by the world's best fighters are undergoing a profound revolution. Back in the early 1990s, when the UFC first came on the scene, martial artists represented their respective traditions and trained exclusively using the methods of their particular fighting system.

All that went out the window when the specialists started getting beat up by the cross-trained MMA adherents.

If a martial artist was a judo man and refused to learn boxing, if a boxer refused to learn ground fighting, if a wrestler refused to learn how to apply submission holds, then those one dimensional martial artists were inevitably and eventually beaten by the *mixed* martial artists. Those who adapted and broadened their approach thrived; those who insisted on staying loyal to a particular school or discipline were swept aside. In the year 2007 fighting has truly become an amalgamation of fight styles. Those that are well rounded fighters become the champions and those who are doggedly and dogmatically one-dimensional don't make the cut.

A similar phenomenon has occurred in the *training* of the mixed martial artist. Initially there were a lot of non-weight trainers. They began getting overpowered, manhandled and beat down mercilessly by heavily muscled men like Ken Shamrock, Mark Coleman, Mark Kerr, Randy Couture and Tank Abbott. Those big, strong, powerful men were knocking smaller men unconscious with six inch punches or effortlessly body slamming weaker opponents. In the year 2007 resistance training is practiced by every MMA in every weight class: it's not an option, it's a necessity. At the top levels everyone is skilled, that's assumed. It's the weaknesses that determine who loses. Top fighters never play to the opponents strengths, they exploit their weaknesses. Why box a boxer? Why wrestle a wrestler? If a man is physically weak, physically overpower him.

If you are skilled and weak, expect to be overpowered by Rampage Jackson and be prepared to be unceremoniously body slammed. If you are strong, but lack endurance, be prepared to be run into the ground by a smart, well-conditioned fighter like Matt Hughes. The champions exploit an opponent's weakness and the losers refuse to correct those weaknesses.

Cardiovascular fight training has undergone an evolution. In the beginning, fighters would ride the stationary bike, perform roadwork or skip rope. That was considered all that was needed to create the requisite endurance needed for a fight. What happened was curious and mysterious: men in great cardiovascular shape, men capable of entering a marathon and finishing the 26 mile run in less than three hours were "gassing out" ten minutes into a fight. "What the hell is going on? I can run all day long—yet I get so winded in an actual fight that I can't hold my arms up by the end of a third round."

What the best brains in the mixed martial arts finally determined was that there were different types of cardio endurance. Though a man might be able to run or ride the stationary bike all day, that type of cardio was steady-state cardio. What was needed in a fight was a radically different type of cardio. The type of endurance training needed to train fighters, had to have an element of muscular exertion involved. Top MMA coaches like John Hackleman figured out that they needed to train fighters differently. Continual, unrelenting stress and effort was melded with cardiovascular exercise. The modern MMA fighter might be found at "The Hacks" country training camp picking up heavy objects, lifting them and heaving them for reps and distance. The idea was to stretch and sustain intense physical effort for a protracted period of time.

During a fight extreme physical effort is required to go along with pure cardio: the fighter has to push and tug on an opponent continually. A considerable amount of strength is needed to apply a submission hold or power out of a bad position. The muscular effort needed in a fight makes steady-state cardio, like riding a stationary bike, virtually meaningless. As Mark Coleman pointed out, intense physical exertion combined with extended cardio effort wreaks havoc on blood sugar levels and sends men into hypoglycemic shock.

Fighters needed to create a new type of conditioning in which a strength element is married to a cardio element to create *sustained strength*. Cardio fight training needed to be amended and modified. In order to prevent fighters from fading, deep into a lengthy battle, a new training protocol was devised.

On the TV special, Hackleman's training camp methods was spotlighted. He ran his elite fighters through a series of drills that were illuminating and instructive. In the first series of drills, five fighters stood at five individual stations. Hack would yell "Go!" and for 40 seconds each fighter would attempt to do as many reps as humanly possible at each of the five stations. The stations were: plyometric jumps up onto a 3 foot ledge, speed sit-ups, a row machine, a versa-climber and a treadmill. After 40 seconds, Hack would yell "Stop!" and the athletes would rest for 20 seconds at which point Hack would yell "Go!" Staying at the same station, the fighter would attack the same exercise again for 40 seconds. When Hack yelled "Stop!" a second time he would yell "Rotate!" and the fighters would immediately jump to the second station and without pause he would yell "Go!" They would repeat: 40 seconds all out, rest for 20, then 40 more seconds all out. This was repeated for several "circuits."

Next Hack took his elite fighters, including Chuck Liddell, to his rural training camp. Here similar methods were used, but of a slightly different flavor. He started the six man squad off by flipping over a giant 500 pound tire for distance. Immediately after tire flips, each executed 50 speed punches. They all grabbed a sledgehammer and pounded the giant tire repeatedly. They pushed wheelbarrows loaded with dumbbell plates up a steep hill and as soon as they dropped the wheelbarrows they began medicine ball drills. They started off by throwing them to one another. Then each man would fling a medicine ball overhead as high as possible before letting it crash to the earth. They would do a squat thrust, pick the ball up and hurl it overhead again. This went on for many minutes. Then they threw medicine balls at a wall for five straight minutes. Finally they were rotated through parallel bar dips and pull-ups. Once they were done with this hellish session, they jogged to an outdoor cage and began nonstop wrestling and submission work. This was just another day at the office for this crew, nothing special for the cameras.

This type of training builds the sustained strength needed to keep from gassing out deep into a fight. By infusing extended cardiovascular effort with intense muscular effort, an entirely new type of endurance-strength is built. Interestingly Hack's approach is strategically similar to the kind of training Len Schwartz, Ori Hofmekler and John Parrillo advise their students to do in order to build additional mitochondria and create cardiovascular density. Each man recommends differing training strategies that ultimately do two things: build sustained strength, as opposed to absolute strength and build mitochondrial density into muscles subjected to each man's particular protocol. Is it better to lift 100 pounds 40 times or 400 pounds 1 time? (The correct answer is, better to be able to do *both*).

If the goal is to construct mitochondria, cardio training needs to have an element of muscular effort. Cardio density is also improved by this type of training, creating additional blood vessels and larger blood vessels. More blood vessels mean nutrients are able to be rushed to muscles faster and waste products removed far more quickly. By developing cardiovascular density, by building more mitochondria, nature's natural genetic limitations are extended and expanded. Schwartz's Heavyhands, Hofmekler's Controlled Fatigue Training or Parrillo's 100 rep Extended Sets are specific exercise protocols designed to build more mitochondria. All three methods fuse intense effort with prolonged effort and resemble the methods used by Hackleman.

It is intriguing that elite fight trainers are independently developing training regimens remarkably similar to those used to build 3rd Way hybrid muscle. Hack simply wants to keep fighters from gassing late in a fight—mitochondria building is the furthest thing from his mind—yet his methods, and the methods used by Mark Coleman, are building mitochondria and cardio density as surely as the methods of Len Schwartz, John Parrillo, or Ori Hofmekler. They say that great minds think alike and never was that hackneyed cliché more appropriate than in this particular instance. 3rd Way cardio training deserves a seat at the training table. Be sure and include it your cardio rotation. Start slinging some heavy weighted implements around for extended periods.

IN PRAISE OF STEVE JUSTA SUSTAINED-STRENGTH GRAND MAESTRO

One of my strength heroes has never won a single lifting title in any strength sport and has no plans to compete. Steve Justa is a strength philosopher who resides on a farm in rural Nebraska. His forte is sustained strength feats and his book, *Rock, Iron, Steel: The Book of Strength* is perhaps the best book on or about sustained strength ever written. Steve uses Mid-America plain-speak with a word economy that would do Anton Chekov proud. His words are so clear I am backing out now to let him talk to you direct...The man needs no interpreter.

> ***"Once I saw a guy do eight reps with 500 pounds in the bench press at a seminar. He was huffing and puffing into the microphone for the next 30 minutes trying to get his wind...now how much good is strength like that going to do you in real life survival situations? What good is strong if you can't summon the strength over and over again?***

Right on! This guy would see eye to eye with Ori, Hammer and John Hackelman. Justa's personal lifting records are awe inspiring...

- Dragged a 540 pound railroad rail backwards for 1/8th of a mile in 25 minutes
- Lifted the same railroad rail from the ground, shouldered it and walked with it for 30 feet
- Picked up a 4 foot tall 315 pound barrel and carried it 1/8th mile

- Carried a 220 pound rock for a mile in 90 minutes
- Deadlifted a 250 pound barbell without straps and then carried it in the completed position for a mile
- Made a chain mail vest, loaded it up to weigh 200 pounds and walked with it on for two miles in 50 minutes.
- Walked for 25 steps though mud with an 800 pound barbell on his back. He sunk up to his ankles on each step and called this "the most dangerous lift I've ever attempted."
- Without the mud, he once walked 40 steps with 1200 pounds on his back in street clothes.
- Worked on farms his entire life. On one occasion for fourteen straight days Steve threw and stacked 1500, 80 pound hay bales.
- Jerked a 250 pound barbell overhead and then walked with it on extended arms for 100 steps.

> ***"Walking with a heavy vest or pack builds super endurance. I once wore a 100 pound chain mail vest every day to work for 8-10 hours a day for a month straight. I wore this vest while I walked through a building full of corn. I would scoop corn and rake corn wearing my vest. When I wasn't in the buildings full of corn I was doing other duties for my job wearing my vest...***
>
> ***I remember {that during the period}...I entered a basketball tournament. The vest work really paid off. I was doing things on the basketball court that I never had done...I was inflicting my will on everyone...I remember dribbling down the court and this big 275 pound guy planted himself in front of me. I just ran over him like he wasn't even there. I bet he slid 20 feet."***

Steve Justa is the personification of sustained strength. No doubt if muscle biopsies were performed on his massive muscles they would be infused with tons of mitochondria. His approach builds 3rd Way Hybrid Super Muscle, though he'd never call it that. His approach to lifting big and getting strong for extended periods of time brings into bold relief an entire new universe of strength training potentialities. Justa is one of a kind, a sustained strength prophet before his time. He is the archetypical Purposeful Primitive. Get his book. www.ironmind.com

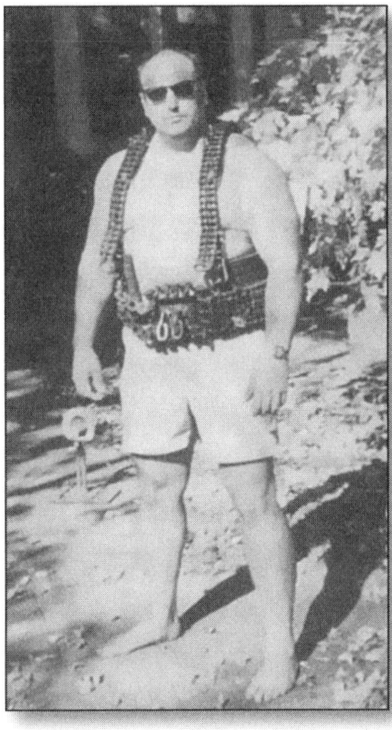

The 100-pound Chain Vest: "What do you want done next Boss?"

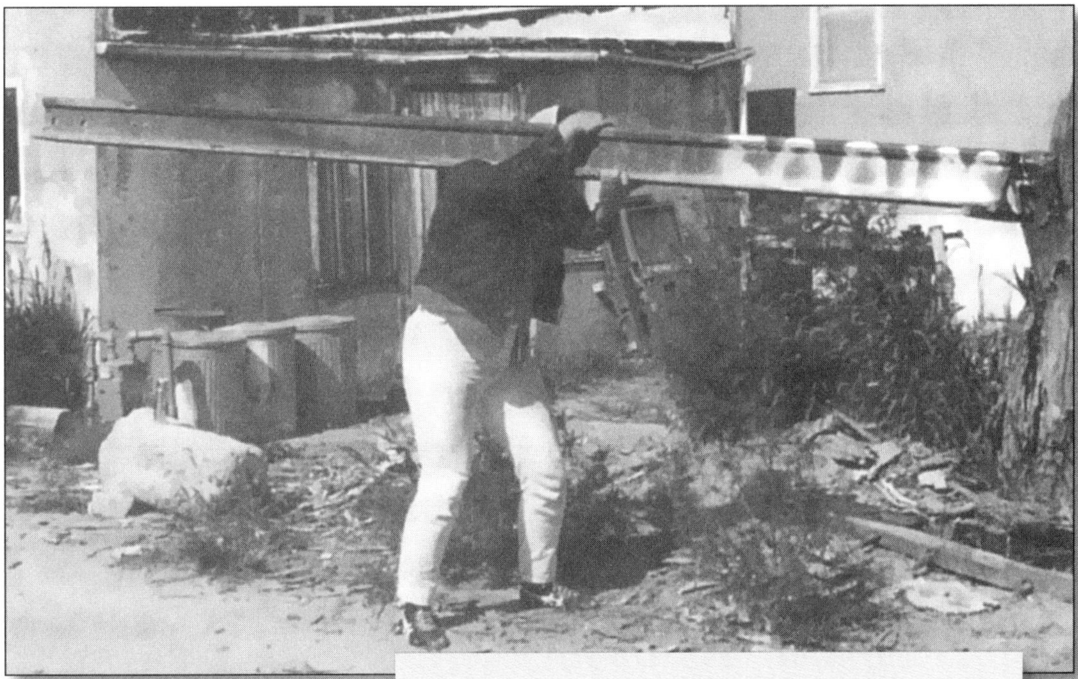

540-pound Rail: walk it for 30 feet, then drag it 1/8th of a mile

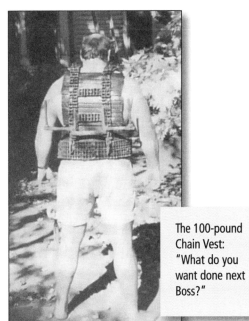

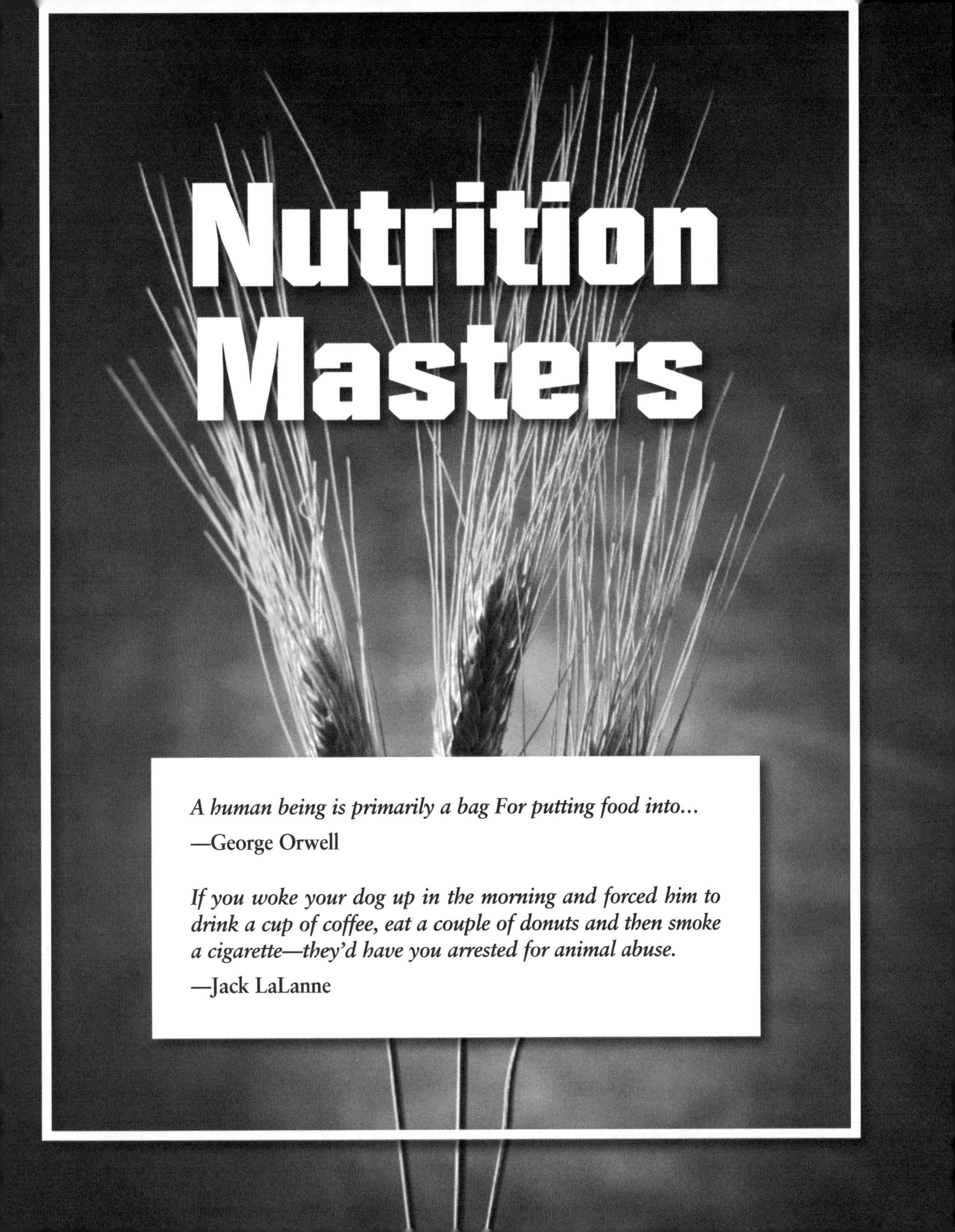

Nutrition Masters

A human being is primarily a bag For putting food into...

—George Orwell

If you woke your dog up in the morning and forced him to drink a cup of coffee, eat a couple of donuts and then smoke a cigarette—they'd have you arrested for animal abuse.

—Jack LaLanne

No Need to Square the Nutritional Circle

When it comes to fitness-related nutrition, things are made way more complex then they need to be. What should be the ultimate goal of a nutritional game plan?

The studied use and diligent application of applied nutrition should enhance the user's ability to build new muscle and aide in the mobilization and oxidation of stored body fat. That's the irreducible goal of Purposefully Primitive nutrition.

I champion two diametrically opposed nutritional approaches: the classical Parrillo Nutritional Program and the deservedly popular Warrior Diet. It would be impossible to find two more dissimilar approaches towards the studied use of food and drink. I feel absolutely zero compunction about squaring this nutritional circle: to me each dietary approach represents a mighty tool in the nutritional toolbox—in fact, likely the only two dietary tools you'll ever need. Both approaches are effective arrows in the nutritional quiver. Both methods work—of this there can be no doubt. There are far too many flesh-and-blood examples of transformed adherents…elite athletes, military Special Forces members, regular people, the obese...literally legions of adherents have used each dietary approach and reaped incredible benefits.

A sound nutritional plan magnifies and amplifies the exercise effort. Expert use of nutrition revitalizes and regenerates the body. Proper nutrition provides the body the ample amounts of beneficial nutrients needed for the construction of new muscle tissue. The expert usage of targeted nutrition accelerates the healing and recovery process. Food (and rest) helps dampen the after-training body shock, the self-inflicted physical trauma that envelops an athlete after a hardcore weight training session or an intense aerobic workout.

I recommend two diametrically opposed nutritional approaches: each one successfully stakes out a logical dietary extreme. In relation to one another, these two strategies are black and white, thesis and antithesis, Yin and Yang. The Parrillo approach is based upon bodybuilding methodology and its philosophy of food relies on the continual consumption of meals throughout the day. The Warrior Diet has a military pedigree and its philosophy of food is to eat a single, major daily meal. I think you would agree that that is one hell of a philosophic chasm.

The Parrillo nutritional system requires the individual eat selected foods in a continual stream of calorically equalized mini-meals. The meals are consumed at equidistant intervals throughout the day. In bodybuilding, at all levels, this approach (or structurally similar nutritional plans) is used to near exclusion. The Parrillo system demands tremendous attention to detail: foods are often weighed or measured and detailed exercise and nutrition logs are kept. Intense physical training is integral to the Parrillo nutritional philosophy. Precision eating actually amplifies training results. Athletes today are demonstrably larger and stronger than in decades gone by, due in large part to a superior understanding of the role of nutrition. Used correctly, nutrition can make a fat person lean, a thin person muscular or a good athlete great.

The Warrior Diet protocol is based on the principle of "intermittent fasting." The goal is to awaken long dormant primordial hardwiring by detoxifying the body. The Warrior Diet creates a daily *anabolic burst*. Daytime fasting is followed by nighttime feasting. Warrior protocol insists followers *do not* eat after awaking from the sleep cycle. The previous night's sleep is actually the start of the next day's fast. Not eating breakfast allows the Warrior Dieter to continue the nighttime detoxification process nature has already set in motion. By not eating during the day, the poisoned body is allowed to detoxify itself. By not eating, primordial defense and survival mechanisms are reawakened. Eat all natural foods and if possible, eat organic. Low-glycemic, chemically-free foods are used whenever possible. Detoxification is a huge part of the Warrior Diet philosophy: Ori Hofmekler presents a compelling case that we are a poisoned race in need of remedial detoxification.

Each of these two magnificent nutritional systems is rooted in science, biology and logic. Both have hordes of transformed followers. The Parrillo nutritional system came out of the elite competitive bodybuilding tradition while the Warrior Diet emerged from an austere military tradition. Each approach is admittedly extreme. If mild methods worked we'd all be lean and muscular. Each approach has proven itself effective at forcing and tricking the body to mobilize and convert stored body fat into energy to fuel physical activity. Both approaches proclaim that regimented eating and intense physical training are inseparable. Food is used to nourish and heal a body continually reeling from the bone-crushing, hypertrophy-inducing weight workouts and the near daily cardio sessions both systems insist on.

Fad diets live in a vacuum. Regimented dieting without a coordinated exercise regimen will only take you so far. Fad diet books place all the emphasis on food content and not enough on dietary *structure*. Almost every diet plan spends an inordinate amount of time telling you what you can and cannot eat. Few food strategies take into account meal size, meal timing, how different foods interact with one another, when eaten in combination, or the impact of intense exercise on the overall dietary effort.

Both Parrillo and Warrior recognize and purposefully create *windows of opportunity*. These windows are fertile metabolic states created by using a specific set of diet and exercise procedures. Create the window then take advantage of this contrived physiological anomaly by consuming a precise combination of nutrients. Periodization principles are applied to weight training, aerobic training *and* nutrition to create physical momentum.

Our Purposefully Primitive approach is to select one of these terrific nutritional systems and give it a test ride for a protracted period. Purposeful Primitives apply periodization principles to both exercise and nutrition, enabling the user to stair-step upwards towards a predetermined physical goal. Elite athletes always have a goal. So should you. Place the goal within the context of a periodized timeline. How do you eat an elephant? You eat the elephant one bite at a time. We transform the body one periodized step at a time.

If the Parrillo Nutritional Program were to be encapsulated in a single sound-bite, it could be: *eat seven times a day.*

If the Warrior Diet were to be encapsulated in a single sound-bite, it could be, eat *seven times a week.*

The philosophical differences could not be more profound. My sound-bite encapsulation of each system is a purposeful oversimplification. Within each system exists a universe of nuanced exceptions, subtleties, shades of grey, provisos and adaptations to the general rules, all based upon particular or peculiar individual situations. As with any fluid philosophy, success is based on the individual's ability to adapt the general guidelines.

Now for a reality check: There is no sense getting fired up about using the Parrillo Nutritional System if circumstance prevents you from preparing and eating multiple meals. There is no sense becoming enamored with the Warrior Diet approach if you cannot or will not limit daytime eating.

John Parrillo has guided thousands of competitive athletes through his process over the last three decades. Ori Hofmekler has an army of adherents. Both men have infused their respective approaches with a streak of practicality that comes from having obtained real results for real people in real life situations. These men do not live in a vacuum: they make their livings transforming people. Both are extremely successful because they are extremely adept at what they do.

How can I recommend two systems so diametrically opposed? Extreme opposites set up the tantalizing possibility of cyclical rotation. Both inventors would disagree and rightly state that enough contrast and variation exist within each system to ensure year round use without any need to resort to any other dietary approach. If your personality, needs or sit-

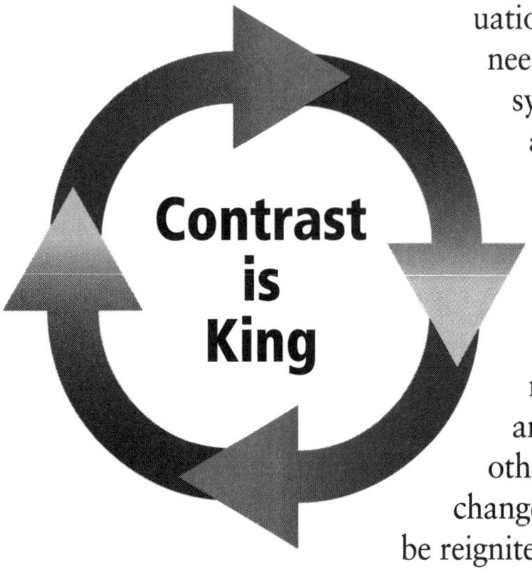

uation are such that one system or the other is all you need or want, then by all means, stick with that lone system in perpetuity. On the other hand, to use another hackneyed yet appropriate analogy, variety is the eternal spice of life.

Because of the immense chasm between the two approaches, a profoundly beneficial possibility emerges, that of dramatic *contrast*. If the chosen nutritional system is eventually neutralized by the amazingly adaptive human body, then leaping to the other extreme could jolt the body back into motion. If change sufficiently contrasts the status quo, progress can be reignited.

These two systems are the epitome of thesis and antithesis. The contrast between the two systems could not be greater; they differ to such a dramatic degree that their periodic rotation could be used to create a cyclical synthesis.

Do you *have* to rotate these systems? No. As a matter of fact each man behind his system would recommend you not do so. As a battle-scarred Purposeful Primitive I know that no one system trumps all others and that every mode and method, no matter how clever or sophisticated eventually ceases delivering results. The founders of each of these systems have addressed the issue of contrast within the confines of their particular system: I periodically choose to step completely outside of whatever nutritional or exercise box I am currently in. I have found that periodic dietary rotation can be beneficial. Necessary? No. Mandatory? No. However I could think of no better alternative system to take up, were I using one system and it ceased delivering results. Eat seldom or eat often, but do so in a regimented fashion. Clean up the food selections and learn how to prepare your own food. Learn how to infuse taste into "diet foods" and learn how to be patient and methodical. Four weeks is a reasonable amount of time to commit to for a nutritional test ride. If mild methods produced radical results we'd all be ripped: radical methods yield radical results. Time to get nutritionally radical.

JOHN PARRILLO

John Parrillo is a true master of bodybuilding nutrition. John is the steadfast revolutionary. Brilliant, iconoclastic, intense, enigmatic, articulate, occasionally abrasive, Parrillo is above all else an innovator. Radical postulations come easy to this guy. Back in the late 70s Parrillo became enamored with the idea that a competitive bodybuilder, seeking to grow as large and lean as humanely possible, should eat *massive* amounts of quality food on a consistent daily basis. Massive caloric intake would "underpin" the blisteringly intense weight training and savage cardiovascular training that he routinely proscribed. Parrillo's postulations were considered heretical when he first presented them. At the time, the late 1970's and early 1980's, bodybuilding was having an identity crisis: men like Frank Zane and Chris Dickerson, small guys with lots of defined muscles, were winning the biggest titles in bodybuilding. In the early 80's Chris Dickerson won the Olympia one year with a 16.5 inch arm! Parrillo, a native of Cincinnati, Ohio was a powerlifter dumbstruck by the gargantuan physiques of the oversized, brutish lifters. John marveled at the elite lifters' sheer size. How did they get so big? He wondered. He noted that humongous powerlifters hoisted huge poundage for low reps in a limited number of basic barbell exercises. They trained infrequently. Their training sessions were extremely heavy and extremely intense. Afterwards top lifters would rest for days. Parrillo also marveled at how much food these men ate—their appetites and capacities were gluttonous.

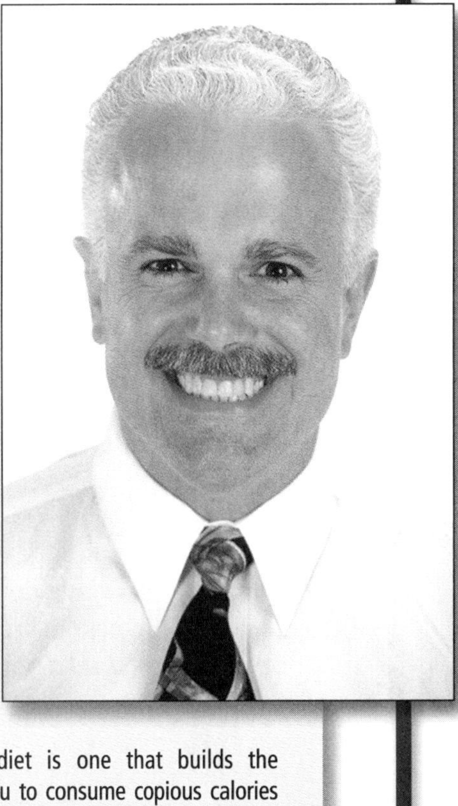

John at 60: He's dedicated his life to bodybuilding and sports nutrition.

"The solution to losing body fat—and keeping it off—will totally amaze you. The solution to losing body fat lies not in cutting calories but in increasing them! My three-stage 12-week fat loss program has been used by competitive bodybuilders to acquire single-digit body fat percentiles for decades. The ideal bodybuilding diet is one that builds the metabolism. This allows you to consume copious calories yet still burn off body fat. Crash diets are disastrous. Denied food, the body begins to feed on the protein in the muscles. Muscle is the human body's most metabolically active tissue; depleting it, cannibalizing it, retards the body's ability to burn calories."

Parrillo deduced that extremely heavy weight training combined with extremely heavy eating (powerlifters ate thousands and thousands calories at a single sitting) would result in tremendous gains in muscular size and strength. On the downside, the indiscriminant consumption of calories was a health catastrophe: pizza, pasta, cheese, fried foods, saturated fat, sugar, Jack Daniels and beer were seemingly the staples of the powerlifter's diet. Massive caloric intake combined with hardcore power training built massive muscles: Parrillo pondered long and hard on how best to improve and refine upon this profound premise.

Bodybuilders of the day turned up their collective noses up at the idea that there might be anything of the slightest interest to be learned from thuggish "power oafs." Parrillo thought that shortsighted and mused, "What if bodybuilders expropriated the training tactics of the powerlifter and copied their massive ingestion of calories? How do we replicate the powerlifter's massive muscle size - yet somehow manage to stay lean and fat free?

At the time top bodybuilders engaged in endlessly long weight training sessions using light weights and high reps. Sessions were long and drawn out. The standardized training protocol was to perform 20 sets per body part. This, it was thought, would sculpt and refine muscles. The elite bodybuilders weight trained *twice* a day, six-days-a-week, using the mind-numbing "double split" routine. Parrillo thought this training approach was a physiological dead end. What if bodybuilders were to cut back on training volume while radically upping the poundage? Reduce the reps, start slinging some serious iron and after these bar-bending sessions ended, feed the body huge amounts of food—good food, beneficial foods. Instead of eating all the day's calories in two or three mega-meals, spread the calories out, eat 5-7 times a day, and reduce the caloric intake at any one time. Eat equalized mini-meals spaced at periodic intervals throughout the day.

What if, Parrillo postulated, instead of consuming gobs of calorie-dense saturated fat, insulin-spiking sugar, refined carbs galore and beer by the case—what if food selections were limited to "quality" food sources? Lean fat-free protein, fibrous vegetables, starchy carbohydrates—and little else. Eat massively but eat "clean," a descriptive adjective denoting a food or beverage devoid (or nearly devoid) of saturated fat, sugar, or insulin-spiking tendencies. A chicken breast is a clean food whereas a fat-laden piece of prime rib is "dirty." The food selections become more discriminating: Dirty calories are replaced with clean calories.

Heavy power training would stimulate muscular growth and the consumption of copious clean calories would accelerate recovery and trigger anabolism. The only foods allowed would be those foods preferentially partitioned into muscle construction or used for energy production. Parrillo would have his trainees eat big, but avoid foods preferentially partitioned into body fat. The goal was to create a new generation of gargantuan bodybuilders: 250 pound monsters with single digit body fat percentiles. Parrillo proceeded to change his own eating and training habits. In no time at all his body exploded with growth: by combining heavy power training with clean mini-meal mega-eating, he transformed his own physique in a matter of months. He set state powerlifting records. The bodybuilders that trained at his gym wanted to know what he had done to trigger such a dramatic transformation in such a remarkably short period of time. He soon found himself in the role of a muscle guru, structuring the diets of competitive bodybuilders. Being detailed by nature, he began systematizing his embryonic philosophy.

Every single time a bodybuilder working under John's auspice fully adopted the Parrillo approach, the bodybuilder became significantly larger and significantly leaner. By the early 1980's Parrillo's "bodybuilder preparation" services were in tremendous demand. Bodybuilders were beating down his door seeking his services. He would design the bodybuilder a customized pre-contest nutritional game plan. In some instances he oversaw training sessions. He became a master at plotting progress and making critical in-flight adjustments and course corrections. Men that had been stuck at a particular level of physical development for years, men consigned and resigned to placing in the middle of the pack at state and regional competitions, suddenly added 30 pounds of muscle while simultaneously *losing* body fat.

Losers became winners.

The word spread as Parrillo's fleet of bodybuilders began wiping the floor with the competition at the local, regional and national level. Soon IFBB professional bodybuilders began seeking his dietary counsel. Several Olympia winners surreptitiously used his products and sought his nutritional guidance. This was on the QT as the Olympia winners were all under exclusive endorsement contracts to giant supplement makers. They endorsed products they did not use. Word spread to the muscle magazines: there was talk of a mystical muscle guru who was using natural methods to obtain supernatural results for men already at 98% of their genetic potential. The underground magician went mainstream. He began penning a column in one of the world's premier bodybuilder publications. The word was out and a revolution gained traction.

Parrillo received a lot of flack from defenders of the status quo. Not everyone was enamored with the idea of 260 pound mega-monsters with 4% body fat percentiles. Bodybuilding opinion makers were fine with the idea of a diminutive David being judged a better bodybuilder than a Farnese Hercules. Eventually the bodybuilding public grew restive and demanded changes in judging criterion. Up until the revolt, massively developed, ripped to the bone bodybuilders like 250 pound Bertil Fox were relegated to sixth place, losing to men Arnold once described as "chickens with 17" arms." All this changed when the fans essentially took to the streets to demand change.

The era of the muscle monster had arrived and John Parrillo was Doctor Frankenstein.

Bigger and Leaner

More Calories/More Training/No Excuses

Parrillo is an odd mix: simultaneously a cutting-edge revolutionary and an Old School throwback. He is a revolutionary in that nothing in the world of bodybuilding was ever the same after his high calorie thesis took root. He boldly proclaimed that an athlete could "build the metabolism" and teach the body how to handle ever increasing amounts of calories and do so without getting fat. He was immediately set upon by the bodybuilding ruling class. They labeled his pronouncements about being able to eat upwards of 10,000 calories a day and not get fat as "Insane!" It defied the laws of thermodynamics, they screamed, to insist that anyone could eat that much food and not have vast portions shuttled into fat storage. Had it been the Middle Ages, this heretic would have been burned at the stake.

Parrillo's pronouncements were greeted with the equivalent of the Bronx cheer by defenders of the prevailing orthodoxy. In assembly-line fashion he just kept churning out bigger and leaner bodybuilders. The professional bodybuilders took notice and were a lot more receptive to Parrillo's ideas than the opinion makers, the supplement manufacturers or the magazine article writers. Athletes continually seek out new avenues of progress and elite athletes will try any crazy substance, training tactic, idea or approach they believe might give them a leg up over the competition. The Parrillo precepts made sense to them. Top competitive bodybuilders noted that after having starved down for a competition, (the accepted contest preparation orthodoxy of the time) when "regular" food was reintroduced into their post-competition eating, after being so drained and depleted for so long, they blew up, often gaining 10-20 pounds within 36 hours of the competition-without any loss in muscle clarity, definition or delineation.

The "super compensation" phenomenon was widely noted among the elite and tied in nicely to Parrillo's talk about "windows of opportunity." The elite bodybuilders were equally receptive to Parrillo's theories about elevating the metabolic thermostat using specific combinations of nutrition and exercise. Parrillo had confirmed the elite bodybuilders' unarticulated suspicions. John Parrillo had bottled bodybuilding lighting: he had figured out how to manipulate the metabolism through the expert use of regular food.

Build the Metabolism

Eat More to Lose Body Fat

Parrillo preached that to ratchet up the metabolism the bodybuilder should eat 5 to 8 times a day. Multiple meals, "feedings" should be spaced at equidistant intervals and only approved foods should be eaten. These foods would be eaten in certain combinations. The continual intake of quality nutrients would stoke the fires of the metabolic furnace. Over a protracted period of time, more calories could and would be consumed at each feeding. Mini-meals were to be eaten every two to three hours. The idea was to never overload the digestive system at any one meal. By spreading the day's calories out in a never ending succession of mini-meals, the bodybuilder's digestive system would become adept at digesting, distributing and utilizing quality nutrients. Parrillo pointed out that the metabolism accelerates when forced to digest certain foods. i.e., lean protein and fibrous carbohydrates. The conscientious consumption of ample amounts of lean, fat free protein and fibrous carbohydrates form the backbone of the Parrillo nutritional approach. Saturated fat, sugar and alcohol are eliminated under Parrillo guidelines. Foods that spike insulin are verboten. The highly systematized Parrillo nutritional approach is disciplined, demanding and effective. The bodybuilders of the 1980's loved it: the orthodox dietary procedure of the day was to starve. Now they were told to eat and eat a lot. They were gleeful and ecstatic.

By eating throughout the day the bodybuilder established Positive Nitrogen Balance and stayed in a state of perpetual anabolism. PNB is created by eating an ample amount of calories. While in PNB muscle growth is possible—not that it occurs in and of itself, but the growth field is made fertile. If while in PNB an intense weight workout is undertaken, hypertrophy occurs. To spike the metabolism consume multiple mini-meals comprised entirely of quality nutrients. Avoid high glycemic foods and avoid refined foods and man-made foods. Engage in intense exercise. Over time the metabolic set-point will be ratcheted upward. "Building the metabolism" is the central tenet of the Parrillo Philosophy. The best analogy for building the metabolism is building and maintaining a blazing fire. If dry hardwood logs are used (quality food fuel) the fire burns hot and intense. If every few hours new hardwood logs are thrown onto the already blazing metabolic fire, the fire is kept blazing and all the logs are burned completely. The hotness of the fire ensures no partially burnt logs remain.

The metabolism is ignited in the morning by eating a quality food meal. The metabolism is then kept blazing throughout the day. The competitive bodybuilder teaches the body to expect food every 2-3 hours. By never overwhelming the digestive system at any one time, by using foods difficult to partition into fat storage, by eating foods difficult to digest, the metabolism is forced to periodically elevate. Intense exercise elevates an already elevated metabolism. The bodily thermostat is raised repeatedly by ingesting specific foods at specific times and by engaging in intense weight training and intense cardiovascular exercise. The metabolism is stimulated in some manner or fashion every few waking hours.

Champion bodybuilders can consume 8,000 calories a day, spread over five to eight meals, and not gain an ounce of fat. They have worked up to this massive caloric intake over a protracted period of time. They avoid foods that deaden or make the metabolism sluggish and eat upwards of 50 mini-meals each week. Every two to three hours the body burns through its current supply of food/fuel and the bodybuilder becomes ravenous for more food/fuel. Over a protracted period of time the size of the meals is imperceptibly increased. This enables the bodybuilder to grow additional muscle without adding body fat in the process.

It is far better, Parrillo postulates, to ingest 5,000 clean calories per day spread over seven meals of 700 calorie apiece than to consume 3,000 dirty calories eaten in three 1,000 calorie chunks at breakfast, lunch and dinner. Parrillo bans nutrients easily and preferentially partitioned into body fat. The multiple-meal eating schedule uses only approved foods. He insists that each of his students have a long-term nutritional game plan and track progress daily by logging each meal they consume. Parrillo has competitive bodybuilders weigh their food, counting grams of protein, carbohydrate, fat, sugar and sodium. Food intake is tweaked and manipulated to an infinitesimal degree. .

Parrillo created the *BodyStat Kit*—a nine-point skin-fold pinch test used to determine body fat percentiles. The kit consists of a set of skin-fold calipers and log sheets. Each week the bodybuilder checks his/her body composition: the fat to muscle ratio. To maximize increases in muscular size and stimulate decreases in body fat, adjustments are made weekly in both diet and exercise. The BodyStat results act as the ultimate weekly benchmark. While skin-fold calipers might not be 100% accurate, when used properly the body fat measurements obtained using calipers are quite accurate and more importantly create a terrific benchmark for week to week comparison and analysis.

In 1985 Parrillo began producing potent, customized supplements for his growing army of competitive bodybuilders. The supplements of the day were pathetic. Weak, lacking potency, loaded with sugar to make the wretched concoctions palatable, Parrillo devised an armada of powerful supplements: his goal was potency. He needed powerful natural products to augment the training and nutritional efforts of his competitive bodybuilders. His nutritional system continued to evolve as he worked with an ever wider range of clientele: athletes from different sports, all with differing needs and goals; Bodybuilders at every level were seeking Parrillo's counsel. They wanted to learn how best to maximize muscle mass while melting off body fat. Regular people began using modified versions of his elite methods with great results.

Thirty years down the road and Parrillo has become an institution. His corporate headquarters are sleek and expansive. His supplements are manufactured onsite. He has an onsite research lab and custom mixes and constructs his products. He exerts maximum control over the integrity and potency of his already potent products and this allegiance to product potency has created a legion of fans and followers. He remains as inscrutable and innovative as ever.

A Day In The Life Of A Parrillo-Style Dieter

John's advice is unbending and consistent: eat lots of clean, quality calories that contain extremely low levels of saturated fat. Eliminate sugar and alcohol and high glycemic foods. Train a lot. Train intensely in both weight training and cardiovascular training. Settle in for three full months. Let us set up a hypothetical situation to illustrate how a full-bore Parrillo nutritional game plan would lay out and look on paper. We will assume our hypothetical athlete is intent on adding muscle mass and has the time and inclination to commit fully and completely to the comprehensive Parrillo approach. In the perfect Parrillo World, the athlete wakes up early and before breakfast performs aerobic exercise for 40 to 60 minutes, five or six days a week. The athlete weight trains in the evening for 50 to 70 minutes, four to six times per week.

Three times a day (with meals) he ingests the following Parrillo pills and tablets: Beef Liver Amino tabs, Vitamin C & E, Mineral Electrolyte, Essential Vitamin formula, Muscle Amino capsules and Creatine Monohydrate. The Parrillo MCT oil, CapTri is used to kick up the "clean calorie" count of each meal. The athlete trains hard and eats often, consuming loads of lean, low fat protein. A portion of fibrous vegetables is eaten with every food meal, as is a portion of starchy carb. Fiber consumption dampens the insulin spike associated with starch. Protein intake is pegged at 1 to 1.5 grams of protein per pound of body weight *per day*.

Our hypothetical athlete weights 200 pounds and intakes 200 to 300 grams of protein each day in order to "support" intense weight training and cardiovascular training. Cardio is done first thing in the morning to create a fat burning window of opportunity. The window opens upon waking and stays open until food is eaten. Another window of opportunity opens after intense weight training and lasts roughly one hour. A smart-bomb shake, Parrillo 50-50 Plus, is consumed after training. Every 2-3 hours nutrients are consumed to stoke the already blazing metabolic fire.

Time	Description
5am	Wake up – All Protein shake (no carbs)
6am	40 – 60 minute cardio session followed by Optimized Whey shake
7am	Oatmeal - one cup 10 egg white omelet with green peppers and onions
10am	Parrillo Protein Bar, Hi-Protein shake
1pm	Chicken breasts, brown rice, green beans, Parrillo Muffin
4pm	Weight training followed by 50-50 Plus shake, Parrillo Energy Bar
7pm	Fish or shrimp, potato sautéed in CapTri, broccoli, Parrillo pudding
Total	**Seven feedings: three food meals, three supplement meals.**

Parrillo On Manipulating The Insulin/Glucagon Axis

Muscle gain and fat loss are controlled by hormones, i.e. chemical signals sent out by the endocrine glands. These signals direct and control the body's metabolism. The hypothalamus gland has a regulating "set point" that decides how much body fat we will carry. Insulin is the body's most powerful anabolic hormone and transports glucose and amino acids into cells. Insulin is required to trigger muscle growth and its hormonal opposite is glucagon, a protein hormone secreted by the Islets of Langerhans. Glucagon increases the content of sugar in the blood by increasing the rate of breakdown of glycogen in the liver. Glucagon moves glucose and amino acids out of the liver and into the bloodstream when blood sugar plummets. These two pancreatic hormones work together to provide uniform blood glucose levels.

The good news is that the respective levels of insulin and glucagon, the insulin/glucagon axis, are determined solely by diet. We can exert an amazing degree of control over each of these hormones through modification of our dietary habits. The Parrillo Performance Nutritional Program is designed to take advantage of this fact and keep insulin and glucagon at precise levels to ensure maximal muscle acquisition and maximal body fat oxidation. Insulin can be a powerful stimulus for body fat accumulation by storing fat inside cells as well as storing protein inside cells. In the Parrillo approach, meals are constructed in such a way as to release carbohydrates into the bloodstream slowly. Lowered insulin minimizes the accumulation of additional body fat.

While glucagon stimulates body fat breakdown (lipolysis) its actions are mostly confined to the liver. Glucagon is released from the pancreas and transported to the liver via the portal vein. Glucagon is not a potent stimulator of lipolysis in peripheral body fat storage compartments. However when intense exercise is introduced into the hormonal equation, epinephrine, also known as adrenaline, is secreted. Epinephrine is the body's most powerful stimulus for fat breakdown. We keep the insulin/glucagon ratio in check through precision eating. Intense exercise causes epinephrine to surge into the system, mediated by a sympathetic discharge in the adrenal medulla. This mobilizes fat from adipose tissue to provide energy.

Under normal conditions epinephrine is delivered to fat cells by direct innervations of fat cells by the sympathetic nervous system. Epinephrine release is increased dramatically during intense exercise. Epinephrine binds to receptors on fat cells and generates a metabolite called "cyclic AMP" or cAMP. This binding causes AMP to activate an enzyme called protein kinase—which in turn activates another enzyme known as Hormone Sensitive Lipase. HSL breaks down triglycerides (the molecular form in which body fat is stored) into free fatty acids (FFAs) and glycerol. The FFAs leave the fat cell and are carried by the blood to the muscle where they are burned for energy. We keep the insulin/glucagon axis under control via precision eating and use intense exercise to mobilize free fatty acids. If you were to lose weight strictly by cutting calories precipitously, half the weight loss would be muscle loss!

ORI HOFMEKLER

In the continually shifting and expanding universe of performance-related nutrition, Ori Hofmekler offers up a nutritional philosophy unlike anything I have ever encountered in my 40+ years of study on the role of food in the transformational process. Hofmekler contends that we eat the wrong foods at the wrong times. He further postulates that as a species we have never "adapted" to the manufactured foods that so dominate modern man's diet. The human body was never designed to utilize the detrimental types of foods we routinely consume. Ori asserts we are a poisoned species, at least in the Western World, and detoxification is critical. He melds his unusual nutritional theories with an equally unusual approach towards exercise: his is an ambitious exercise protocol aimed at transforming the actual composition of muscle fiber. Ori Hofmekler is a visionary and a thinker; his writings on optimal human archetype are fascinating and thought provoking. He is part anthropologist, part military historian, part scientist, part soldier and part artist.

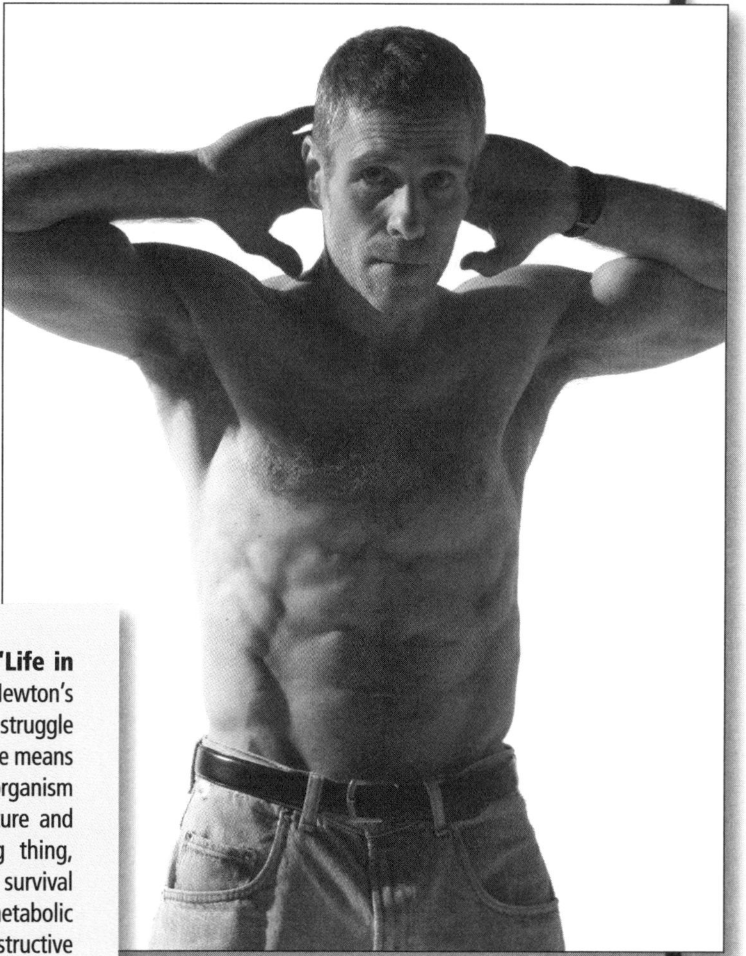

Ori at age 55: ripped and ready to roll. "Life in Paradise should be rugged!" "According to Newton's third law of thermodynamics, life is a constant struggle against the universal forces of entropy. Without the means to resist these forces of degradation, any living organism will lose its ability to sustain its integral structure and consequently will cease to exist. Each living thing, including the human species, carries inherent survival mechanisms that when triggered will induce metabolic actions that will protect the body against destructive forces that cause disorders, disease and death…food provides us the fuel for the survival machine. Anything that threatens the integrity of our nutrition is detrimental to our very existence."

Ori has made a lifelong study of how best to renovate the human body. His is extremely knowledgeable and opinionated on the subject of food toxicity and how best to detoxify. Much of his approach is about recreating and reintroducing primordial physical attributes we as a species have lost. He reaches back in time; back into man's evolutionary past, searching for clues and methods. Ori has done extensive research on primordial man's food selections and dietary habits looking for answers to modern maladies. Is it a coincidence, he asks that man stopped evolving as a species in about the same time that modern agriculture was introduced? Modern agriculture led to the widespread consumption of high glycemic foods. For the first time in human history farm-raised grains were configured and eaten in a variety of ways. Ori points out that as a species we never "adapted" to high GI food. Any time we consume insulin-spiking nutrients it produces a detrimental effect on the body.

Ori contends we compound continual caloric overload with chemical poisoning. Artificial, chemically-drenched foods devoid of quality nutrients make up a large part of the modern American diet. Highly glycemic foods pickled in chemicals are not merely empty calories they are toxic calories. The over consumption of impure foods interferes with the human body's inherent cleansing and fat burning mechanisms. Ori outlines the problems and offers tough love solutions. As you might expect from an ex-Israeli commando, his physical and nutritional solutions are not for low-pain tolerance, politically correct sissies.

Ori writes at length on what he believes is a huge undiagnosed societal problem: estrogenic poisoning. A fast food outlet recently introduced a single sandwich containing 1400 calories and 100 grams of saturated fat. The cumulative effect of eating highly processed, highly estrogenic foods is not a pretty sight. Go to the food court at any local mall and observe the preponderance of obese, obviously sickly individuals… men… women… children. Innumerable modern maladies can be traced back to the artificial, highly processed, chemically-loaded foods we eat and the sedentary lifestyles we lead. Is it any wonder, Hofmekler asks, that obesity, cancer, diabetes and heart disease are epidemic? Is it any wonder that for the first time in American history, children, on account of their dietary habits and sedentary lifestyles, are not expected to live as long as their out-of-shape parents? His messianic-tinged prophetic postulations are a natural outgrowth of his eclectic background.

Ori Hofmekler is an iconoclastic eclectic by any yardstick or benchmark you care to apply. Raised in Israel, he was identified as a child prodigy-a painter. He pursued art and was touted and awarded at every stage of his artistic career. As a teenager, he joined the army and became a Special Forces commando. After his military service, he pursued his passion for art while simultaneously obtaining a degree in biology. His art career took off and his work was soon featured in *The New York Times, US News and World Report, Rolling Stone, Time, Newsweek, Der Spiegel* and *Playboy*, to name but a few. *Catch 22* author, Joseph Heller, labeled Hofmekler, "The world's foremost political satirical painter."

In a cruel twist of fate, Ori's art career was derailed when (Beethoven-like) he began to lose his eyesight. He was forced to quit painting or risk permanent blindness.

Since childhood Ori has been fascinated by the exploits and attributes of ancient warriors. He was enthralled by ancient military cultures and studied the lifestyles, physical abilities and the training techniques of ancient warriors-particularly the Roman Legions at the apex of their military dominance. After years of intense study on the Roman Warrior culture, Ori came to a counterintuitive conclusion that the ancient fighters would best our modern soldiers were head-to-head military competitions possible. How had he arrived at this strange conclusion? Ancient warriors possessed rare skills and physical attributes. Their physiques and capacities were built as a direct result of their daily routines and dietary habits. Ancient warrior skills were broader then the specialized skills of the modern elite athlete.

Ori developed a unique approach towards training that actually sought to replicate the physical abilities and attributes possessed by ancient Roman Legionaries. He melded modern tools with esoteric exercise protocols to create *Controlled Fatigue Training*. CFT was designed to recreate ancient warrior capabilities and capacities.

Hofmekler's optimal physical archetype is a *military* archetype, not an *athletic* archetype, and while there are many similarities between the optimal athlete and the optimal soldier, there are considerable differences in both capacity and capability. Ori's optimal military archetype developed a functional physique, shaped in response to the daily demands placed on the foot soldier forced to carry heavy armor and weaponry for long distances. Ori's CFT training improves specific capacities in order to improve overall function: his training seeks to meld strength with endurance. Training for sustained strength results in the formation of additional mitochondria within the working muscle Hofmekler's ultimate goal, the construction of a retro military archetype, is in dramatic contrasted to the "vanity motivation" common to mainstream fitness.

> ***"Fitness cannot and should not be about simply seeking to look better in the mirror. Nor should it be solely about feeling better or adding muscle for the beach. Nor should it be about losing body fat to attract members of the opposite sex. Fitness-related endeavors and efforts should be directed towards creating a functional body, one with enhanced survival skills. As a species we are degrading and degenerating. "***

His initial efforts and postulations were met with intense skepticism by the fitness establishment. However, the amazing results obtained by individuals who followed his comprehensive system generated widespread interest among elite athletes, law enforcement officers and military professionals.

Ori Hofmekler's contentions and assertions flew in the face of every prevailing fitness and nutritional orthodoxy. Philosophically, his was an entirely new approach on how best to favorably alter and reconfigure the human body. His prototypical archetype was a throwback, a purposefully primitive replication of what we *were* (in a heartier age) as a species. Warrior attributes could and should be built using modern methodologies. His throwback methods were designed to construct a modern man able to function and flourish in our pressurized, industrialized society. A man with superior capabilities and capacities; a detoxified man, a man possessing ancient warrior attributes: a formidable man by any measure

"I was always interested in ancient warrior archetypes. I was convinced the ancients were superior in many ways to modern man and that as a species the ancients were better survivors."

Hofmekler developed highly formalized ideas about what we should eat, when we should eat, and how much we should eat. We cannot gorge for years (or decades) on artificial, processed, highly refined foods containing noxious elements, without consequence. If fed a continual diet of food garbage, over time we destroy ourselves: Super Size Me. Ori takes aim at everyone and everything: he feels soy products (flooding the market today) are toxic, worse than processed foods. Soy, Ori contends, causes the body to over-produce estrogen. Too much estrogen in the body creates a variety of health problems, including cancer and obesity

Estrogen infects and poisons much of our food sources. Estrogen thrives in our toxic environment. The rampant use of petroleum-based pesticides, according to Hofmekler, "has castrated our soil and water." The plants and animals we feed on now are pale imitations of the potent produce and chemically-free live stock consumed prior to 1950. Ori feels estrogenic poisoning of our food, water and environment potentially threatens our future existence as a species. Female infertility and male impotency rates have skyrocketed since 1950. In the industrialized Western World estrogenic poisoning, according to Ori, is a widespread yet relatively undiagnosed societal malady.

He wrote *The Anti-Estrogenic Diet* to help people suffering from undiagnosed estrogenic poisoning. He devised an entire food philosophy designed to lower estrogen. He identifies estrogenic foods and identifies anti-estrogenic foods. Ori shows those suffering from Type II diabetes, hypertension, digestive disorders, cardiovascular disease and insulin-related blood sugar problems how to alleviate their condition through the use of precision nutrition. Hofmekler identifies an arsenal of estrogenic inhibitors including flavonoids and mysterious plant compounds that have been shown to possess powerful anti-oxidant/anti-carcinogenic/anti-estrogenic properties. Conjugated linoleic acid, indoles and lignans shift estrogen metabolites into the production of anti-estrogenic metabolites.

Ori approaches food from a completely unique angle: while the rest of the civilized world says, "Breakfast is the most important meal of the day." Ori says, "Bah Humbug! Breakfast sucks! Don't eat it! Allow the natural detoxification process that commenced the previous night to continue on into the next day." Eat little if anything during the day. Avoid breakfast, particularly a chemically-laden breakfast of highly estrogenic and high glycemic foods. Allow the body to continue the natural detoxification process already underway. Then at night eat a single major meal, a veritable feast, with ample amounts of low glycemic, all natural, preferably organic food, food free of petroleum-based pesticides and chemical preservatives. If the body is allowed to operate without being continually overloaded or poisoned, primordial protective mechanisms are reawakened and allowed to work as Nature intended. Body fat is used for energy, detoxification occurs, metabolic balance is established and the body reestablishes ancient circadian rhythms and patterns. Modern man needs to reawaken dormant, primitive, protective circuitry and hardwiring.

In *The Warrior Diet* and *The Anti-Estrogenic Diet* Ori contends we should eat far less food and eat natural foods free of chemicals and preservatives. Regular exercise amplifies results. He contends that we should consume foods, "lower on the food chain," foods eaten by man before our evolutionary apex was reached. Ori suggests that nuts, seeds, fruits and vegetables were a large part of the primordial man's diet and are extremely beneficial for modern man. He recommends a heavy intake of cruciferous vegetables: broccoli, cabbage, collards, kale, rutabaga, Swedish turnips, seakale, turnips, radishes, rapeseed, cauliflower, canola, mustard, horseradish, wasabi and watercress—along with fibrous vegetables such as asparagus, green beans, carrots, bell peppers, onions, cucumbers, egg plant, lettuce, spinach and Zucchini squash. Seeds and nuts are also highly recommended. Organic meats and free-range fowl trump steroidal-infused beef and poultry. Low glycemic foods are always preferred. All natural and (if possible) organic foods should replace artificially produced, chemically-loaded foods. He views refined carbs as mildly poisonous.

Ori's ultimate human archetype is a warrior archetype possessing a certain combination of physical attributes. Acquiring these attributes results in the construction of a certain type of physique. CFT training is designed to create such a physique. The Hofmekler protocol purposefully blends strength training with endurance training. His physical ideal possesses ancient warrior attributes. Warriors were required to exert sustained strength for extended periods of time during hand-to-hand combat. Warriors needed endurance to engage in forced marches for long distances while carrying heavy weapons and armor. They needed foot speed to quickly charge or retreat, as the battle situation demanded. On average, Roman warriors weighed 140 pounds and carried 50 pounds of armor and weaponry. They routinely marched for 20 to 30 miles a day and ate once, at night. They possessed 7% body fat percentiles and were remarkably adept at fighting or fleeing. Ori has no interest in building humongous muscles. His interests lie in building functional muscle. He has devised a training system that, over an extended period of time, reconfigures the composition of muscle fiber. Hofmekler's training regimen morphs muscle fiber into a hybrid type that possesses a balanced blending of both fast twitch fibers (optimal for strength) and slow twitch fibers (optimal for endurance). Ori labels this particular muscle fiber amalgamation, *Hybrid Super Muscle*. The hybrid super muscle is the end product of his unique training protocol: Controlled Fatigue Training.

His CFT training methodology is designed to increase mitochondrial density within a targeted muscle. CFT seeks to replicate the muscle fiber type ancient warriors possessed. The hybrid super muscle possesses an ability to generate significant strength and sustain that strength output for a protracted period of time. Ori's CFT produces the abilities that Danish Olympic coach Kenneth Jay referenced when he wrote,

> ***"Back in ancient Greece...the human race had superior genetics when compared to us. Exercise physiologists, engineers and historians from several European universities set out to determine the level of conditioning {ancient warriors} possessed. Historical analysis of information on ancient training and their ability to sail ships and cover great distances on foot {while wearing armor} showed that it would be hard if not impossible to find men today who could replicate the ancient's feats. The scientists wrote: 'It would be hard today to find enough world class athletes in the entire world to row a single copy of ancient battleships at the same speeds and for the same durations as men in the past were able to do. We would not stand a chance against these men."***

Ori Hofmekler seeks to replicate the physical traits the ancients possessed using a modern exercise protocol of his own invention. He integrates a unique nutritional philosophy with an equally unique training philosophy. Those who adhere to his precepts construct unique, functional, fat-free physiques. His military archetype stands in stark contrast to the orthodox athletic archetype. He offers a stunning alternative to the lock-step, group-think of conventional fitness. Ori Hofmekler is a true nutritional Master, an iconoclastic innovator by any benchmark.

The Warrior Diet Template

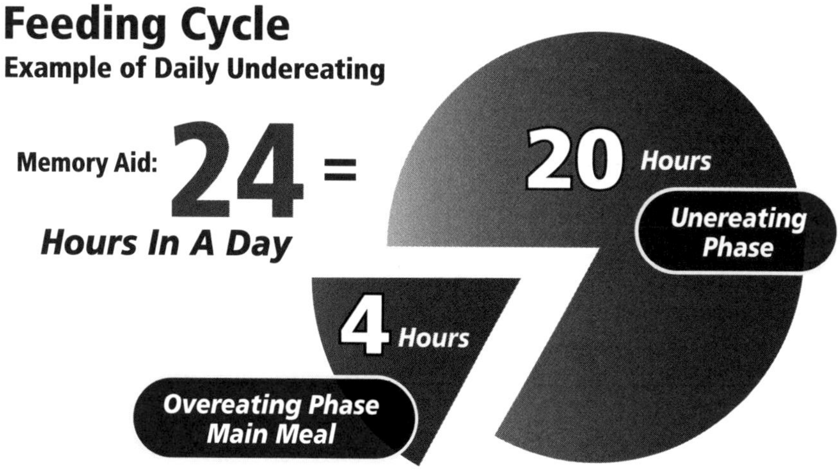

The Warrior Diet is based on a daily feeding cycle that uses under-eating during the day and over-eating at night. The under-eating phase maximizes the Sympathetic Nervous System's (SNS) 'fight or flight' reaction to stress. Under-eating promotes alertness and generates energy while igniting the fat-burning process. Triggering the SNS improves the capacity to endure physical stress.

The nightly over-eating phase can last up to four hours. The goal is to maximize the Parasympathetic Nervous System's (PNS) recuperation effect on the body, thereby promoting calmness and relaxation. Digestion improves, as does the utilization of nutrients for repair and growth. The nightly "feast" stimulates the production of cellular Cyclic AMP or GMP, which stimulate hormone synthesis and fat burning during the day. Growth hormone release occurs during deep sleep.

"Avoid Extreme Low Calorie Diets."

"People who lose weight need to keep their metabolic rate high. Think of the metabolism as the body's thermostat. We want to keep the thermostat set high in order to burn calories. When the metabolic thermostat is set low, weight gain is all too easy and fat loss becomes physiologically impossible! When a dieter goes on a highly restrictive

low carb/low calorie diet they often shatter their metabolism. The body reacts in accordance to the amount of food-energy you put into it.

Using the Warrior Diet and the Anti-Estrogenic Diet, we input most of our food-energy at night, eating large meals that spike the body's metabolic rate every night. This nightly overcompensation shoots the metabolism into overdrive. During the day you under-eat while pushing a lot of energy out. You burn off body fat stores in the process. Nonetheless, by the end of the day you need to recuperate and replenish energy stores and that is where the Warrior Diet/Anti-Estrogenic Diet procedure of nighttime feasting comes into play. Another bonus to eating large nightly meals is the correlation between ingesting high calorie meals and the resultant thyroid hormone boost; a stimulated thyroid increases body heat and elevates the metabolism. There is also an undeniable correlation between high calorie meals and boosting testosterone levels. Three things can drop your sex hormones level and shut down your metabolism: low calories, overtraining (too much exercise), and ingesting chemical additives."

"Detoxify the Body"

"Another major cause for metabolic shutdown is food toxicity. Avoid refined, overly processed, chemically preserved foods such as 'fast foods' and, ironically, chemically-loaded, commercial 'health supplements' such as low carb products and diet products. The chemicals in foods and nutritional supplements shatter the metabolism by interrupting the body's hormonal balance. The typical, low carb nutritional supplement, be it a sport nutrition bar, a protein shake or a diet 'health food' snack are so 'dirty,' so chemically loaded, that their toxicity overwhelms the body, counteracting the body's command center: the neural, glandular and hormonal system.

Chemical additives are known to cause estrogenic problems: petroleum-based chemicals mimic the female hormone estrogen causing undesirable weight gain and metabolic disorders such as female disorders (PMS, fibrocystic disease, etc), softening of the male body, prostate enlargement and potentially cancer among men, women and children. Chemicals cause excessive strain on the liver, which leads to insulin resistance, elevates blood lipids and cholesterol, and causes a total metabolic decline. The way to stop this vicious cycle that causes metabolic shutdown is to eat a sufficient amount of food: low glycemic, all natural, "clean" foods that don't tax the liver; foods that help the body generate energy, burn fat, build up muscle and recuperate quickly from exercise; foods that support the body's metabolism."

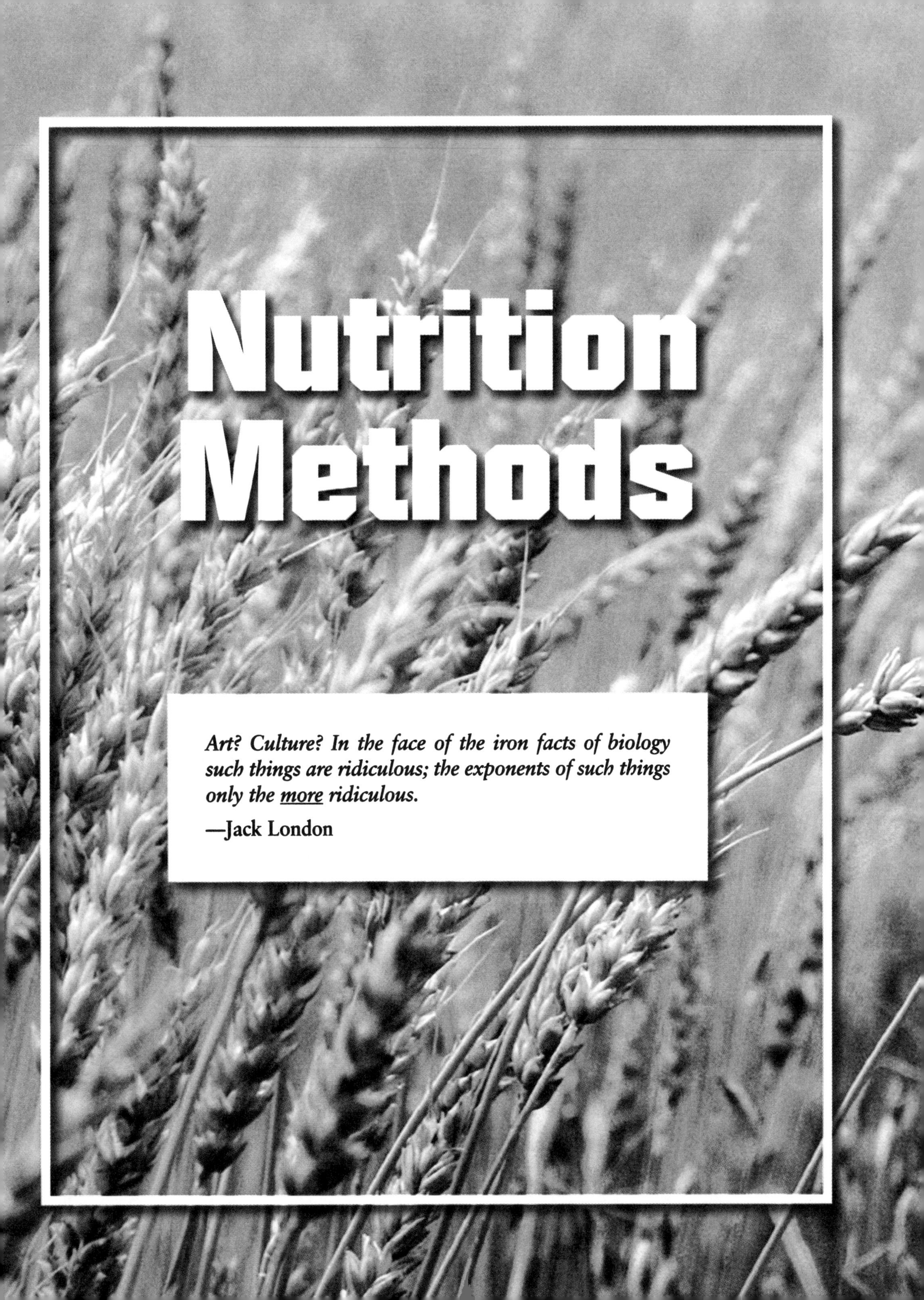

Nutrition Methods

Art? Culture? In the face of the iron facts of biology such things are ridiculous; the exponents of such things only the more ridiculous.

—Jack London

THE NUTRITIONAL AMALGAMATION

Which Nutritional System Trumps the Other?

More often than not, after I outline both the Parrillo nutritional approach and the Warrior Diet approach, my listener inevitably asks, "So which system is better? Which one trumps the other?" That is the wrong question. It is like asking does a shovel trump an axe? Does a screwdriver trump a hammer? Dietary strategies are nutritional tools, nothing more, nothing less. Each of the systems I recommend works spectacularly if implemented completely and comprehensively. The procedures are exacting and need to be executed with disciplined diligence. If you do as each dietary strategy dictates, the body will build new muscle and give up its stored body fat. Both methods have philosophic gravitas and time-tested pedigrees. Each has been delivering significant benefits to diligent adherents for decades. Each system flat out works: the only wildcard, the only variable is you.

There is an old dietary adage that goes, "All diets work!" Regardless the foods selected, if you burn off more calories than you eat, on a consistent daily basis, you will lose *body-weight*. As Purposeful Primitives we are concerned about losing body *fat*. The Parrillo approach and The Warrior Diet represent tested strategies. Each system utilizes dietary procedures that allow the dieter to maintain muscle tissue despite purposefully plunging into Negative Energy Balance. Losing body fat requires we operate in NEB. How do we lose body fat without losing muscle? This is the eternal conflict, the Zen dietary Koan. Both systems offer up comprehensive methods designed to resolve this seemingly irresolvable physiological contradiction.

Both Parrillo and Warrior recognize and seek to create "windows of opportunity." Create the window (through the expert manipulation of exercise and timed nutrition) then take full advantage of the newly opened window. In order to force the body to give up body fat, the idea is to straddle the caloric cusp, the tipping point that separates anabolic from catabolic. After maneuvering to the cusp, use intense exercise to create a catabolic state. Body fat is preferentially burned to fuel the exercise. Fat calories are mobilized and oxidized at an accelerated rate if intense exercise is performed in a glycogen-free metabolic state. When the session is over, take in a specific amount of specific nutrients and purposefully morph from catabolic to anabolic. The Window is created catabolically and closed anabolically.

How can two such diametrically opposed nutritional strategies peacefully coexist in our Purposefully Primitive Universe?

The seasoned Purposeful Primitive is always on a search to find effective *extremes*. You would be hard-pressed to find more contrast: one system says "eat often" while the other system says "eat seldom." The Parrillo Nutritional System and The Warrior Diet peacefully coexist within the primordial world of the Purposeful Primitive because these two approaches are effective extremes, profoundly different, yin and yang, thesis and antithesis. The contrast between the two systems could not be greater and this creates the exciting possibility of cyclical rotation.

We have far too much respect for each system to tamper with the integrity of the respective protocols. Each system stands alone and each system can be used exclusively and in perpetuity just as they are. I choose to periodically *rotate* the two systems and create a rotational *synthesis*.

The Right Tool for the Right Job at the Right Time

For a person intent on revamping their current ineffectual approach towards nutrition, there are three preliminary questions that need to be answered...

1. What is the physical goal?
2. Can you prepare your own meals?
3. Are you situationally and psychologically able to commit to a 4 to 12 week process?

Where is your physical starting point? Are you clinically obese and desperate to lose weight? Are you an underweight athlete seeking to add muscle to improve sports performance? Are you ready, willing and able to prepare your own meals? Are you unable or unwilling to make your meals? Do you work a lot of hours? Are you able to eat properly at appointed times? Success is dependant on having a life situation conducive to sustaining a prolonged and exacting regimen of diet and exercise.

The first step in designing a customized nutritional program is to establish realistic physical goals. Select a dietary plan. Select a resistance and cardio exercise program. Periodize the exercise and periodize the dietary approach. Break the overall goals down into weekly mini-goals. Each successive week the trainee achieves that particular week's mini-goals. There are many weekly mini-goals. A comprehensive training and nutritional game plan will have predetermined weekly poundage and rep goals for each resistance exercise; cardio goals will revolve around frequency, duration, intensity and number of calories burned per session. Predetermined nutritional benchmarks could include weekly bodyweight goals, daily caloric or protein goals, increasing or decreasing carbohydrate intake. Over time the continual attainment of modest mini-goals results in the ultimate attainment of the final physical goal.

Which Way to Jump?

Let us assume that you are ready, willing and able to embark on a battle campaign designed to jar your complacent body out of its current stagnant physical status. Let us further assume you have the time, the situation and the inclination to commit to a twelve week renovation process. The first order of business is to set some goals. Realistic goals...

What is you starting point? Are you an athlete seeking to increase size and strength? Are you a competitive bodybuilder in the off season? Are you a thin person seeking to become significantly more muscular? Are you looking to "muscle-up," i.e., grow a significant amount of muscle while staying lean in the process? Are you desirous of radically increasing your base strength and raw power?

If the answer is 'yes' to these questions then it would be impossible to top the effectiveness of the Parrillo nutritional system. Parrillo adherents eat lots of "clean" calories in an unending series of daily mini-meals. These smallish feedings "build the metabolism." Parrillo insists precision eating be combined with intense weight training and intense cardiovascular exercise. The Parrillo approach requires *time.* Time to prepare food ahead of time, time to stop and eat 5-7 times a day seven days a week; time to weight train 4-6 times a week, time to perform cardio 5-6 times a week. The Parrillo route, a classical bodybuilding template, requires a heavy time investment. It requires a lot of discipline and commitment. If you select the Parrillo approach, be aware that critical mass is achieved through strict adherence to a very exacting set of protocols and guidelines. Use a fully implemented Parrillo approach for a protracted period and the results are positively astounding. If you have the situation and the motivation, the Parrillo nutritional approach is pure perfection.

What is your starting point? Are you are significantly overweight or obese? Are you an athlete needing to stay light to compete in a particular weight class? Are you afflicted with blood sugar disorders? Are you an older trainee with limited time to train? Are you unable to prepare meals ahead of time? Are you cursed with excessive estrogen and in need of detoxification? Are you in a situation that makes it impossible to eat with any regularity during the day?

If the answer is yes to these questions then it would be impossible to top the effectiveness of the Warrior Diet. In our manic, frantic, modern world, *time* seems to be our most precious commodity. The Warrior Diet is the ultimate in ease—no fuss, no muss, no bother—little if any eating during the day and then eat once at night, consuming hearty amounts of nutritious, natural foods. If you select the Warrior Diet approach, be aware that critical mass is achieved through strict adherence to a very exacting set of protocols and guidelines. To repeat what we said about the fully realized Parrillo approach: the tenacious implementation of a full-on Warrior Diet for a protracted period results in dramatic physical improvement. The Warrior Diet nutritional approach is also pure perfection, perfection in a different flavor.

Both systems boldly proclaim that you must eat *more* (of the right stuff) in order to lose body fat. Ponder that for a minute. That is a profound and counterintuitive assertion: eat more to lose body fat! How is that possible? Hofmekler and Parrillo both concluded that intense exercise amplifies dietary results and conversely, timed and targeted nutrient intake actually amplifies workout results. In both the Parrillo and Warrior approach diet and exercise are inseparable.

Jumping into the Deep End of the Pool

Be aware that there is an inherent rigidity within each of these two nutritional approaches: both systems have specific guidelines and are quite formalized and nuanced. The best approach is to make a two week commitment during which you will follow every rule and guideline of the chosen system. Experience has shown that a 14 day trial period will bring to the forefront one of two possibilities: that the system selected can and will meld with the realities of your life—or that there is no realistic way at this point in time that you will be able to use the selected approach. A 14 day test period done with diligence, regardless the system selected, will yield tangible results. Often, after only seven days, the trainee becomes so fired up by the preliminary results that they undergo a wonderful psychological transformation. Those initial seven days produce such rapid and radical results that the trainee receives a psychological jolt, an infusion of exuberance that morphs into genuine procedural enthusiasm. Real progress fires up the trainee like nothing else and causes the individual to exert an ever greater degree of disciplined commitment. Time and again I have seen quick results catapult a stagnant individual into a growth spurt that borders on miraculous. It's a wonderful thing to see. The secret to triggering near instantaneous progress is to lock down all aspects of the selected program fully, completely and simultaneously-right from the proverbial 'git-go'.

A Hypothetical 12 Month Rotational Nutritional Macro Cycle

Weeks	System	Goal
1-12 (January thru March)	Parrillo	Add 12 pounds of mass
13-30 (April thru July)	Warrior	Drop 5% body fat
31-43 (August thru October)	Parrillo	Go to 220 bwt maintaining 9% fat percentile
44-52 (November thru December)	Warrior	Cleanse and detoxify as preamble to anabolic burst

The Psychology of Taste

Sensual gratification is a dynamic, often overpowering human urge. Many of us are slaves to gratifying one sense or another. The most overlooked aspect of disciplined eating (dieting) is the psychological aspect. Food consumption is based on personal habits, likes and dislikes. Modifying habits is self-administered behavioral modification. The mind needs to be reconfigured a bit if we are to successfully adopt a new relationship with food—assuming the relationship we currently have with food (and drink) isn't working. First we must recognize that Taste is King. Food and drink habits are directly related to sensual gratification. We all have highly individualistic taste likes and dislikes.

Taste gratification is a major driving force in all of our lives.

Most diets attempt to suppress or ignore the power of taste. Suppression is another form of willpower and all acts of will are finite. Rather than attempting to suppress taste we need to recognize and come to grips with taste. Do not pretend it doesn't exist, do not deny its impact, or, worse yet, satiate it in a way that undermines the "cleanliness" of the Parrillo approach or the "detoxifying/all natural" tenants of the Warrior Diet. Can we successfully satiate powerful, primordial taste cravings and still stay true to the clean food precepts of the Parrillo and Warrior nutritional approaches?

We all have certain foods that we like to eat and that also happen to be good for us: acceptable foods under either the Parrillo or the Warrior approach. We need to identify those acceptable foods and construct our dietary approach, be it Parrillo or Warrior, around the consumption of these acceptable foods. Make tasty, acceptable foods, food you find tasty, the backbone of your nutritional effort. Often professional bodybuilders will eat the same acceptable foods many times over the course of the day. Often Warrior Dieters will eat the same feast meal three or four times a week. If you like it, if it's acceptable and beneficial, give your self permission to eat it—often.

Addiction to sweets and sugar is another major dietary stumbling block. Rather than attempting to suppress a sweet tooth, let us find potent nutritional supplements that satiate and satisfy sugar cravings. Both Parrillo Performance Products and Defense Nutrition make excellent nutritional supplements designed to nourish and enhance our dietary efforts. A person with a sweet tooth can overcome detrimental sugar binges via the purposefully primitive "substitution principle." When a sugar craving hits and a binge is about to happen, instead of eating candy, pie or ice cream, substitute an "engineered food," a food that tastes sweet but is in actuality a beneficial nutritional supplement that contains no sugar. We trick the taste buds. Don't try and suppress a sweet tooth—satiate it!

Creeping Incrementalism is another helpful psychological tactic—be aware that as the dieter delves deeper into the process they gradually, naturally, *incrementally* tighten up the food selections and amounts in direct proportion to their degree of success. The deeper into the process they are drawn, the more results they see and the more they commit. Initially the mildest of dietary changes reaps tremendous results and this ignites enthusiasm, a self-sustaining mental propellant. Over time tangible physical results spur the dieter to become far more discerning, selective and disciplined. Creeping incrementalism enables the trainee to induce further progress by gradually tightening down protocols and procedures on an ongoing, across the board basis.

A profound psychological metamorphosis occurs when "dieting" is no longer viewed as dieting.

As long as we view dieting as an odious task of self-denial, a repugnant and extended exercise in stressful willpower, we will never turn the corner. Tangible results generate genuine enthusiasm for the process. When exercise becomes enjoyable and dieting becomes effortless, enthusiasm has supplanted willpower. Enthusiasm is an infinite mental propellant and can propel the process indefinitely.

Where and How to Start

Be Hot or Be Cold! Avoid Lukewarm!

Plan ahead. Regardless of which nutritional direction you decide to head in, make a real commitment. If you choose to head in the Parrillo multiple-meal direction, you need to determine the acceptable foods that you like. Assemble the lean proteins, fibrous and starchy carbs that you intend on using. Prepare food ahead of time, on the weekend. Consume the pre-made foods during the week, Come to grips with food preparation. If you decide to embark on The Warrior Diet, brush up on the rules. You may eat during the day. Not a lot, some low glycemic fruits, raw vegetables, light proteins, salads are okay. Both systems insist you "smart bomb" after a training session: drink a potent protein/carb liquefied drink immediately after every workout.

Both men correctly insist dietary results are amplified dramatically by combining right eating with intense exercise. Pick a plan and execute it with the requisite gusto. If you eat and train correctly, after seven days you will gain a toehold; two perfect weeks nets you a foothold; three weeks without a back slide and you establish full traction. Synergistic momentum kicks in within a month; when that occurs the process achieves critical mass. There is nothing like dramatic results to fire a trainee up and cause them to redouble their efforts.

Purposefully Primitive Performance Eating

Eat like a Man, even if you're a woman. Do not, as author Jim Harrison once noted, "Approach a meal with the mincing steps of a Japanese Geisha."

There are more nutritional theories than there are stars in the sky and one seemingly contradicts the next. As soon as you buy into one dietary theory, you come across another one that blows the underpinnings out from beneath the one you just finished accepting and embracing. As the old saying goes, all diets work. If you eat more calories than you burn off, you will not lose weight no matter how sophisticated the food selections or how sophisticated the dietary philosophy. If your caloric breakeven "zone" ranges from between 2,000 and 2,300 calories per day and you eat 3000 calories, it becomes a thermodynamic impossibility for you to lose weight. On the other hand if your caloric norm is 2,300 calories per day and suddenly you drop to 1,000 calories per day for a protracted period, regardless if those calories are derived from ice cream or chicken breast, you will lose body weight.

Not all calories are created equal. Some calories have a detrimental effect on the human body while other calories have a beneficial effect. Obviously, for muscle building or fat-melting purposes, a wonderfully grilled cod fillet trumps a serving of pecan pie—despite the fact they both might have an identical number of calories.

In the ridiculous world of mainstream fitness, an "expert" publishes a diet book that gains traction and becomes all the rage. Draped in pseudo science, the fad diet book trumpets one food nutrient over all others. If the fad dieter consumes fewer calories, regardless the type of nutrients consumed, the dieter loses body weight. The dieter mistakenly attributes their weight loss to the dietary uniqueness of the fad philosophy. In fact their weight loss is entirely attributable to calorie reduction. Fad strategies only work if the user tips the energy balance equation to the negative. Fad diets turn adherents into crash dieters. The crash dieter loses an unacceptable amount of muscle tissue during the weight loss process and feels drained and exhausted all the time. They eventually quit. Let us be done with the fad diets.

Thermodynamic Reality Check

Pick a Direction and Commit

The prime directive of any intelligent nutritional game plan is to stimulate the oxidation of body fat and/or accelerate the acquisition of new muscle mass. Saying "I want to add muscle and lose body fat simultaneously (do both at the same time) betrays rookie ignorance. Elite athletes go in one direction or another. The athletic elite alternate directions, they swing pendulum-like between the two extremes: they pick one direction, add muscle or lose body fat, and then focus 100% of their efforts towards the attainment of that goal. Goals are always set into timeframes.

- If the goal is to *add muscle*—consume more calories than you oxidize on a consistent daily basis. Adding muscle mass requires you to stay in a calorie-surplus state. The Energy Balance Equation (EBE) must be tipped to the plus side. Simple as that: no new muscle can be built if you are not in a caloric-surplus status. More calories need to be ingested than oxidized in order to supply enough excess food/fuel to support the construction of additional muscle tissue.

- If the goal is to *reduce body fat*—burn more calories than you consume on a consistent daily basis. The Energy Balance Equation must be to be tipped into the negative. Stored body fat cannot and will not be mobilized and drawn down until activity exceeds the available energy pool of calories.

- To attempt to melt off fat while simultaneously building muscle creates a thermodynamically irresolvable dilemma. The Energy Balance Equation cannot be tipped both directions at once. Pick one of two directions: add muscle <u>or</u> burn off stored body fat. Head in the selected direction, commit to the process fully and completely for 30 to 90 days.

Used singularly or in continual rotation, the Parrillo Nutritional System and The Warrior diet are each effective dietary systems, despite being light years apart philosophically. Each system is effective and each can stand alone. You may at some point choose to toy with the Purposefully Primitive rotational synthesis of these two dissimilar approaches.

Periodized Nutritional Rotation

	Phase I Beginner	Phase II intermediate	Phase III advanced
Parrillo Thesis	4 meals – Food from grocery store	5 meals – plus Parrillo supplements	7 meals - plus Parrillo supplements
Warrior Antithesis	Light day foods or Warrior supplements Night eating 4 hours	Less day food Warrior supplements Night eating 3 hours	No day food; Post-workout consume Warrior supplements Night eating 2 hours
Rotational Synthesis	4-12 Weeks Warrior Diet	4-12 Weeks Parrillo Diet	4-12 Weeks Warrior Diet

Parillo Nutritional System Synopsis

The Parrillo Nutritional system has general guidelines that stay constant regardless if the goal selected is to add muscle mass or become as lean as possible. Protein intake is kept high year round, regardless the direction selected. Parrillo is a great believer in consuming lots of lean protein as protein "spares" muscle tissue during the fat burning process. Fiber carb consumption is also kept high, regardless the phase or direction. Starchy carb intake is manipulated depending on the goal—less for fat loss, more starch during mass building phases. Supplements are used to augment the Parrillo nutritional approach. Supplements make hitting make hitting daily protein and carb goals much easier: you don't have to cook and eat every bite! His engineered foods can be used by those wanting to wean themselves off sweets. Powder mixes are used to create cakes, cupcakes, muffins and pancakes. His line of sport nutrition bars provide sweet treats devoid of sugar. These are powerful nutritional tools for use in the battle against sugar addiction.

1. Pick a goal: either add muscle mass or reduce body fat.
2. Establish a multiple-meal eating schedule with feedings 2-3 hours apart.
3. Meals should be relatively equal in the caloric sense.
4. Three to four meals (or more) should be regular food meals.
5. A food meal consists of a portion of lean protein, a portion of fiber and starch.
6. One to three meals may be "supplement-only" meals.
7. Daily protein intake should be a least one gram per pound of bodyweight.
8. Fibrous carbs are eaten with every food meal to dampen insulin.
9. Starch carb intake is dependent on the goal: less to lean out, more for mass.
10. Goals are set into a 4-6-8-10-12 or 16 weeks timeframe.
11. Weekly target goals are established and achieved in systematic fashion.
12. The scale, skin-fold calipers and a tape measure are used to access progress.
13. Saturated fat is limited to 5% of caloric intake; sugar and alcohol deleted.
14. Parrillo sport bars, cakes, muffins, etc, are used to satiate a sweet tooth.

WARRIOR DIET SYSTEM SYNOPSIS

The Warrior Diet adherent eats little or no food during the day. The exception to this rule is the Warrior Dieter who will eat or supplement immediately after an intense training session, regardless the time of day. At night, the Warrior Dieter engages in "feasting," a 1 to 4 hour period of nutritional super compensation. Night feasting creates a miniaturized anabolic burst. Daytime fasting allows the detoxification and fat-burning process (begun during the sleep cycle) to continue. The day fast creates a window of opportunity and eating ample amounts of approved food at night kicks the metabolism into overdrive. After an intense exercise session Warrior Supplements are consumed to take advantage of the post-workout window of opportunity. Healing, regenerating nutrients are absorbed and distributed far faster and far more efficiently when the post-workout window is open. Warrior supplements are used to overcome sweet cravings.

1. Only all natural, low glycemic, organic food is consumed.
2. Eliminate manmade foods and foods and beverages loaded with chemicals.
3. The principle of intermittent fasting is used.
4. Daily windows of opportunity are created: after intense exercise; after fasting.
5. During the fast, detoxification and fat burning occur.
6. During the fast, the body's enzyme pool is reloaded.
7. During the fast, insulin drops and the fat-burning hormone glucagon increases.
8. If you must eat during the day, eat a bit of raw food, i.e. fruits and vegetables.
9. The daily 'overeating' phase occurs late in the afternoon or at night.
10. Start the overeating phase with subtle-tasting raw foods.
11. Move to cooked foods; include many textures, tastes, colors and aromas.
12. Fasting followed by overeating accelerates the metabolism.
13. Fasting followed by overeating replenishes glycogen.
14. The Warrior Diet uses foods and supplements to satiate a sweet tooth.

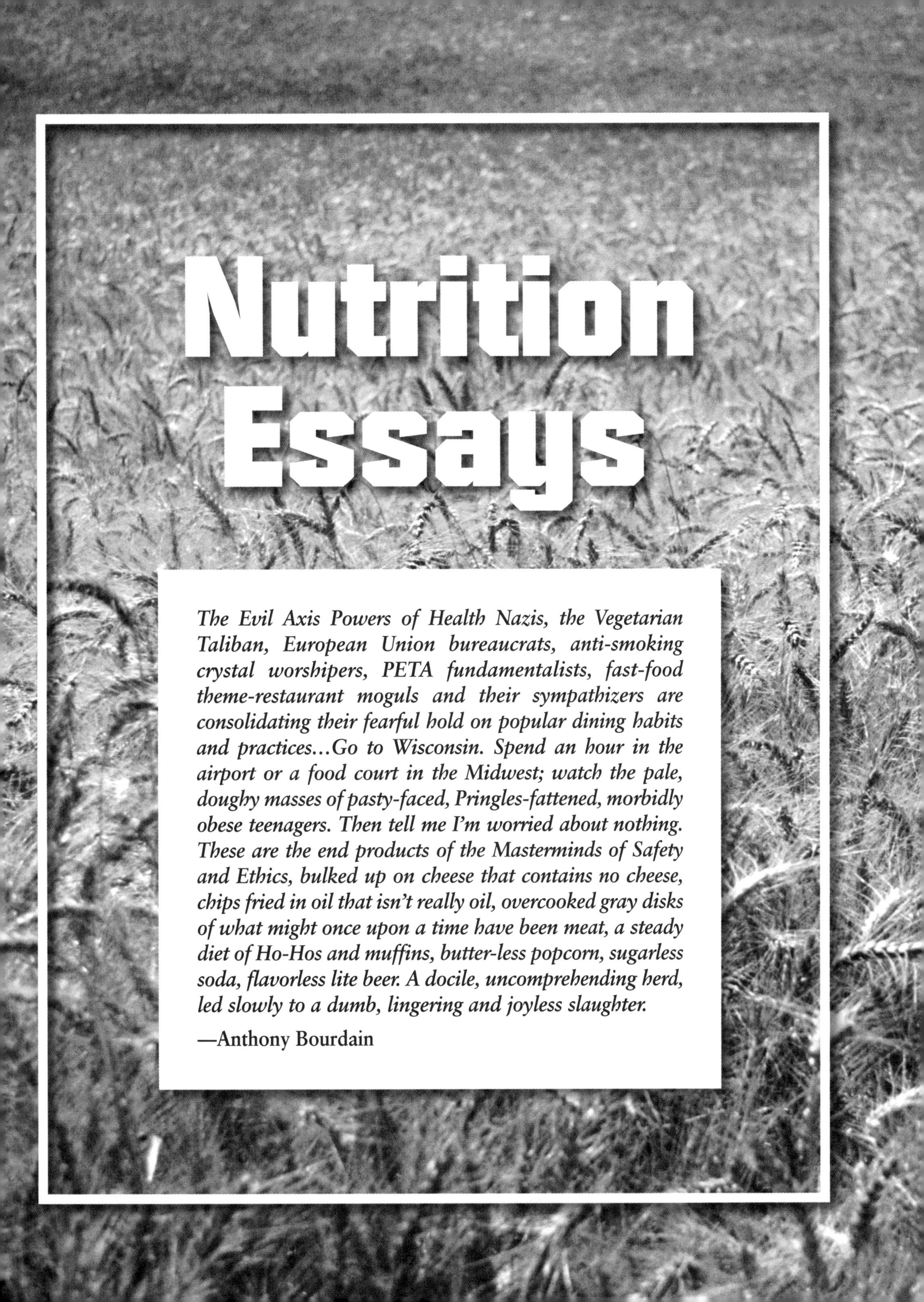

Nutrition Essays

The Evil Axis Powers of Health Nazis, the Vegetarian Taliban, European Union bureaucrats, anti-smoking crystal worshipers, PETA fundamentalists, fast-food theme-restaurant moguls and their sympathizers are consolidating their fearful hold on popular dining habits and practices...Go to Wisconsin. Spend an hour in the airport or a food court in the Midwest; watch the pale, doughy masses of pasty-faced, Pringles-fattened, morbidly obese teenagers. Then tell me I'm worried about nothing. These are the end products of the Masterminds of Safety and Ethics, bulked up on cheese that contains no cheese, chips fried in oil that isn't really oil, overcooked gray disks of what might once upon a time have been meat, a steady diet of Ho-Hos and muffins, butter-less popcorn, sugarless soda, flavorless lite beer. A docile, uncomprehending herd, led slowly to a dumb, lingering and joyless slaughter.

—Anthony Bourdain

THE ANABOLIC EFFECT OF FOOD

Anabolism is a good thing. Metabolically speaking, when a person is anabolic, muscle growth is possible. Anabolism is such a good thing that medical people invented anabolic steroids as a way to artificially induce anabolism. Elite athletes and cutting-edge coaches understand that by creating an anabolic environment and then subjecting the anabolic individual to a high intensity weight workout, new muscle is constructed. The natural way to establish anabolism is to consume a lot of calories. The way to create anabolism—and not add body fat—is to obtain those calories from quality food sources.

It is easy to establish anabolism: eat lots of calories from indiscriminate food sources. Fat calories pack a wallop: 9 calories per gram. Protein and carbohydrate deliver 4 calories per gram. Eat a lot of fat calories and establish anabolism quicker than you can say, "Pass the Prime Rib." To grow muscle and not add adipose tissue during the growth process requires discrimination and restraint. Athletes that overeat not only induce anabolism and grow muscle they also construct new fat cells. Excessive calories not used for the production of muscle tissue or used for energy (or passed through the digestive system and excreted) are converted into fat and stored away for future use. Optimally, the person intent on establishing an anabolic toehold will consume enough calories to trigger anabolism—yet not consume an excessive amount of calories as excess is shuttled to bodily fat storage depots.

How do you know when you've tipped the energy balance equation to the plus side and established anabolism? How do you know when to stop taking in calories? The answer is best arrived at by approaching the problem from a different direction. Train like hell and afterwards consume an ample amount of beneficial foods. Avoid detrimental foods altogether. That would make for a superb start. Do this for a week. Fine tuning can occur when we do things on a regularly reoccurring basis. Certain foods are extremely difficult for the human body to convert into body fat—not impossible, but damned difficult. By consuming calories derived from these foods, the anabolic margin of error is dramatically increased. Lean protein, protein with a minimal saturated fat, has been the staple bedrock nutrient of elite athletes for 50 years. Why? You can eat a mountain of *lean* protein and not add to fat storage—assuming you train with intensity sufficient enough to trigger hypertrophy. Lean protein is difficult for the body to break down and digest. As a direct result, the body kicks the metabolic thermostat upward to break protein down into subcomponent amino acids. That's a good thing.

We use the thermic effect of food to goose the metabolism. We use intense weight training to goose the metabolism. We use hard cardio to goose the metabolism. After a few weeks of continually goosing the metabolism it *stays* goosed—permanently amped up: you have successfully reset the metabolic thermostat upward. Quite an amazing feat, actually.

When a healthy, rested muscle operating in the fertile field of Positive Nitrogen Balance is suddenly subjected to a high intensity weight workout (then fed and rested) that muscle grows larger and grows stronger. The muscle must be adequately stressed to induce growth, stressed to such a degree that the 'adaptive response' is triggered. The adaptive response occurs when the athlete trains with a training intensity sufficient to trip the hypertrophy switch.

Muscle tissue needs to be fed to stay alive. If you shatter a muscle in training then starve that muscle, the muscle shrinks and weakens. Instead of the wonder of anabolism, catabolism takes root. Catabolism (simplistically speaking) is muscular cannibalism. During catabolism, the body can eat its own muscle tissue. When catabolism takes root the body will strip the amino acid content off muscle walls to fuel caloric shortfall. This in an attempt to ward off perceived starvation. The human body seeks to preserve stored body fat at all costs. Stored fat is like money in a savings account. The body views stored fat as the last line of defense against starvation. If overworked and under-fed, the body will preferentially eat muscle tissue to save its precious body fat. Too much training and not enough food produces the catabolic horror of self-inflicted muscular cannibalism. Slash calories for a protracted period and trigger a metabolic freefall.

Obese individuals that engage in crash diets and precipitously slash calories always end up as miniaturized versions of their old fat selves. They might lose 100 pounds of body weight yet still appear fat. Why? Because they are still fat! Despite reducing their weight from say 350 pounds to 250 pounds, the body has cannibalized as much or more muscle tissue than body fat during the reduction process. Though the individual might weigh 100 pounds less, they still might possess a 40% body fat percentile. Obese individuals that choose to starve the weight off lose unacceptable amounts of muscle mass (not that they had any to spare to begin with) during the weight loss process.

How do you avoid the metabolic shutdown associated with crash dieting? Don't crash diet.

Choose the right fuel sources. Never starve yourself. Use a slow downward glide-path when whittling off body fat. The Basal Metabolic Rate (BMR) is "the amount of energy expended while at rest in a neutrally temperate environment." The BMR is the metabolic thermostat and denotes the rate at which our body consumes calories while at rest. Digestion of certain, hard to digest nutrients naturally elevates the BMR.

- Lean protein is difficult to break down. Amino acids are needed to heal, recover, repair and construct new muscle tissue. Lean protein is the bedrock nutrient in the physical renovation process. It feeds muscle tissue battered by high intensity weight workouts and extended cardio sessions. Purposeful Primitives need lean protein and lots of it.

- Fibrous carbohydrates, carrots, broccoli, green beans, bell peppers, spinach, cauliflower, onions, asparagus, cabbage, salad greens, Brussels sprouts and the like are nearly impossible for the body to convert into body fat. Certain fibrous carbs require almost as many calories to digest as they contain. A green bean or baby carrot might contain 10 calories and the body will expend nearly that much energy to break down and digest these rugged vegetables. Fiber is critical!

Protein and fiber are the central foods in the Purposefully Primitive Performance eating approach. Elite athletes make protein and fiber the foundational backbone of their nutritional regimen. So should you!

Fibrous carbohydrates have a wonderful roto-rooter effect on the body's internal plumbing. As fiber carbs work their way though the digestive passageways, mucus and gunk is scraped off intestinal walls and sludge buildup is kept to a minimum. For this reason fibrous carbohydrates are the perfect complement to a diet rich in lean protein. Fiber is the Yin to protein's Yang. Both protein and fiber have a beneficial dampening effect on insulin secretions. It is no accident that competitive bodybuilders, the world's best dieters, men capable of reducing body fat percentiles to 2% while maintaining incredible amounts of muscle mass, construct their eating regimen around the copious consumption of protein and fiber.

The goal of the bodybuilder in the weeks leading up to a competition is to melt off as much excess body fat as possible while maintaining the mountainous amount of muscle built up in the "off-season." In their pre-competition phase a professional bodybuilder will consume lots of protein, lots of fiber and a wee bit of starchy carbohydrate. A 3,500 calorie pre-contest daily meal schedule might be broken down into five 700 calorie feedings spaced two hours apart…or perhaps seven 500 calorie meals. The competitive bodybuilder eliminates all food sources that contain calories easily converted into body fat. Refined carbohydrates, sugar, alcohol, etc. are tossed when the pre-competition process commences. Saturated fat intake is kept to a minimum. Optimally, smaller meals of relatively equal size, comprised exclusively of foods hard to convert into body fat, are eaten at specified times. By eating every two to three hours, the bodybuilder refuels in about the time the nutrients from the previous meal have been expended.

Every time the bodybuilder eats a protein/fiber/starch mini-meal they elevate their metabolism and reestablish anabolism. These mini-meals give the body lots of practice at assimilating and distributing quality nutrients. Increases in body heat associated with food digestion create a phenomenon known as *thermogenesis*. The metabolism gears up to digest hard-to-digest nutrients creating a thermic effect. Meals are used to spike the metabolism. A competitive bodybuilder deep into contest prep has their metabolism jacked up to such a degree that they will break out in a sweat as they consume a meal. The introduction of calories causes a dramatic increase in the bodybuilder's body heat.

At the other extreme the crash dieter has succeeded in lowering their metabolic set-point. The calorie slasher always feels hungry, deprived, listless and lacking in energy. Calorie slashing sabotages the metabolism, causing it to nosedive. Once the metabolism is shattered, the body goes into starvation mode and resorts to catabolic cannibalism.

If you are obese, heed this dietary pitfall. Eat more to lose fat.

POST-WORKOUT SMART BOMB

Indisputably Indispensible

There is a rock solid consensus among the iron elite that a physiological nutritional "window of opportunity" opens at the conclusion of an intense weight training session and closes about an hour later. If nutrients are ingested while the window is open; nutrients are absorbed, assimilated and distributed at four times the normal rate. The battered body craves calories after a kick-ass weight training session, specifically amino acids and glycogen-replenishing carbohydrates. By providing traumatized muscle tissue *exactly* what is needed in the post-workout environment, healing and growth are accelerated. Results are actually enhanced.

That's a pretty damn sensational thing when you think about it: by simply eating or drinking a proscribed amount of protein and carbs after a workout, results are amplified; demonstrably superior to results from an identical workout where post-workout nutrients are not consumed. Wow! What could be easier? Simply drink a great tasting shake after working out and increase results derived from that workout. That's a no brainer! Of course this only works if sufficient training intensity is achieved and the proper nutrients are ingested within the designated timeframe. Unless the workout is intense enough to trigger hypertrophy, post-workout supplementation is superfluous; yet another excuse for the over-eating under-trainer to consume more self-indulgent calories.

Be aware of digestive lead times. While eating a chicken breast and a serving of brown rice after a workout might be providing the battered body exactly the nutrients it requires, these foods require time to digest. Allow a sufficient amount of digestive lead time to break down and distribute whole food. If foods are ingested near the end of the window timeframe, the recuperative fuel could reach the devastated muscles too late. If the post-workout nutrients are in liquid form, the digestive process is greatly accelerated. Liquefied nutrients reach their ultimate destination, devastated muscle tissue, far faster than solid food. The liquid post-workout drink is known as a *Smart Bomb* and is consumed on a widespread basis by elite weight trainers.

I personally prefer a liquid Smart Bomb that provides a 50/50 combination of protein to carbohydrate. I use a powdered mixture that I activate with cold water. My protein/carb drink provides me with tons of high biologic-value protein and glycogen-replenishing slow release low glycemic carbs. Because it is liquefied, my Smart Bomb goes to work instantaneously. This potent potion tastes great and I actually consume my mixture about 2/3rd's of the way into the workout. I have a problem with energy nosedives towards the end of a session and find that my performance improves appreciably if I Smart Bomb while the session is still underway. I place my dry powder in a half-quart Tupperware container and throw it into my gym bag. When I'm ready to activate the mixture, I walk to the water fountain, unscrew the top, add water, replace the top, shake the tar out of the container and drink it. My Smart Bomb provides me a minimum of 30 grams of high BV protein, 50 grams of low glycemic carbs, no sugar and a few grams of beneficial, benign fat. My liquid concoction is pure perfection and designed specifically to provide battered muscles precisely what they need to heal, recover and (ultimately) grow in the post-workout environment.

I unreservedly recommend that all hardcore, purposefully primitive weight trainers consume a protein/carbohydrate Smart Bomb shake as the workout winds down. Feel free to also eat a sport nutrition bar. I try to have a regular food meal 1 to 3 hours after working out. The meal should contain a lean protein source and a quality carb source or two. Portion size will depend on the size of the individual and I tend to err towards eating more, not less, in that first real food meal after a savage workout. I'm famished anyway. About the worst thing you can do is to train like a demon and then starve yourself. I use Parrillo 50-50 Plus, a mix of protein and carb powder designed specifically for post-workout replenishment. Typically, I will double or triple the recommended serving size. I want to make sure I take full advantage of that elusive open window of opportunity. Ori Hofmekler makes a highly recommended all natural, organic Smart Bomb concoction combining three powders, Warrior Milk, Warrior Whey Protein and Colostrum.

Don't be a dumb ass! Smart Bomb!

ORI'S TAKE ON THE WINDOW OF OPPORTUNITY

Exercise, when done intensely, is a form of physical trauma. In order to recover from the traumatic and destructive effect of exercise on muscle fibers, the body induces awesome *compensating mechanisms* that involve anabolic growth promoting stimulatory actions. These actions enhance tissue rejuvenation and activate compensating mechanisms that have been shown to improve insulin sensitivity. Body fat is used as fuel for energy. These compensating mechanisms increase nutrients assimilation within the muscle. Nonetheless, as critical as this portion of the recovery process is, it is only the beginning—we are only dealing with the initial phase of recuperation. The final results of post exercise recuperation (increased strength gains, increased muscular development) depend on the completion of the recovery process in its entirety. The ultimate fate of optimal recovery lies in the very beginning of the recuperation process, right after the workout.

A post-exercise period lasts between 30 minutes and 4 hours and is known as an "open window of opportunity." This is when the body's growth promoting hormones reach peak levels and insulin reaches peak sensitivity. *The recovery meal should be ingested immediately after a workout.* Timing is everything. The capacity of a meal to promote recuperation and muscular development follows a formula: consume the right nutrition at the right time and reap maximum recuperation and rejuvenation. *When* you eat makes *what* you eat matter.

Post exercise, carbohydrate ingestion promotes swift Insulin-like Growth Factor-1 (IGF1) action within the exercised muscles. Post exercise, increased levels of muscle IGF1 are believed to be the most important factor in triggering muscle hypertrophy. What is the recommended amount of carbohydrate to consume after a workout? 10 to 30 grams Carbs should come from a low glycemic, complex fibrous source to avoid over-spiking insulin and thereby creating undesirable blood sugar fluctuations. Having said that, one trick of the trade is to purposefully trigger a *slight* insulin burst, just enough to take advantage of the anabolic properties of some insulin being introduced into the bloodstream after an intense workout.

A small amount of simple carbs from natural, low glycemic source, preferably a fructose-free source such as rice, malt or maple syrup, may induce a beneficial, immediate, short-term insulin spike. A spike is required to facilitate an immediate post-exercise anti-catabolic effect. 5 grams of simple carbohydrate will do the job. Any excess of sugar may cause insulin resistance, hypoglycemia and undesirable fat gain. It is imperative to incorporate meals that provide long-term support to the actions of these anabolic hormones.

Protein with maximum biological value containing a blend of fast and slow releasing proteins is considered optimal. You could combine fast-acting whey with slow-acting milk protein; whatever the choice, the nutrients should be consumed immediately following an intense training session. The amount of protein per serving should be between 10—30 grams, depending on the intensity and volume of the training. The fast releasing proteins will help boost an immediate post-exercise protein synthesis while the slow releasing proteins will help sustain the already established anabolic state. Carbohydrates, consisting of a blend of fast and slow releasing carbs, should be used to maintain an optimum level of blood sugar. This customized blend will induce an instant insulin spike, followed by a steady and slow carbohydrate release, required for stabilizing insulin levels. Insulin sensitivity increases immediately after intense training. Incorporate a post-workout recovery meal. Take advantage of the anabolic effect of insulin. Post-exercise, fast releasing carbs (simple carbs) will immediately inhibit muscle protein breakdown. Then slow releasing carbs (complex or fibrous carbs) will help maintain anti-catabolic activity in the muscle tissue for a longer period of time.

GETTING IN TOUCH WITH HUNGER

"Unless that apple tastes like the best apple you've ever tasted in your life, unless a pear or an orange tastes fabulous—unless the slightest deviation in your diet tastes like a dish prepared by a professional chef—you aren't going to achieve the sub 5% body fat percentile needed to win. Unless you are always on the brink of hunger, hunger so deep and intense that eating a single piece of fruit, or having a bagel with a hint of jelly is a fantastic taste experience, than you need to redouble your dietary effort. There comes a point in deep dieting where the slightest stray from your day to day eating routine results in what I'd call amplified taste."

This statement was made by a well known professional bodybuilder I interviewed just prior to his competing in The Arnold Classic. At the time he carried a 4% body fat percentile weighing 211 pounds with 19 inch arms and a 30 inch waist. He took 6th place.

"I would love just one sip of that beer...but of course that is ridiculous; I cannot have even one sip of that beer. Not that it wouldn't be incredible...that sip would taste so incredible... As soon as this competition is over, in three days, I can have all the sips of beer I want—and I shall!"

This man won the Mr. Olympia competition within a week. Denial and discipline are Old School dietary progress levers. An overlooked aspect to successful dieting is the acquirement of the "amplified taste phenomenon" that arises out of fasting and deprivation.

When Douglas McArthur liberated General Wainwright's survivors of the Bataan death march in 1945, they treated the emaciated survivors to a banquet consisting of the first real food these men had

eaten after four years of brutalization and starvation. A major literally fainted away and fell to the floor in a fit of taste euphoria after he took a single sip of cold, whole milk.

—William Manchester, *American Caesar*

Hunger and heightened taste are inexorably linked. You can improve your quest to effect a total physical transformation by purposefully getting in touch with hunger. Okay, so maybe you don't have to take it to the extremes used by those competing in professional bodybuilding competitions, and perhaps you do not need to develop the taste deprivation of a concentration camp survivor, however the missing piece of your dietary puzzle could well be getting in touch with true hunger, deep hunger. Hunger, deprivation and taste amplification are interrelated and acquiring taste amplification (through purposeful deprivation) could be just the thing needed to bust you through to the next level of physical development.

Carefully consider the relationship between taste and hunger. Can you use hunger to your advantage? Can hunger reactivate long dormant primitive hardwiring? Can deep hunger be used to our benefit – instead of its usual role as a detrimental binge trigger?

The first step is to stop eating. At least for a little while.

Eventually deprivation reawakens deadened and desensitized taste buds. Taste amplification arises out of the depths of true and prolonged hunger. Amplified taste becomes another valid arrow in our nutritional quiver. Another productive tool. In this day and age of plenty, taste buds are deluged and deadened with an unending barrage of overly sweet, salty, bitter, savory, chemically-drenched food and drink. We are taste junkies. We are used to eating what we want when we want. Our taste buds are overwrought and overwhelmed. Only the most extreme foods are able to push their way through to the forefront of our overwhelmed palettes and make any kind of taste impression.

Our taste receptor sites are clogged. Hunger cleans out these sites. Taste sensation reemerges in direct proportion to how long we abstain from food. Fasting is one way to make a clean break with the detrimental foods we are so addicted to.

Let us go cold turkey... Let us reestablish taste reality.

True hunger amplifies the sense of taste and makes us appreciate what we get when we get it. Hunger makes everything taste better. Hunger is multi-leveled and multidimensional. Hunger can be used to reestablish nutritional sanity.

We are continually assaulted by Carnival Barker diet hucksters, each screaming for our attention, each demanding our money in return for a Golden Calf dietary solution. Don't be fooled as this is old wine in new bottles. Flee the carnival madhouse of food addiction. You need purchase nothing!

Simply stop eating.

What could be simpler? Stop eating. Detoxify the body and simultaneously detoxify the taste buds. The most elemental way to induce heightened taste sensibility is to purposefully induce intense hunger: simple fasting works best. Stop eating for a few days. Acquire an amplified sense of taste via fasting then carefully preserve this newfound heightened taste sense. Once our vibrant taste sense is reestablished, we find we appreciate the subtler tastes associated with healthier foods. We appreciate sensible, beneficial foods prepared tastily. A binge, post-fast, (still maintaining a heightened sense of taste) becomes eating a perfectly prepared fish filet with a serving of farm fresh fiber vegetables. It used to be, a binge was devouring an entire pint of ice cream covered with a pint of chocolate syrup. In the post-fasting amplified taste state, eating the ice cream and syrup would likely result in a violent physical reaction.

Once you have fasted and induced heightened taste, reintroduce natural foods back into your diet one at a time...slowly and carefully...savoring each...appreciating each, never overwhelming the taste buds and never exceeding the now reduced consumption capacity. By following this "slow walk" procedure, the amplified taste sensation can be prolonged indefinitely.

Take three days. Start on a Thursday afternoon and by 11 am Friday morning gradually, imperceptibly, eliminate solid food. From that point forward drink fruit juices and protein shakes on an as needed basis. Adhere to this liquid fast as long as is prudent, sane and rational. Most individuals new to fasting are able to fast for 36 to 48 hours before they feel compelled to reintroduce solid food. After the liquid fasting period has run its course, reintroduce light, potent solid foods one at a time. The Warrior Diet approach is perfect for reentry from a prolonged fast. Start the nightly feast with fruits and raw vegetables. Then move to vegetables barely cooked. Eat light coming off a fast. Don't go crazy. Reintroduce foods slowly, Eat natural, organic foods (if possible) and after a few days of eating solid food, reintroduce exercise—gradually and slowly. Put it all together and you force the human body to oxidize stored body fat in order to fuel caloric shortfall.

Those first foods you taste coming off a prolonged fast should have unbelievable taste intensity. That first piece of fruit you taste coming off the liquid fast should rival the descriptive ecstasy our IFBB pro bodybuilder used when recounting eating his apple. Deprivation heightens taste sensitivity and as long as you don't overwhelm the newly reacquired heightened sense of taste, it will stay with you. Maintain taste ultra-sensitivity; stay hungry. Do not overwhelm the metabolism; a proper combination of calories and activity creates an elevated metabolism. If you allow bad habits to creep back in—by recklessly consuming excessive calories derived from impure sources (saturated fat, sugar, refined carbohydrates, alcohol)—the body's delicate metabolic gyroscope will be knocked off its pivot point. If overwhelmed, the metabolism will become sluggish and inefficient once again. Get back in touch with hunger on a periodic basis. Eliminate the sluggish metabolism by cleaning out the system. In doing so reestablish a magnified sense of taste. Take a tip from the pros and self induce the amplified taste syndrome.

Ori Hofmekler's Warrior Diet turns intermittent fasting into high art. His approach is pure genius. By creating a fast condition on a daily basis and super-compensating at night, he creates taste deprivation that keeps our taste buds sensually attuned while allowing the empty body to detoxify. Day fasting—a continuation of the sleep fast—triggers primordial internal defense mechanisms. The nightly "feast" creates an "anabolic burst" and super-compensates muscles. Over time detoxification occurs and in a sensitized primordial state, taste amplification is ever present. Once the physiological phenomenon of taste deprivation takes hold, it continues until the individual does something to derail this marvelous heightened state. Warrior Diet adherents and professional bodybuilders purposefully put themselves into this amazing state and stay there for weeks on end, resulting, ultimately, in a body that is virtually fat-free, while still retaining 90% of hard-earned gym muscle. Let's expropriate the amplified taste tactic for our own purposes. Give yourself permission to stop eating. Let us stop poisoning ourselves, let us reawaken deadened taste buds, let us get in touch with hunger—let us stop the insanity!

MY MEAL WITH MONGO

A Truly Memorable Meal—For All the Wrong Reasons

I had a tragic dinner with a well-meaning friend the other day.

The man is a great athlete and a truly horrendous cook. The food he served would have caused a prisoner riot in a forced labor camp.

His foray into food prep provided me with sudden insight that served to amplify and clarify why proper food preparation, *tasty* food preparation, is critically important for those serious about triggering true transformation. Once we learn how to infuse diet foods with taste, the nutritional portion of the fitness battle is all but won. But what happens when you are Mongo and have the culinary acumen of an over-sexed thirteen year old boy fully infected with attention deficit disorder? Effort, my friends, is no substitute for culinary success. My friend's culinary offering was a total disaster on a multitude of levels. The meal was what happens when laziness is combined with ignorance and compounded with a total lack of taste. (A riddle wrapped in an enigma tucked inside a paradox wrapped around a bonehead?)

The first course was salad-in-a-bag. I use the stuff myself in the wintertime when local produce is unavailable, but bagged salad has to be eaten quickly and for that reason I buy small bags; Mongo had bought a monster bag from Sam's Club and kept it in the moisture retaining plastic bag for over a week before we got around to using it.

The salad was reduced to one vast, tasteless mound of gooey fiber: the lettuce was starting to tinge brown around the edges, the individual flavors had dissipated into nothingness, the shredded carrot tasted the same as the pepper slivers and time and moisture had reduced the components into an indecipherable mass of moist blandness.

My wife grows yellow and red peppers and when she plucks a ripe one off the vine, the vibrancy of flavor is astounding. It is an object lesson on why top chefs insist on farm fresh produce; a just-picked pepper has an intense flavor that shines though whatever dish you use it in; assuming you don't cook it to death.

Our soggy salad was topped with giant orange croutons that tasted like square cubes of those salty BBQ potato chips my teenage daughter loves. Our dressing choices came in 3-for-$2.00 plastic bottles. We could have French dressing that tasted like liquefied orange candy, blue cheese that contained no blue cheese, or oil-and-vinegar that seemed as if it were mixed with crankcase oil instead of extra virgin olive oil.

"I'm not too big on salad." I lied as I slid my caustic concoction to one side.

Being a powerlifter, my pal poured the entire contents of a 12 ounce blue cheese bottle over half a box of croutons and then asked if he could eat mine. "Salad is good for you!" He mumbled semi-coherently between bites. As he pawed at his salad, a dribble of blue cheese dressing ran down his chin; he put me in mind of Anthony Quinn's portrayal of Mountain Rivera in *Requiem for a Heavyweight.*

Done with the first course he bought out the vegetables: steamed broccoli, steamed green beans and steamed asparagus. He announced, for no particular reason, "Call me a slob or call me dumb...Say what you will about me Mart—but I eat *healthy*!" He was quite proud of the fact that in order to "save time and be efficient" he had steamed all three green vegetables at the same time in the same steamer basket. He'd purchased a monster rice streamer that held enough rice to supply a Vietnamese village for a month. Into a steam bath that could have powered a locomotive or have melted paint off wood, he had dumped all three vegetables. The succulent tips of the asparagus had melted; the tender broccoli crowns had been reduced to a soft blur and the green beans were emulsified at the ends yet remained raw in the middle. All the nutrients from the asparagus and broccoli had been leached out and lay in the green water at the bottom of the steamer. The green water he threw down the kitchen drain contained far more nutrients than the "green vegetable medley" he piled high on our plates.

Every bit of flavor had been blanched out of each veggie, yet my power-pal ate everything with relish and zest. The way he went at the vegetables, you'd have thought Jacques Pepin had just served us delicate white asparagus topped with a luxurious crème sauce. "Nothing like a home cooked meal—here have some more!" He ladled more soylent green onto my plate before I could mount a protest. It occurred to me that he had steamed the greens as if he were trying to decontaminate someone who'd been exposed to massive amounts of radiation.

He then produced a pile of baked potatoes. In hindsight this was easily the culinary zenith of the meal. He loaded up his two baked potatoes with a half stick of butter and a half a container of sour cream—each. Bye, Bye butter stick, Bye Bye quart of sour cream. "I LOVE freaking potatoes!" He yelled as he proceeded to grind his potatoes into a butter/sour cream/potato mush. He mashed and ate the spuds using a special oversized wooden spoon he fetched from the kitchen, specifically for this course. His spoon was the size of a child's beach shovel and fit his mouth perfectly. It allowed him to shovel calories into his pie hole with much greater efficiency.

The spoon put me in mind of an Elvis story: supposedly Elvis' favorite breakfast concoction was to have his cook make a huge mound of mashed potatoes then mix the spuds with copious amounts of white pepper gravy and a pound of crispy bacon, complete with the bacon grease drippings. Elvis would have his cook mix all the ingredients, spuds-gravy-bacon-bacon grease together in a blender. She'd throw in an entire stick of butter and some whole milk to liquefy the goop. The King would eat the resultant goo with an oversized spoon. I could imagine the King and Mongo, elbow to elbow, each ravenously chowing down their starch goop with child-like glee. They'd probably hi-five each other as they ate; then take a nap. Later they would head out in one of the King's pink Cadillacs with Sonny and Red and pick up some dancers at a Memphis topless bar. So much for my Elvis fantasies.

Mongo got up with great flourish and said, "I can't wait to show you our main course!" Now came the culinary star of the show. He described his piece de resistance as, "Grilled flank steak—just like the *freaking Mexicans make it!*"

Flank steak is a tough, brutal cut of meat and requires the deft skills of a celebrity chef to prepare properly. Tough and stringy, the optimal way to prepare it is either fast and quick over blazing hot coals for a brief minute, or slow and carefully for a long, long time.

This poor cow must have had a tough life.

Mongo had tossed the meat onto a super hot propane grill and burned it to a cinder. Not quick and fast, not long and slow, but blast furnace hot for a long, long time. "I like my meat *crispy*!" He related over his seventeenth lite beer. I asked why he incongruously drank lite beer. He didn't seem the type. "I'm on a *gawd damned diet!* Doctor says my blood pressure is about to blow my *freaking head clean off my shoulders! Can you believe THAT!*" He was yelling again. He flexed a 20 inch biceps for my inspection. He kissed it before heading into the kitchen to retrieve the incinerated cow.

The charred, already tough cut had been cooked with the equivalent of a blow-torch. Any residual hint of moisture had been roasted dry. Tableside presentation was done with great flourish and lots of machismo posturing. The beef, still smoking, appeared to be some unidentifiable part of a hapless forest creature struck by lightning.

He started to carve, but had to stop. "Hmmm..." He mumbled as the meat shot off the platter and onto the rug. Wordlessly he picked up the meat and headed back into the kitchen. He obtained a sharper, sturdier blade. The knife he'd first selected was not nearly up to the task and bowed like a hillbilly musical saw when he attempted to cut me a slice. The downward pressure kept making the meat slide off the plate. He relocated to the kitchen where he could place the charred cinder on a wooden board for better cutting traction. I saw him break out a meat clever that looked like something from a horror movie and heard rapid-fire chopping interspersed with cursing.

He hit the meat one time and it flipped into the air and onto the kitchen floor. Unperturbed, he then took a pronged fork and nailed the meat to the cutting board. "There...That's better!" He then got out an electric knife and surgery continued. "Do you like yours well done?" He asked rhetorically. After a few minutes he reappeared tableside, beaming like Wolfgang Puck. He heaped two slices on my plate. He placed six slices on his own plate and began eating his charred carcinogenic cinder with cannibalistic gusto. I marveled at his jaw strength and reckoned that in a street fight this man could bite off both your ears and your nuts in four seconds flat.

He ate at least 24 ounces of toasted shoe leather while I sat chewing like a cow on its cud on my first and only bite.

I understand Plains Indians in the 19th century would chew on buckskin to ward off hunger during times of starvation. I mulled this over as I chewed his "grilling masterpiece. Suddenly he erupted in another of his Tourette's Syndrome outbursts. "This steak is *great*! This steak came out *way better* than the one I grilled a couple weeks back when Granny broke a tooth off." When he wasn't looking I slid my bite full out of my mouth and into my napkin. Per usual he finished his and then ate my leftovers. "You can't beat steak fresh off the grill—can you Mart!" He was ecstatic. The meal was past perfection to his way of thinking.

For desert he brought out a giant pecan pie he bought from the grocery store and ate the entire thing when I begged off, saying I was too full. "I'll work the pie off at the gym tomorrow." He said between pie bites and beer chugs. I reckoned the pie alone contained 2000 calories and at 10 calorie per minute burn rate he would need to jog for four straight hours just to cancel out the pie. I didn't even calculate the caloric content of the 18 lite beers he guzzled in three hours. He seemed sober as a judge.

I looked at my watch and said, "Wow! Look at the time! Can you believe it? Time flies when you're having fun." In actuality I'd been there less than an hour. "I hate to part good company, but I have to see my accountant at 1 pm. I need to talk about upping my IRA contributions." He jerked upright, got super serious and said, "I know you're Irish and all, but I wouldn't be giving any IRA Irish terrorists money contributions if I were you Mart. The feds might be tapping your phone. I think they're tapping mine—hold on a minute while I pack you a doggie bag."

As I burned rubber down the gravel road that led away from his mobile home in the trailer park back to the highway, I threw my doggie bag out the window at a rabid looking wolfhound that was chasing my car. I watched the dog out my rearview mirror as he pulled up and began pawing the bag apart to get at the meat. Would the starving canine eat or reject the steak? It was inconclusive: he grabbed it between his jaws and ran off into the woods. I hoped he wouldn't break off any teeth like poor granny.

So what does this culinary Chernobyl have to do with fitness?

In order to really get your hands around the throat of the critical nutrition leg of the transformational process, you have to come to grips with food preparation, make that tasty food preparation. You cannot depend on mom, the wife, the girlfriend, boyfriend or power pal to prepare your meals. Ideally you should develop a large arsenal of healthy, nutritious dishes for your culinary repertoire...dishes that you can prepare. We all have our food preferences and the smart trainee identifies and doubles up on the consumption of acceptable foods. Jettison foods that retard or derail our efforts. Once the good stuff is identified, learn how to prepare it and prepare it with such a degree of competency that we actually look forward to eating it. Check out the Food Network. The food prep tips are invaluable. Shows like "*Boy Meets Grill*," "*Molto Mario*" and "*Good Eats*" can take the mystery out of meal making. Once you come to genuinely enjoy the taste of the foods that you make, beneficial foods instead of detrimental foods, the dietary campaign of the fitness war is all but won. Let Mongo's memorable meal serve as a lesson: taste is in the mouth of the beholder and insanity can take many forms and guises.

The Diesel Leads the Way

The Procedural Consensus of the Bodybuilding Elite for Shedding Body Fat

Over the past twenty years a procedural consensus has emerged from within the ranks of the elite bodybuilding community on precisely what modes and procedures should be used to become as lean and fat-free as possible. What modes and methods best melt off body fat while (and this is critical) retaining as much existing muscle mass as possible? Anyone can slash calories, stop eating and lose body*weight*—the bodybuilding elite have developed a consensual system that burns off the body *fat without burning off the muscle.*

Across the nation and the world, bodybuilders are lifting weights, hitting aerobics and eating with incredible precision. They might fight like cats in a sack over the details, but competitive bodybuilders will agree on the universally accepted core preparative modes and principles.

The pre-competition goal of the competitive bodybuilder is to melt off as much body fat as possible without losing hard earned muscle mass in the process. Competitive bodybuilders agree on the need to lift weights, perform cardio and eat using a disciplined and regimented multiple-meal schedule. The elite might quibble over specific weight training tactics-but there would be no disagreement that weight training is absolutely critical. They might argue over food selections-but there would be no argument over the applied use of the multiple meal template. They might argue over which cardio mode is superior-but no one would argue that cardio was critical. There would be uniform agreement on the *overall training template* and uniform agreement on the *overall nutritional template.* Differences of opinion would arise in the various subcategories and details. To create maximum muscle, lift weights and feed the body afterwards. Ample lean protein intake spares muscle tissue. To melt off fat maneuver the body downward to the caloric breakeven point and use exercise to create a temporary energy deficit.

Lose body fat in a slow, sustained and protracted fashion. Pros look to lose fat at a rate of about one pound per hundred pounds of bodyweight per week: a 200 pound man would seek to drop bodyweight at a rate of two pounds per week; a 145 pound woman would seek to lose bodyweight at a rate of 1.5 pounds per week. Less is hardly worth the effort and losing weight faster runs the risk of burning off muscle tissue.

The flat fact is that a radically lowered body fat percentage can be obtained by anyone who has the know-how and the requisite maniacal discipline. Lift weights with ferocity, blast away at metabolism elevating cardio, preplan every bite of food you will eat. Eat what you are supposed to when you are supposed to. Keep up the fierce lifting, the intense cardio and the perfect eating without break or respite for a prolonged period of time, say 60 to 120 days. Do so diligently and results are flat guaranteed. The pros know that when a tight system is in place and locked down real results will begin appearing within fourteen days, mind-blowing physical changes appear by day 30; utter and complete physical transformation is a foregone conclusion for anyone with enough guts, tenacity and grit to keep up this kind of ferocious effort for 90 days. No brag. Proven fact. Proven by thousands of local bodybuilders, men who routinely achieve sub 8% body fat percentiles while maintaining 90% of their incredible muscle mass.

That's the good news.

The bad news is that to acquire a sub-10% body fat percentile you must be in total control of yourself, your environment and your life-circumstance. To lose fat while maintaining muscle mass requires that precision eating be combined with intense exercise. The methods used are not magical: they work every single time. The procedures used are (nowadays) common knowledge. But knowledge and tenacious application are two entirely different things.

Even at the local level competitive bodybuilders are routinely achieving sub-10% body fat percentiles. It's no big deal. Go to any jive little local bodybuilding competition held at the high school, the Mr. Suburban Colossus competition. Even at these entry level bodybuilding competitions, dozens of local yokel bodybuilders will exhibit sub-10% body fat percentiles. Thirty years ago only elite bodybuilders attained the magical sub-10%. What happened? The information revolution revealed to those in the know the procedural consensus of the Iron Elite.

While the preening peacock aspect of bodybuilding might be off-putting to John Q. Public, expropriating bodybuilder tactical procedures for melting off body fat is a terrific idea. To win at bodybuilding, above all else, you must be lean. If you are not lean you are damned to nothingness. Unless you are carrying a less-than 10% body fat percentile (for a man) don't even consider entering a *local* bodybuilding competition—you'll get blown into the weeds! In the bodybuilding world it's assumed everyone is lean, otherwise they wouldn't be there. The winners are those who have muscle mass and symmetry in addition to the prerequisite single digit body fat percentile. So how is it that bodybuilders, even at the local level, routinely acquire 5% body fat percentiles, a degree of physical condition once considered unreachable by all but elite professional bodybuilders?

The information revolution coincided with a coalescing of consensus. The once tightly held methods and procedures used by the bodybuilding elite finally filtered down to the masses. Protocols and procedures have gotten better and more sophisticated with time. We are six generations into this system and the tactics have become more refined with each succeeding generation. Since the end of WWII bodybuilders have been honing and refining their lean-out tactics. Top bodybuilders have long compared notes on eating and exercise. There have been several significant "breakthroughs" over the years that contributed to the effectiveness of today's consensual method.

A leanness quantum leap forward occurred when bodybuilders began regimenting their nutrition to an infinitesimal degree. Top bodybuilders *weigh their food.* As they prepare foods ahead of time for storage and consumption later in the week, they will weigh pre-cooked portions on a food scale that measures in grams. This cumbersome procedure provides them a heretofore unimaginable degree of exactitude. Do you have to weigh your foods? No, if getting down to 9% or 10% body fat percentile is acceptable; for a competitive bodybuilder wanting to whittle down to 2-5%, weighing every bite is mandatory.

We are much more knowledgeable and sophisticated about nutrition nowadays than we were in the 60's and 70's.

Leanness took another quantum leap forward when bodybuilders began systematically including cardiovascular exercise into their training template. Up until the 1980's it had been assumed that cardio exercise would "tear down" muscle. That was factually inaccurate. Cardio not only burns extra calories, cardio builds cardiovascular density and improves endurance. Improved endurance allows the bodybuilder to train harder, longer and more often. Intense and repeated cardio makes the human machinery far more efficient. Cardio kicks the metabolism through the roof and improves nutrient assimilation. John Parrillo was an early and articulate champion of aerobic inclusion into the bodybuilding template. John was recommending cardio before cardio was cool. Per usual, he took a lot of heat from critics back in the beginning. Now cardio is SOP.

The final leap forward in the modern bodybuilding era occurred when amateurs and professionals began dramatically increasing their off-season bodyweight. By pushing their bodyweight upwards in the off-season, they were able to present a larger final finished physical product. By commencing the lean out cycle larger and still relatively lean, onstage, at the end of the process, they would be significantly larger yet still able to retain their previous degree of conditioning and muscularity. The new muscle, theoretically, would be strategically added onto weak or lagging muscles to smooth out asymmetrical disproportions. Eating massive amounts of clean calories in the off-season became an accepted practice. The calorie crazy bodybuilders didn't get fatter they actually got leaner. Thus the new breed of muscle monster was born: massively muscular-yet (incongruously) leaner than earlier, smaller, lighter champions.

It was discovered that lots of calories could be eaten as long as the caloric intake was spaced out and food was derived from approved sources. Cardio and clean calories allowed bodybuilders to become larger and leaner. The inclusion of aerobics into the training template proved to be the last missing piece to the fat burning puzzle.

Top pro bodybuilders were routinely eating 6,000 to 10,000 calories per day in the off season and staying relatively lean. Dorian Yates would whittle down from an off-season bodyweight of 295 pounds, carrying an estimated 10% body fat percentile. On contest day he would weigh a ripped-to-the-bone 255 pounds carrying a 2% body fat percentile. He would gradually reduce his calories from an off season high of 6,500 a day to 3,500 a day. He never dropped below 3,500 as that might degrade muscle: he used a slow reduction process to spare muscle in the face of declining calories. He might take 12 full weeks (or more) to strip off forty pounds of body fat, a 14% reduction from his starting bodyweight. If he dipped below 3,500 calories a day, hard-earned muscle would evaporate. Famous for lifting bar-bending poundage, his food selections were surprisingly normal. His pre-contest meal plan was sanity cubed.

Dorian Yates Daily Meal Schedule Pre-Competition Phase

3,500 calories
Nutrient percentiles: 50% - 55% carbs, 30% protein, 15% - 20% fat

Time	Description
7am	500 grams oatmeal, 6 egg whites w/ 2 yolks, 2 slices wheat toast, banana
10am	40 grams of protein (powder mixed with water), 300 grams potato
1pm	200 grams chicken breast, 100 grams rice, 100 grams mixed vegetables
4pm	40 grams of protein, banana
6pm	Post-workout 70 grams of carbohydrate powder, 30 grams of protein powder
7pm	200 grams of extra lean beef, 300 grams baked potato, 200 grams broccoli
10pm	40 grams of protein powder, 50 grams oatmeal

Yates ate seven times a day, starting with his initial, post-cardio meal at 7AM. He would eat his final meal at 10 PM. Four full food meals were augmented by three supplement meals: note that the supplement meal always included a carb, a fruit, vegetables or oatmeal. Other than his post-workout Smart Bomb shake, he made it a point to eat real food with every 40 gram protein shake.

This meal plan is the very definition of rationality-particularly when compared to the ridiculous extremes to which many of his competitors were subjecting themselves. His food selections allowed the inclusion of whole wheat toast, lean beef and fruit. This represents strict eating, yet his menu hardly seems inhumane. Interestingly, while John Parrillo recommends an optimal 1.5 to 1 ratio of carbs to protein to optimize the insulin/glucagon ratio, (and thereby maximize fat burning) Dorian prefers a slightly higher carb/protein ratio 1.7 to 1 for optimization of the insulin/glucagon ratio. Dorian allows far more saturated fat into his dietary template than Parrillo. Dorian's daily fat intake could run as high as 20%, a whopping 80 grams of fat per day. This is a gargantuan amount in the restrictive, fat-phobic world of international level bodybuilding. It is also noteworthy that Yates' moderate approach resulted in a final finished physique that was always the leanest, most fat-free physique onstage. One would think that extreme deprivation would be needed to create the leanest body, yet here stood Yates, eating 3,500 calories a day and consistently able to come in as hard and lean as any of his competitors.

Yates would continually fuel himself with wholesome nutrients, eaten at equidistant intervals throughout the day. He maintained his sanity by eating fruit, beef and potatoes, hardly gulag fare.

The Mighty Diesel points the way. You would do well to mimic his patience with the process, his savage work ethic in the weight room, his realistic and humane dietary approach and his studied use of cardio. He successfully combined and balanced the elements to create a superbly effective approach. If you have the circumstance and the discipline, a milder, detuned version of the Diesel's approach could work wonders for you. Expropriate the bodybuilder's nutritional template for your own fat-loss aspirations. Bodybuilders give the phrase, nutritional discipline a whole new meaning: they weigh their food in order to establish exactness and uniformity. Should you do the same? A lot depends upon your psychological makeup. Anal retentive types love the exactitude of the food scale. Precision portion control makes charting and logging easy. Those who abhor the idea of measuring every bite can get very close by "eye balling" portions. This approach will certainly get you 90% of the way to the ultimate physique. Unless you are planning on entering a bodybuilding competition, a 10% body fat percentile is realistic for those who eyeball. Male bodybuilders nationwide are routinely obtaining single digit body fat percentiles using highly regimented procedures. Expropriate the bodybuilder's protocols and procedures for you own use. You now have the roadmap.

HOLIDAY HEDONISM SETTING UP THE ANABOLIC BURST

An Amazingly Persuasive Rationale for "Sanctioned Gluttony" to Take Advantage of Temporary Metabolic Amnesia

I continually receive correspondence from folks fretting over the fact that they might binge a bit over the holidays. They tell me all about their elaborate plans to avoid anything on the "banned list" at the beach, or during Thanksgiving, or over the Christmas/New Year Holidays. My advice is so shocking to them that you'd have thought I asked them to have carnal relations with a farm animal.

I echo the message football iconoclast John Riggins related to Supreme Court Justice Sandra Day O'Connor as he lay inebriated on the floor of the National Press Club at an important charity/award function. Riggins looked up from the floor, drunk out of his mind, winked at the grey haired Supreme Court justice and said, "Sandy! Can you hear me GIRL! Look it Sandy, I *like you*—but you are *way too tight*! You're gonna *blow a gasket*—you gotta *loosen up* Sandy BABY!" He closed his eyes to take a nap complete with loud snoring. Later that month he set a Super Bowl rushing record.

My advice to those who relate the extremes they intend to resort to in order to forgo a single piece of pumpkin pie, three Christmas cookies or a serving of mash potatoes with gravy is this...Loosen up people! You are way too tight! I say—train hard and eat strict *in anticipation of* the holidays then eat, drink and be merry! Get back into the fitness saddle immediately afterwards. C'mon people, loose the robotic tendencies! A terrific rationalization/argument could be made on behalf of sanctioned gluttony.

Are my hedonistic, Mad Irish tendencies showing? You bet. Here is how we rationalize sanctioned gluttony. Train intensely and eat in restrictive fashion leading up to the holiday/vacation. After a period of prolonged deprivation, a short, sudden, massive reintroduction of calories, calories of an indiscriminate nature, will trigger the mythical "Anabolic Burst." This results in a significant increase in *lean* muscle mass, literally overnight. A successfully executed Anabolic Burst requires a protracted period of highly restrictive eating followed by an all out, no regret, unapologetic food binge.

Leading up to the holidays eat light and eat strict. Utilize the highly disciplined Parrillo pre-competition lean-out approach or the intermittent fasting approach of the Warrior Diet. Augment the highly controlled eating with a lot of volume-biased weight training. Perform lots of cardio in the lead up. Tight diet and extensive exercise done for a protracted period sets up the appropriate pre-conditions for a successful Burst. Exert extreme iron discipline for three to four weeks leading up to the holiday. Then once you arrive at the vacation destination, BAM! IT'S ON! Eat anything and everything (including cocktails and adult beverages) for the next 48 hours.

The result is something called "super compensation." When depleted muscles are suddenly force-fed a massive amount of calories the muscle cells volumize and swell to unimagined size without any loss in leanness and muscularity—for a while.

The trick is you have to stop the binge after 48 hours or you'll blow the whole deal and experience something called "spillover." Get off the binge before spillover occurs and all is right with the world. The Anabolic Burst produces a dramatic increase in muscle-building hormones. A veritable anabolic cocktail is created by the sudden introduction of massive amounts of calories into a severely depleted body. Such a body is literally *unable* to properly process strange nutrients, i.e. saturated fat, sugar and refined carbohydrates—for a little while.

Denied these substances for weeks and weeks leading up to their reintroduction, a small window of opportunity is created wherein the body is unable to shuttle these nasty nutrients into fat storage. The body has "forgotten" how to process these detrimental nutrients. I call this phenomenon *temporary metabolic amnesia*. When Super Compensation occurs muscle fibers swell to unimaginable size in a matter of hours. The secret lies in the sparse, light eating and the intense exercise *leading up to* the Anabolic Burst. The body scrambles to relearn how to process the bad stuff. The trick is to back off the binge before the body remembers how to properly process fat, sugar and bad carbs.

When spillover occurs the body regains its fat/sugar/refined carb compartmentalizing bearings. Until that point, all calories are sucked into depleted muscle cells, until saturation occurs. Until that spillover saturation point is reached, any nutrients not used to supercompensate muscles are passed in urine/feces or used for energy. None are stored as fat. During the lead up phase, when calories are clean and nutrients are pure, enzymes that promote fat storage efficiency decrease in activity. Enzymes control the metabolism of fat and carbohydrate and for a short time nitrogen balance can be manipulated to our benefit.

In one study entitled "The Hormonal Response to Overfeeding" scientists started off with a highly restrictive "maintenance diet" and coupled it with a vigorous exercise program. The test subjects then had their respective daily caloric intakes doubled (love it!) and everybody experienced significant increases in lean body mass. Once the body "adapts" to the over-feeding, the proverbial party is over. From that point forward the body converts all excess calories into fat faster than you can say "pass the pie!" The trick is jumping off the caloric party train before spillover occurs. Empirical experience has shown that 48 hours is plenty short enough to avoid spillover. Some bodybuilders have gone for as long as five days before hitting spillover. I know what you're thinking but let's not get greedy. Be safe and jump back on the wagon within two days.

I like to start my burst on a Friday afternoon, go all day Saturday and back off Sunday evening. By Monday morning, I'm ready to get back on the straight and narrow path. Trust me, 48 hours is plenty enough time to indulge in every form of food and drink porn imaginable. You'll likely make yourself sick—but that's okay—revulsion makes it easier to jump back on the wagon.

Be good in the weeks leading up to vacation then have your very own Bacchanalian Festival upon arrival. It's sanctioned and approved. If you are sufficiently and properly depleted, a 48 hour Anabolic Burst will cause your muscles to explode; they swell like a dry sponge immersed into a pail of warm water. After two days of partying like a rock star, lockdown the tight eating and resume weight training and cardio. Big men have been known to gain 10-25 pounds of muscle in 48 hours.

I once had to diet down 22 pounds in 34 days to lift at the National Master's Powerlifting Competition. I made weight on Friday afternoon at 1 pm, weighing in at 218.5. I was starved and famished and felt like a wolf crawling out of a hibernation den at the end of a long winter. I began eating and by 2 pm the next day I weighed 234 pounds. I had gained 16 pounds, all of it muscle. I was gargantuan in comparison to my competitors and squatted a national record in my age group 44–49 weight class 220 pound, 704 pounds. My tale is not out of the ordinary, rather a fairly representative example of a successfully executed Anabolic Burst in all its resplendent glory.

How fanatics spend their holiday—a cautionary tale of the ridiculous extremes some bodybuilders will go to:

I once knew a professional bodybuilder who proudly told me in a *Muscle & Fitness* interview that he used to pack his own food in Tupperware containers when he went home for Thanksgiving. He referred to himself in the third person. "Tommy (fictitious name) tells mom and dad and the relatives that Tommy needs his own food at Thanksgiving. Tommy's only got 19 weeks until the Mr. Olympia contest and Tommy don't eat no turkey or mashed potatoes, that trash will make Tommy fat!" So Tommy would pack a half dozen skinless chicken breasts, steamed broccoli and dry rice and break them out after grace was said and proceed to eat his gruel at the table while everyone else ate the holiday fare in the festive spirit. He'd make small talk about himself to whomever would listen, "Tommy's gonna win the Olympia and its only six months away—so Tommy can't be doing anything that would derail Tommy's vision quest!" I kid you not. Tommy was good enough to qualify for the Olympia, but never came within a country mile of finishing in the top ten.

In my mind's eye I always envisioned some wonderful, all-American family, dressed for church, gathered around a terrific spread of delicious home-cooked Thanksgiving food, grandma in her apron, the men in ties and jackets, the kid's at the little card table—and this steroid freak in baggie workout pants, a skin tight tank top (in November in the Northeast) wearing a do-rag continually fumbles and jostles with a mountainous stack of Tupperware containers, piled up next to his seat at the table—with nothing to talk about other than himself and his "career."

Tommy eventually had to have a liver transplant. Tommy pumped so much steroidal poison through his body that Tommy melted Tommy's guts. Now Tommy uses a wheelchair and sits quietly at that Holiday table dressed like everyone else.

Enjoy the food, the drink, the company and the holiday vibe. Monday will be here in no time. Use the Anabolic Burst. To make the burst work, do your work ahead of time. And in the immortal words of that iconoclastic football Purposeful Primitive, "Loosen up people! You're way too tight!"

What's the Biggest Myth in ALL of Fitness? Spot Reduction!

The Lie That Will Not Die

The biggest fallacy in all of fitness is the unchallenged contention that abdominal exercise melts off the layer of fat that lies atop the abdominals.

They say that inside every fat man there is a thin man yearning to escape so I suppose beneath every beer gut there is a ripped six-pack yearning to be exposed. Body fat reduction, not abdominal exercise, is the key to developing a crisp, delineated, defined waistline. Excess body fat keeps the six-pack abs blurred and indistinct.

If someone were to invent a magical fat-dissolving ray-gun, you could arbitrarily aim it at any human waistline, pull the trigger and guess what? Every ray-gun victim would have defined abdominal muscles, even those that had never done a single rep of abdominal exercise. Unlike a bicep or thigh muscle that looks scrawny when undersized, the gut is different: magically melt the fat that obscures the waist muscles and anyone's abs will look absolutely fabulous. No need to do any ab work whatsoever: simply oxidize the thick layer of lard that lies atop the ab muscles and presto! Ripped abs, gloriously displayed!

True, from an aesthetic viewpoint a fat-free 29 inch waistline will be visually more attractive than a fat free 40 inch *distended* beer gut. Regardless the circumference of the gut, melt off the fat and we <u>all</u> have a delineated waistline hidden away somewhere. In my admittedly heretical opinion, there is *no need* to endlessly train abdominal muscles, performing set after set, endless rep after endless rep. There is no need for exotic ab machines or devices. If the Purposeful Primitive is training and eating according to the prescribed dictates, body fat will melt and the abdominal muscles (that we all have) will eventually emerge.

Abdominal exercise does not, can not, and will not preferentially melt off the body fat that lies atop the abdominal muscles.

Gut muscles are worked hard by heavy squats and deadlifts and with far more intensity then effete crunches or ineffectual broomstick twists. Bio-mechanically, a properly performed deadlift is in actuality a weighted reverse sit-up. The waist muscles activate to an incredible degree in order to maintain an upright torso while performing a proper squat. Ab device product pushers perpetuate a myth that there is no need for diet or cardio; simply engage in endless ab exercise, usually using some sort of abdominal device. "Use the Sonic Gut-Buster and waistline fat is magically melted!" If only that were true—we'd all have ripped guts!

Personal Trainers worldwide routinely recommend abdominal work galore. This exercise prescription is expressly for "chiseling, defining and revealing the waistline." Why are multiple sets of high reps proscribed for the abs and not all the other body parts also awash in a sea of excess body fat? How come women with saddlebags thighs aren't made to perform hundreds of endless high rep sets of squats or leg extensions? If high rep ab work spot reduces the body fat overtop the ab muscles, why isn't this same methodology carried over into other regions? Extending this faulty logic, why not utilize dozens of sets of 100 rep curls and 100 rep triceps extensions to melt body fat that covers chubby female upper arms? Man boobs? Let's do dozens of 100 rep sets in the decline bench press. Physiologically speaking, specific deposits of body fat cannot be targeted or "zeroed in on." There is no way that by working the hell out of a particular muscle the fat that lies atop that muscle is preferentially dissolved. Body fat is kept in fat storage depots that dot the body's landscape. Men usually have their fat storage depots atop the frontal abdominal, pectorals and external oblique region. Women have their largest fat storage depots atop the buttocks, upper arms and upper thighs. Spot reducing fat is another example of George Orwell's "smelly little orthodoxies." The rationale for perpetuating the myth of spot reduction is simple: it sells products.

Where Body Fat Is Drawn Down From Is Beyond Your Control

Excess calories turned into body fat are stored away in random fashion. Science has never been able to say definitively that there is a discernable pattern as to how the body stores fat, or how the body draws down from those fat stores. There is no specific pattern that stays constant, human to human, though empirical evidence tells us that each of us have certain fat storage depots that are preferentially used and therefore larger than the other depots.

Body fat is excess energy tucked away for emergency use at some point in the future. Stored body fat is used when the Energy Balance Equation (EBE) tips into the negative. Obviously if a person consumes more calories than they oxidize over the course of the day, the EBE never goes negative. Unless energy demands outstrip available calories, stored body fat is never mobilized to cover caloric shortfall—because there is no caloric shortfall. If a person is in continual caloric surplus there is never a reason for the body to call upon its strategic fat reserves.

There exist fat mobilization strategies used by the athletic elite to *trick* the body into mobilizing stored body fat, this despite the fact that many of these athletes are ingesting 5,000 calories or more per day. How can an athlete eating 5,000 calories a day actually burn fat? They are able to do so because they have jacked-up their metabolic burn rate through a strategic combination of exercise, activity and calorie selection. Think of the metabolism as the body's thermostat. If the thermostat in your house is set at 32 degrees very little fuel is burned, if the thermostat is turned up to 95 degrees, lots of fuel is needed. An obese person has their metaphorical thermostat set at 32 degrees and needs very few calories to maintain. A professional bodybuilder has reset their caloric burn thermostat to 95 degrees and loses fat by *only* eating 3,500 calories a day!

Want a Ripped Waist? Reset the Metabolic Thermostat

Professional bodybuilders intent on achieving 2-6% body fat percentiles (while retaining 250 pounds plus of muscle mass) eat foods difficult or impossible for the body to convert into fat. They break their calories into roughly equal size meals and eat every few hours to trigger thermogenic attributes associated with digestion. They perform torrid cardio before breakfast to take advantage of the benefits of doing aerobics in a catabolic, post-sleep, glycogen-free environment. In the absence of glycogen the body is forced to burn body fat. Some will perform a second cardio session late in the day.

Muscle requires calories to exist. By building muscle the body demands more calories simply to breakeven. Adding ten pounds of muscle jacks up the daily metabolic breakeven point by 300 to 400 calories. Combine specific training tactics with specific eating procedures and over time the metabolic rate is elevated to stratospheric levels. A muscle-laden body needs thousands of calories just to maintain. When the muscleman cranks back their massive caloric intake ever so slightly, a caloric deficit is created and even though they might still be eating six 800 calorie meals a day, this might be a significant reduction from six 1,000 calories meals. Enough to tip the EBE into the negative. This slight 200-calorie per meal reduction might seem negligible, yet cumulatively, spread over six meals nets an impressive 1,200 calorie a day reduction.

Slashing calories drastically derails the metabolism and triggers dormant primordial hard-wiring: the body, sensing starvation, becomes obsessed with hanging onto body fat at all costs. To fuel any caloric shortfalls bought on by crash dieting, the body's alarm goes off and the body eats muscle to save precious body fat. The body "spares" fat by cannibalizing muscle tissue. Lovely.

Ab Exercise Heretic

We have no say in how the human body preferentially draws down its strategic fat reserves. There are no known procedures or tactics that can force the body to draw down from a specific fat storage depot. To oxidize stored body fat we first need to create an energy deficit. Optimally a balanced combination of precision eating (first and foremost) is closely coordinated with a specific exercise protocol that emphasizes cardio exercise—not abdominal exercise.

In the Purposefully Primitive approach we recommend very little direct abdominal exercises. Heresy? Absolutely! Cardiovascular exercise, done in close coordination with a tight diet, is far, far more effective use of training time if the goal is to attain a fat-free body. Nutrition is the biggest single factor in lowering body fat. When the athlete successfully pulls all the right physiological triggers, then and only then will the body mobilize stored body fat. The fat burning prerequisites need to be recognized and attended to: how are you going to burn fat if you are over-eating the wrong foods? That's a deal breaker: bias food selections towards foods that are difficult to convert into body fat. Break the daily caloric intake into smaller amounts. Or use the Warrior Diet approach. Try performing pre-breakfast cardio. A sluggish metabolic rate makes it impossible to "get underneath the caloric ceiling" and cut calories further in order to reduce body fat. How does someone whose metabolism is slowed to a crawl and existing on 1,000 calories a day going to cut calories further to lose more fat?

The Caloric Cost of Exercise is Vastly Overrated

How many calories do you suppose it takes to perform 100 crunch reps? It's negligible. Using exercise to tip the energy balance equation is brutal work. The amount of exercise needed to produce a significant caloric reduction requires intense, prolonged effort.

Burning off 900 calories in an hour requires the athlete chug along at a Herculean 15 calorie per minute burn rate. A single ice cream sundae could *easily* contain 1,000 calories. The best way to melt off excess body fat is to stop making poor food choices. It is far easier to not eat the 1,000 calorie sundae than try and burn off 1,000 calories through intense, prolonged exercise. Toss the obvious junk foods and find the caloric tipping point where food intake equals energy expenditure. How to tell? Here's a commonsense solution that requires only one tool: a bathroom scale. Reduce food intake until you drop a pound. Hold this level of food intake level for a few days and see if you stabilize. Then add calories back in until you are able to bump back up a pound. You have now found the caloric tipping zone: clean up the food selections. Use exercise to create a caloric deficit. Lose weight at a rate of one pound per hundred pounds of bodyweight.

Elite bodybuilders whittle fat down slowly, steadily and consistently; they avoid crash diets that "shatter the metabolism" as Ori says. Calorie slashing causes muscle tissue to disappear as fast or faster than body fat.

The Procedural Consensus of the Iron Elite

A procedural consensus, a fat-burning template, has emerged that can and should be used by normal individuals seeking a sleek physique. Use a patient, protracted, cyclical/periodized approach: take 8-12 weeks and reduce body fat using a slow and steady glide path. Pare away 1 to 3 pounds per week, depending on your size. Melt off fat in a systematic fashion, slowly and carefully, thereby preserving muscle tissue in the process. Expropriate hardcore bodybuilder methodology and use their procedures. Toss the fad diets and miracle products that lure you in with the seductive promise of how easy and effortless the fat loss process can be. Fat loss is difficult and should be done over a protracted period of time.

Place your faith in science, biology, intense exercise, elite empirical experience and above all else, disciplined eating. It's a tough love message. As one music critic said after listening to the jarring, disconcerting music Miles Davis was playing in the 70s, "His music is like taking an ice cold shower; immediately shocking and unpleasant; ultimately bracing and invigorating." Be done with spot reducing myths about ab exercise. The best single abdominal exercise is to exert control over your knife and fork. Clean up food selections, maneuver downward to the caloric breakeven point, use the caloric cost of exercise to create NEB. Hold tight for 6-12 weeks. Watch those abs emerge from beneath that sea of lard. Understand the futility of spot reducing. Recognize the inherent falsity of this first-magnitude fitness myth.

Food Tricks

Learn How to Infuse 'Diet Foods' with Taste

As a young athlete I never paid a damned bit of attention to the nutritional content of anything. As I grew older I developed an interest in melding my newfound nutritional awareness with the peasant food preparation skills that I learned from my elderly grandmother. She resided on a spooky farm in the Arkansas delta. Tucked away in Yoda-like solitude, she taught me how to prepare foods I liked and naturally gravitated towards. Her approach was Old School all the way. Farm fresh foods were prepared simply, letting the natural flavor of fresh ingredients shine through. She intuitively laid a table that was a good balance between her garden vegetables (canned in the winter) and local pork, beef and fish. She raised chickens, turkey and geese. Freshwater fish, caught from ponds and the Mighty Mississippi, were plentiful between April and October.

Peasant cooking virtuoso: My grandmother at age 85 at her Arkansas home. She was ¼ Cherokee and her job was cooking for the field hands. Born in 1896, she became expert at preparing local fish, pork, beef and farm fresh produce. The best meals use the freshest ingredients prepared simply. I was addicted to her ethereal cooking. She taught me the food basics I use to this day.

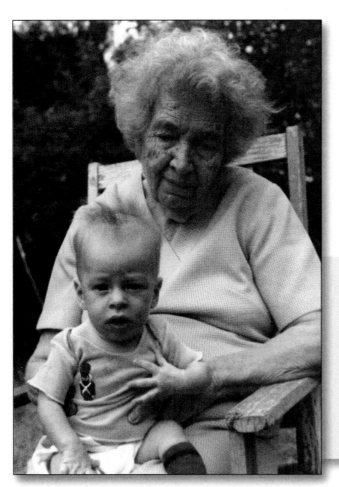

Purposefully Primitive Performance Eating is all about melding great *taste* with great ingredients. When it comes to eating, taste trumps everything. We love great tasting food and hate bland gruel. Learn to prepare foods that are both beneficial for you and tickle your taste buds. Bland food needs to be transformed into tasty food. Creatively prepare acceptable, wholesome, beneficial foods in quantities sufficient enough to keep your refrigerator stocked for 3-7 days. When its time to eat, simply pop the proper portion size into the microwave and two minutes later eat a power-packed, terrific tasting meal. The idea is to create diet meals you actually look forward to eating. It is important that you learn basic food preparation tactics. Come to grips with elemental food preparation. That way you are in control of your nutritional destiny and not preparation-dependant on someone or something. Here are a few classic food preparation techniques.

Grilled Steak

You'd be surprised how many folks cannot grill a decent piece of meat. Nothing is easier, quicker or more delicious. Take the steak out of the refrigerator and let stand at room temperature for at least 30 minutes as this softens the fat. Sirloin, rib eye, filet mignon, strip, T-bone, porterhouse, flank or skirt steak, are best grilled on a red hot grill that has been oiled with olive oil or a piece of steak fat. Generously season with coarse kosher or sea salt and pepper right before placing on the hottest part of the grill. Don't walk away or get distracted; pay attention and flip the meat only once. Leave the 1st side totally alone for 1-3 minutes. You can also use the oven broiler. The length of steak cook time varies depending on size and thickness: if this is problematic use a meat thermometer—120 for rare, 145 medium rare. When done, let the steak stand for five minutes to allow the juices to settle. A properly grilled steak is one of life's true pleasures. My personal favorite is a perfectly prepared cowboy rib steak or a fork tender filet.

Squashed Chicken

Boneless skinless chicken breast is the absolute number one bodybuilding food. White meat chicken is relatively inexpensive and has a high protein/low fat ratio. Preparing a chicken breast that is delectable, moist and tender is difficult.

There is a method that produces absolutely the best breast I've ever tasted. This method of preparation allows you to produce a chicken breast that can be sautéed, baked or grilled to succulent perfection. The breasts can be stacked and stored in the refrigerator for up to one week.

The key is to squash the bulbous breast *flat* prior to preparation.

By eliminating the rotund profile, by squashing the raw breast into a low rider flattened configuration, you can cook a perfectly done, juicy breast every single time. From start to finish it takes less then ten minutes to prepare a squashed breast. I pay a few extra cents per pound and buy organic chicken—not only is it chemically free, the taste of the bird is significantly superior. Set a breast on a cutting board covered with a couple of plastic grocery bags. Flatten the breasts one at a time with a kitchen mallet. The force used to mash a breast is a little too intense to perform on a kitchen counter; the repeated blows could conceivably damage the counter surface. Try placing the cutting board on the floor. I go outside on my deck, use a 10 pound tamp and flatten a dozen breast inside of five minutes. I cover the tamper with layers of grocery bags and cover a small square of plywood with grocery bags. Once the fibrous core is hit square the breast will give way and flatten out nicely. The breast optimally ends up about 1/8th to 1/4 inch thick.

I often store the flattened breast in a Jacuzzi bath, usually a vinegar-based marinade. I use Stubb's Marinade. The squashed breasts marinate until its time to cook them. My favorite method is to dredge the marinade breasts in Japanese Panko bread crumbs and sauté them in olive oil. You can bake squashed breasts by placing them on a wire rack set atop a baking pan. Slide the pan into a 350 degree oven. You can grill them over charcoal or over propane. Flattened bird makes you forget all about Colonel Sanders. A plain squashed breast can be grilled or sautéed and ready to eat inside five minutes.

Oven or Weber Roasted Beef, Lamb, Chicken or Turkey

You can oven roast standing rib roast, leg of lamb, whole chicken, turkey or duck. Roasted whole birds are easy to prepare.

To roast a chicken, turkey or duck wash the bird inside and out with cold running water. Let it drain dry in the sink. If you're in a hurry, pat dry with paper towels. Coat the outside of the dry bird with a light application of salt and pepper. Ditto the cavity. Set the bird on a wire rack inside a pan and roast at 350/375 degrees. Cook until internal temperature (probe inserted at the deepest part of the thigh) reaches 170 degrees. I use a $10 kitchen thermometer that has a long metal braid rope connected to a probe which allows the digital readout to stay outside the oven and can be read without having to open the oven door or lift the Weber lid. No more guesswork. When the internal temp hits 170 an alarm goes off that alerts me that the bird is done.

I pull the bird out when the magic 170 is reached and let it set for a full ten minutes. The final finished result is perfection every time. If you are roasting a leg of lamb the internal temperature of the meat should reach 120 degrees.

For variation I use a Weber grill. I love the taste of wood smoked meat. Place charcoal in a starter tube in the center of the grill. Lightly soak newspaper or paper towels with a little vegetable oil and place the balled up oiled paper underneath the charcoal starter and light it.

In 10 to 15 minutes the coals will be white hot. When the coals turn white, divide them into two equal piles on opposite sides of the grill. In the middle place an aluminum drip pan. This is the indirect method of cooking. I like to place big chunks of water-soaked hickory, mesquite, apple or peach wood on top of the hot coals before setting the top grate in place. Place the protein payload, be it beef, lamb, turkey, duck or chicken in the center over top the drip pan. Put the lid in place and leave it alone. Use the meat thermometer to determine when the protein payload is thoroughly cooked. The same oven roasting temperatures apply to the Weber.

Regardless the protein payload, the final finished product is mind-blowing: succulent, smoke-infused meat, fowl or seafood rendered fork tender and smoky delicious.

Brined Poultry

Brining is a centuries-old method of making fowl tender and juicy by soaking the turkey, chicken or duck in a pail of water containing salt and sugar. The salt water is sucked into the cells and volume-moisturizes the meat. I brine whole turkey and chicken by submerging the bird in a 5 gallon paint bucket lined with a garbage bag. I fill the bucket with warm water and mix in a cup of salt and a ½ cup sugar and let is soak. Most experts say don't brine longer than two hours. I brine a whole birds and sometimes chicken breasts. I find in every instance the brined bird turns out tender and juicy. Brining is particularly appropriate for roasting or smoking.

Fish

Whole fish or filets can be sautéed, grilled or steamed in a matter of a few minutes. Atlantic salmon, steelhead, haddock, cod and trout are my usual fish choices. I can have a perfectly prepared piece of fish ready to eat inside 5-15 minutes using a skillet, a spatula, a little olive oil and some dry spice. Sometimes I'll dredge the trout, cod or haddock filets in Panko bread crumbs. I often sprinkle Paul Prudomme's Blackened Redfish dry rub on fish. I use enough extra virgin olive oil to cover the bottom of a deep, large skillet and sauté the fish. If the fish has skin, place the filet into the skillet skin side down.

I use a relatively high heat taking the oil to just below its smoke point. The smoke point on any cooking oil occurs when the heat from the cooking source causes the oil to burn and evaporate. Extra virgin olive oil's smoke point is around 370 degrees. Hot oil is what we seek—too hot is to be avoided. Don't mess with the fish—let it sit and cook on one side 70% of the way before flipping it over. Turn the fish over carefully using a wide spatula or tongs. I often sprinkle dry rub on fish. Total cook time depends on the thickness of the filet. When complete, remove the fish gently.

Grilling is easy: oil the grate, let the fish cook mostly on side number one. Fish can be baked on a pan or steamed in a bag. To steam, place the fish on a big square of aluminum foil, throw in some herbs, perhaps some thin sliced onions, scallions or ginger. Add a dash of wine, seal the aluminum foil and place it on a cookie sheet. Slide the whole thing into a preheated oven; after 10 minutes check for doneness. The fish steams itself in the bag and this hassle-free preparation method produces a terrific tasting fish dish within 20 minutes of walking in the door after a long day at work. Please avoid battered frozen fish.

Shellfish

Nothing tastes better: shrimp, scallops, crab, squid, lobster, mussels, clams, oysters—the fresher the seafood the more vibrant the taste. Do you live along one of the coastlines and have a fisherman's market or wharf in your area where the locals sell seafood? Frequent it! If you live inland, find where the river fishermen sell their divine freshwater fish. Again, think of the tortured route your supermarket seafood takes....catch it, sell it, transport it, reroute it—all before it gets to you.

According to my nutritional bible, *The United States Department of Agriculture Handbook #8*, a 100 gram portion of shrimp contain 18.1 grams of protein, 0.8 grams of fat, 1.5 grams of carbohydrate and 91 calories—a 100 gram portion is slightly less than ¼ pound. Once you buy it, don't wait to cook it. Everybody steams shrimp and most folks overcook shrimp.

Try this alternative method for shrimp preparation: in a skillet add a slight bit of olive oil and heat the pan to just below the smoke point. Throw the shelled shrimp into the pan and make sure to not overcrowd the skillet. As soon as the shrimp begin to turn pink, within a minute, remove the pan from the heat and turn each shrimp over. The residual heat will continue to cook the crustaceans. Leave them alone until they cool, then peel them one at a time. The shells will come right off. If I intend to eat the shrimp by themselves, I will cook them thoroughly—but not too much. If I intend to use them in another dish I will err on the side of undercooking rather than over-cooking. Nothing is worse than overcooked shrimp as that turns the crustaceans rubbery and dry. If you cook shrimp completely then throw them into another dish, the shrimp will cook further and end up going past the point of no return.

Once you have cooked and shelled the shrimp, you can store them in the refrigerator for future use. Shrimp makes a killer meal and is always a hit when guests drop by. Mixing shrimp with vegetables gets maximum mileage out of this expensive ingredient. Don't purchase the teeny-tiny popcorn shrimp: I like the largest possible crustaceans in the $9 to $14 per pound range and find that a single pound is good for one mega-meal or two normal meals. Let's reconsider shrimp: yes they are expensive when compared to chicken breast and egg whites, but man cannot live by bird and bird eggs alone. As I told one novice trainee who complained that shrimp were too expensive to be included in his dietary game plan, "Sure you can! Take all the money you previously spent on $4 a pint ice cream, buck-a-bar candy bars, donuts, pastries and don't forget the six-packs of Pepsi and beer—redirect all this recovered income towards some fat-free seafood!"

Steamed Rice

A rice steamer is a terrific tool and quite inexpensive. I use the nutty brown rice variations. Keep a cooked supply in the refrigerator ready for instant use. Nothing could be easier than preparing a mountain of rice for consumption in the coming week. Don't overcook rice or it will dissolve into a mound of starchy mush. To make sure the rice is evenly done, I stir the steaming rice with a long handled wooden spoon during the cooking procedure to keep the rice on the bottom from getting over done while the rice on top remains crunchy. I particularly love organic Lunenburg Black Japonica, a gourmet blend of black and mahogany rice: rich, nutty flavored, power-packed and gluten free.

For those intent on building mass, rice rules!

Baked Sweet Potatoes

Nothing tastes better than a baked sweet potato, particularly for someone with a sweet tooth. I like my sweet potatoes baked thoroughly and I bake them until the potato skin seems loose and feels brittle to the touch. This is another taste treat that can be prepared in mass quantities ahead of time. I prefer the smaller sized spuds. Yams and sweet potatoes are interchangeable. Potatoes can also be sliced paper thin and sautéed in olive oil.

Sauteed Fiber Vegetables

I buy raw green beans, bust off the stem end and throw them in a deep skillet with a few tablespoons of olive oil. Dice up few bell peppers and cut a large organic carrot into strips. Let these three fiber veggies sauté for as long as it takes to tenderize the beans. It could take a while. Beans are tough, as are carrots and red, yellow or green bell peppers. Add a large sliced onion and/or broccoli flowerets later in the process. Right before serving put in a pile of raw spinach. Remove from the heat. Sometimes I add goat cheese. Stir periodically with a wooden spoon.

You can create an amazing medley of fibrous carbs that has a multitude of flavors. If you prefer certain fiber carbs and don't like others, add or subtract according to your taste preference. This concoction stores well and I will scoop out a portion to complement my protein portion. I often construct this pan of fiber without the greens beans; this cuts down cooking time dramatically. Other times I will add some thin sliced cabbage and garlic. I eat some sort of pan sautéed fiber concoction every single day.

Salads

Fresh is best. On the other hand, what could be easier then opening a bag of premixed salad and pouring on top some low fat salad dressing? Quick, easy, convenient and effective, try to eat one salad a day. Don't cancel out the benefits by loading up the salad with a high-fat or chemically-doused dressing. I honestly don't eat a lot of bagged salad except in the winter when the local produce is unavailable. For someone looking to throw together a hassle-free meal after work, bagged salad is the ultimate in convenience. Stacy makes excellent homemade dressing: extra virgin olive oil mixed with balsamic vinegar, plain organic yogurt and a little bit of dill.

Farmer Market Foods

Every urban area has a farmer's market. The farmers who live in the region surrounding the city drive into town once a week during growing season and sell their farm fresh wares to the City Slickers. When you go to the grocery store to buy produce, that pepper or onion (or whatever) was grown on a Midwest or West Coast mega farm, doused with pesticides and chemicals to keep the bugs off, picked, trucked to a central distribution hub, placed on trucks and driven to your store. All that takes time: the nutritional potency and taste of a vegetable fades in direct relation to the length of time from when it was picked to when it is eaten. Go to the farmer's market and taste the vibrant flavor of fruits and vegetables picked within the last few days. The taste difference is astounding. Eat what is in season and don't allow it to languish in your refrigerator for too long: cook and eat produce as soon as possible.

So Much More

This is a sparse and meager sampling. The idea behind any Performance Eating plan is to eat healthy and eat foods that actually taste terrific. Unless you have a personal chef on staff, unless you still live with your mother, unless you eat out every night, unless your wife, girlfriend or your "significant other" cooks, you need to come to grips with food preparation. It is easy, creative and fun. Good cooking is a bunch of simple procedures followed in a precise sequence. Taste and diet need not be a contradiction in terms.

Learn how to prepare tasty beneficial foods and you will amplify results obtained from weight training and cardio. When you exercise intensely you need to take in sufficient calories in order to speed up recovery and fuel new muscle growth. Over-exercising and under-eating is a cortisol-inducing, physiological catastrophe. Let's eat smart and eat tasty and eat enough to recuperate and recover. Eating lots of protein and fiber: that's the backbone. Eating copious amounts of acceptable food will dampen a sweet tooth. And if the sweet tooth persists, check out the Parrillo or Warrior line of nutritional supplements; lots of sweet tasting bars and engineered foods that fool the sweetest of sweet addictions – yet these supplemental foods are acceptable and downright beneficial.

MAGNIFICENT MINI-ME!

Miracle Home Smoker

As is my habit when I watch TV and there is nothing really on, I turn to the Food Network. I'm a "foodie" and love to cook— to me it is another creative outlet and I'm usually at my best when I'm involved with something creative and constructive. I like to watch real food pros inventively deal with ingredients. They alert me to new food combinations, techniques and insider tips I'd never thought about.

One day I happened to catch a strange episode of Alton Brown's show *Good Eats*. He is a strange combination of quirky chef, standup comedian, culinary wizard, science geek and food historian. In this particular episode, he ran the voodoo down (as Miles Davis called "truth telling") on meat smokers: he did so from a science and practicality vantage point.

The subject of wood smokers may, at first glance, seem an odd choice for a fitness book. However food plays a *huge* role in the fitness equation. To succeed in transforming ourselves we need break out of our current love/hate relationship with food—which is really a love/hate relationship with *taste*! Imagine a magical world where every diet food tasted as if Iron Chef Mario Batali had lovingly prepared it, especially for you, using gourmet ingredients that you loved. Would not dieting cease to be dieting?

In order to break taste habit-patterns, it is critical to develop a vast and virtually inexhaustible repertoire of *delicious* recipes. The foods need be nutritionally acceptable. The trick is to learn how to infuse a relatively narrow band of food selections with wonderful taste. Is it possible to create a menu of delicious, nutritious, potent, acceptable foods that you can make? Do so (make diet food taste great) and sticking to a diet is no longer problematic.

One way to make meats, fowl and seafood taste succulent, subtle and delectable, is to cook them slow and smoke them. Wood smoke applied to meat, fish, seafood or fowl, infuses and imparts unparalleled flavor into the blandest cut. Slow smoking renders the final finished product tender, succulent, and incredibly delicious. Over the years I've earnestly sought to recreate at home (even to a small degree) the amazing smoked cuisine I've sampled commercially. Until now it's been nothing but fool's gold. Alton Brown explained in five minutes why all my home smokers were doomed and why my frustrations and poor results were to be expected. First and foremost: the commercial smokers I had purchased and used were all made of thin metal and thin metal allows heat to easily escape. Hence thin metal smokers are inefficient and need continual refueling.

- Smoke needs to be thick, concentrated and consistent
- The best temperature for smoking is between 190 and 220 degrees.
- Thin metal allows heat to escape through its thin surface
- Propane burns and emits chemicals that make it slow smoke-unfriendly and odd tasting
- Effective smokers are expensive—cheap ones are ineffective

His solution was innovative and inexpensive. I mimicked his device with outstanding results. His home smoker solution was pure genius: inexpensive ingenuity cubed with great simplicity.

- Purchase a large earthenware terracotta planter pot—mine measured 16-inches at the top
- Purchase a 17-inch terracotta planter base—this is used as a lid. Price for both? $27
- Purchase a single burner electric hot plate—I got mine at Wal-Mart for $8
- Purchase a square wire rack and an 8-inch baking pan—$11
- Purchase a bag of hardwood from Home Depot—$8
- Purchase a cooking thermometer from Home Depot—$8

Place the terracotta pot on two bricks: this creates a gap under the pot. Set the hot plate in bottom of the pot and run the cord through the drain hole. Plug the hot plate into an outdoor extension cord. I set my smoker outside the unheated garage gym. Turn the hot plate on and set it at maximum temperature. Place the baking pan atop the hot plate coil and place a goodly amount of soaked hardwood into the baking pan. I use dry small slivers of hardwood and combine them with larger wet wood chunks. The little slivers get the smoke party started, quickly, and give the big chunks a chance to get rolling.

Place the bent-to-fit wire rack into the pot: I purchased a lightweight wire rack from the kitchen supply bake accessory aisle at Wal-Mart for five bucks. I bent it with my bare hands, no big deal. But then again as a brute, bending things comes easy for me. I bent the square grate so the four corners touched and held when placed inside the pot. Place the meat thermometer in one of the wire rack holes. Alton drilled a hole in the lid of his and sat the thermometer sensor into the newly created hole. I may get around to that someday.

Place the protein payload: the fish, chicken, turkey, lamb, beef, seafood or pork on the rack and cover the whole deal with the 17-inch bottom. The top fits real nice. Within five minutes this weird contraption is generating fragrant wood smoke like crazy. The small internal chamber area creates intense hickory, mesquite, apple or peach wood smoke. The wood chips go a long way. The smoke is contained in this tight little container and the small chamber prevents the smoke from diffusing or escaping. Every 60 minutes (for long cooking meats) remove the top; pull the rack out with the cargo still atop it. Set the wire rack down onto the overturned smoker lid (placed on the ground adjacent to the smoker) and baste the payload.

Add new wood chips replace the rack with the payload back into the smoker and go away. I've had my Miracle Terracotta Wood Smoker up and running for a year and this thing is by far the most effective smoke contraption I've ever used.

Two things make this device trump everything on the market under $1,000: the heat conductor is clay, not metal, and this funky substance holds heat incredibly well: clay reflects the heat inward instead of letting it dissipate through the surface as thin metal does. The smoker is small and miniaturized and the smallness makes it easy to create, contain and control heat and smoke to an exacting degree. To refuel use tongs and lift the pie pan of burning hardwood out and set it somewhere safe. Turn the hot plate temperature control down—or up—if the internal temp is less than 200-degrees.

When this device is up and cranking at capacity, tantalizing wisps of fragrant smoke mix with the meat/fish smell of whatever is being smoked. The smoke slips out from under the lid and smells positively seductive. ("Languid, luscious, lustful.") The drawback is capacity: smallish, not tiny, but small. It takes very little wood-fuel to keep this sucker smoking like a locomotive. The lid fit is heavy and complete; the inner chamber supercharged with intense smoke infused with the wood flavor of your choice. Hickory and mesquite are the most widely available and both are excellent. The device is safe because everything is neatly contained inside the sturdy pot.

Regardless the protein source selected, the procedure is the same: place the food inside the supercharged smoke chamber for as long as it takes to reaches doneness. 120 degrees for lamb, 130 for beef and 170 degrees for fowl. I eyeball seafood. This device is earthen and primitive, one bus stop away from burying pigs in the ground. The cost was under $50. I set my smoker up next to the garage gym so I can tend it during our lifting sessions. I torture and tempt lifters with the smell of the succulent slow-roasting protein. The wood smoke smell drifts into the gym and drives everyone to insane distraction. Food and intense physical training are inexorably related: train hard then eat tasty, beneficial food afterwards. Smoking makes meat, lamb, bird and fish unbelievably tasty. What an easy enjoyable chore it is to produce smoked protein with the Lilliputian Magnificent Mini-Me.

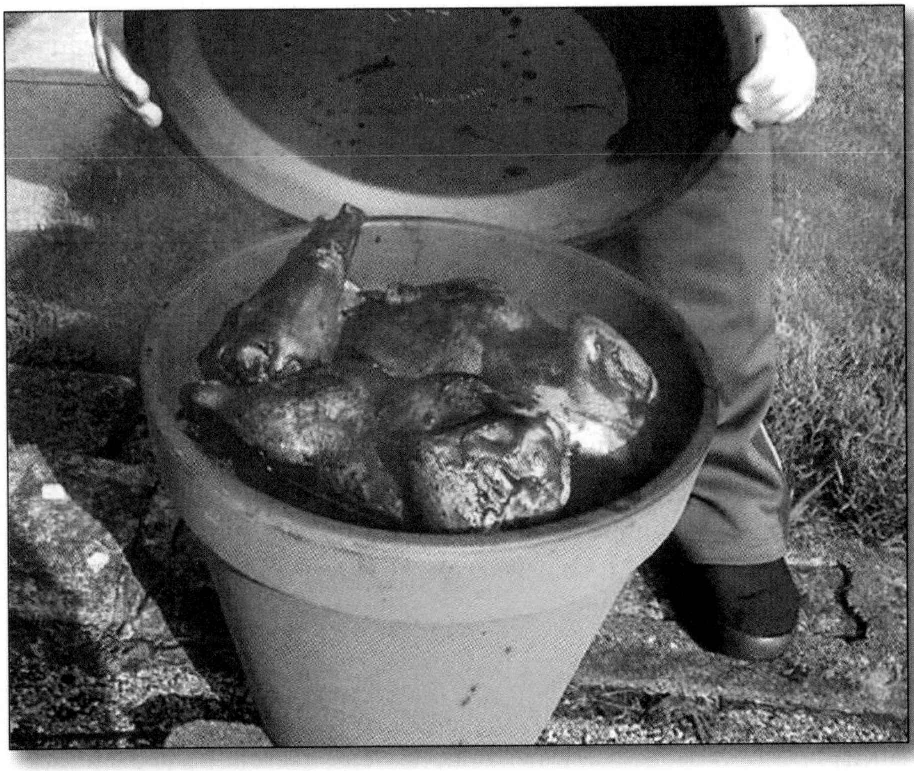

Magnificent Mini-Me in full flight: set up next to the unheated garage gym, I get sadistic pleasure training with muscular no-necks while hickory, mesquite or apple wood meat smoke permeates the gym. At some point the big men break down and literally beg me to invite them to stay and eat. In the photo I am mesquite-smoking local free-range organic chicken parts and some fall-off-the-bone lamb shanks. The device is super simplistic: set a single burner hot plate in the bottom of the terracotta flower pot. Run the cord out the bottom through the drain hole. Set the hot plate on ¾ or high heat and place a 9-12" pie pan atop the hot plate. Place wood chunks in the pie pan. I found a wire grate and bent it to carry the protein payload. The wire mesh sits about 10" above the wood-filled pie pan. I use a terracotta bottom as the lid. It takes less than five minutes for the wood chunks to start smoking. Jumbo shrimp, scallops, salmon, fowl, beef, lamb, you name it and this little smoke machine will make it taste better!

Epilogue

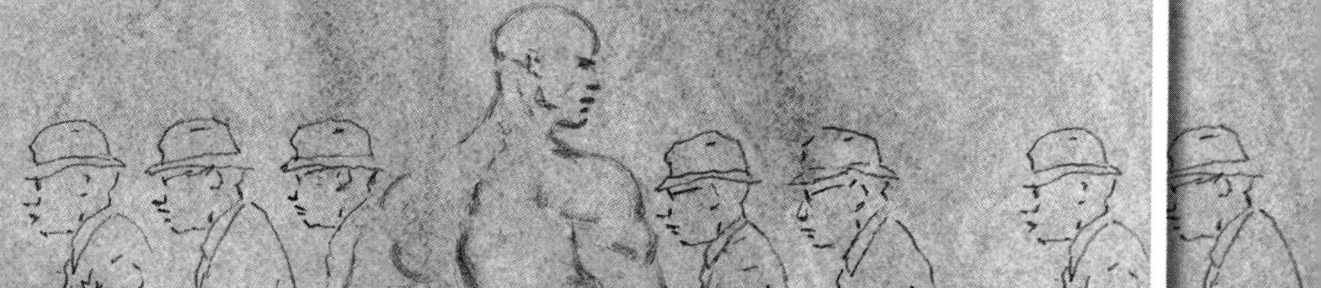

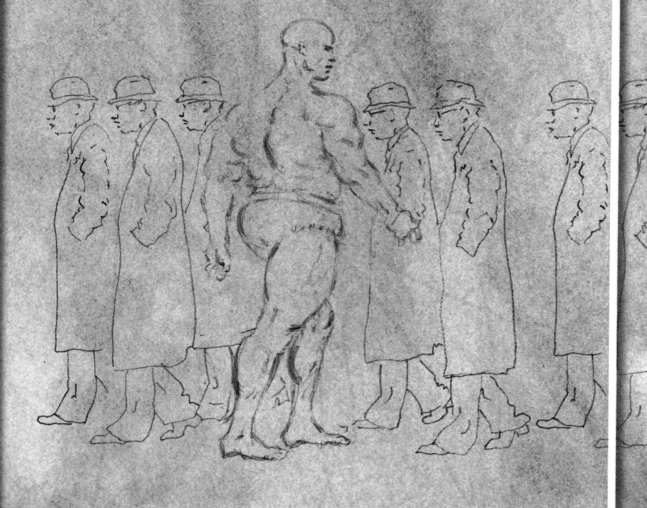

The Purposefully Primitive Manifesto
Doing Fewer Things Better
Primitive Tools and Simplistic Modes are Used to Power Sparse Methods

Executed with the requisite tenacity, intensity and precision, Purposefully Primitive methods can and will favorably alter the compositional makeup of the human body. Primitive tools and simplistic modes are used to power sparse methods. By generating a methodical and sustained physical and psychological effort, the human body is forcibly morphed from what it is into what we want it to become: leaner and more muscular. The human body is not seduced, lured, cajoled, convinced or persuaded to alter itself—it is *forced* to alter itself. We force the body to favorably reconfigure itself by generating physical and psychological fierceness during training. The intense, protracted physical effort is amplified and enhanced by the studied and sustained use of specific nutritional strategies. Commonsense nutritional strategies and Old School training tactics are synchronized and placed within a periodized timeframe.

The three interrelated Purposefully Primitive disciplines (weight training, cardiovascular training and nutrition) need to be regularly and routinely practiced in a balanced and proportional fashion. Lock down all aspects of the program and within seven days of full implementation tangible results appear; by the end of the first month, body composition (the fat-to-muscle ratio) undergoes a dramatic turnaround; those who commit completely for 90 days undergo a total metamorphosis. Does this mean everyone will end up looking like Arnold Schwarzenegger on his best day? No, but no matter how deep a physical hole you are currently standing in, 90 days of maniacal discipline and teeth-gritting effort will enable you to utterly and completely change the shape, texture, efficiency and hardness of your body.

Our Purposefully Primitive Methodology is a loose amalgamation of methods and modes absorbed from genuine Masters. This cumulative, combined knowledge is grouped into one of four categories: Iron, Mind, Cardio or Nutrition. These are the four avenues of transformational progress. The Purposefully Primitive amalgamated philosophy is not time intensive, but it is physically intense: total training time for a beginner or intermediate athlete does not need to exceed five cumulative hours per week—not much time at all when one considers the innumerable physical benefits derived. The caveat is that you must generate extreme physical effort during those five hours. Sub-maximal training yields submaximal results; we consciously and continually push against the lip of the limit envelope because we understand that extreme physical effort is the transformational precursor.

Disciplined nutrition underpins gut-busting training. Eat plentiful amounts of wholesome, nutritious and delicious tasting foods. Bias food consumption towards nutrients preferentially used to build muscle and accelerate the healing and recovery process. Avoid foods preferentially shuttled into body fat storage. Purposefully Primitive training is self-inflicted physical trauma. We need to supply the battered body with ample amounts of regenerative nutrients. Certain nutrients ingested at specific times will accelerate the physical recovery process. Physical recovery is the precursor to actual muscle growth.

Certain foods accelerate results and other foods undermine hard training. We consume foods that amplify our efforts and jettison foods that subvert and derail the transformational process.

Those disciplined few able to attain and maintain that delicate, elusive balance between resistance training, cardiovascular training and precision nutrition, ignite *physiologic synergy*. When synergistic critical mass is attained progress compounds at an astoundingly fast rate; results exceed realistic expectations. The transformational total exceeds the logical sum of the deconstructed parts: 2 + 2 + 2 = 10. A fully instituted Purposefully Primitive regimen *always* transforms the physique. The human body subjected to our peculiar and particular procedures and protocols has no biological choice in the matter: when the human body has been successfully served with certain physiological imperatives the laws of causation must be obeyed. Enact our procedures in the prescribed fashion and muscle *must* be manufactured; stored body fat *must* be mobilized and oxidized.

I have provided you with a series of tried-and-tested tactical training templates. I have provided you with nutritional strategies used on a worldwide basis by the athletic elite. Hopefully I have shed the light of truth on a few basic physiological facts-of-life. There are certain laws of science and biology that are profoundly applicable to the process. All fitness-minded individuals need to understand these facts-of-life if they are ever to gain any traction in their own transformational quest.

I have empowered you with classical knowledge gleaned from true Masters. You now know precisely what procedures and protocols will work. By replicating and instituting Purposefully Primitive training and eating strategies, you will be able to engineer your very own physical metamorphosis.

Your search for effective transformational methods is over.

An Inch Wide and a Mile Deep

> ***Scientists are concerned about discovering commonalties that can be reduced to theorems and laws—the artist is concerned about peculiarities and particulars that can draw distinctions and differences.***
>
> **—Vladimir Nabokov**

A true Purposeful Primitive is both scientist and artist. We are scientists in that we are guided by the immutable laws of biology. We obey the theorems and laws that govern the scientific guidelines of the transformational process. The Purposeful Primitive is also an artist that uses a skillful blend of creative methods to sculpt and mold the human body. We are aware and concerned with the *peculiarities and particulars*. Each of us is unique and has individual idiosyncrasies that need to be taken into account.

The Purposefully Primitive approach flies in the hi-tech face of everything you thought you knew about "fitness." We embrace harsh reality and understand that the transformation process is difficult, arduous and intense; hardly the effortless glide path profiteers would lead you to believe. The athletic elite know from firsthand experience the difficulty of the renovation process; those who have actually traveled the path and engineered their own transformation know what works. They also know that ease, sameness and sub-maximal training deliver negligible results. Those lucky civilians who actually find a sound game plan rarely understand the degree of pure physicality needed to trigger muscular hypertrophy. Nor do they understand the exacting procedural processes necessary to force the body to convert stored body fat into energy to use as fuel. You need more than just an intelligent game plan: you must train exceedingly smart and you must train exceedingly hard.

Physical renovation is a riddle wrapped in an enigma tucked neatly inside a paradox. Taken individually, the various component parts that make up the Purposefully Primitive matrix are quite easy to understand. Someone once said about the poker game, Texas Hold 'Em, "It takes five minutes to learn and a lifetime to master." Ditto the Purposefully Primitive approach. Bach's opening *Aria* in *The Goldberg Variations* lasts one minute and fifty three seconds and could (almost) be played with one finger of each hand, yet to play it with soul and conviction takes a lifetime of study and commitment. So it is with our deceptively simplistic approach.

To achieve synergistic critical mass requires extreme exertion in the gym and disciplined eating 24-7. The process is powered by the continual invocation of certain politically-incorrect psychological traits: tenacity, patience, ferocity, discipline and genuine enthusiasm. The process *is* the reward. Our primitive menu of training and eating is extremely limited yet exceedingly rich in flavor, depth, dimension, detail and texture. Limitless variety can be found within our small exercise and eating menu. Our approach is about doing fewer things better.

Do you want a seat at the transformational table? Then let us put away all the fitness gadgets and toys, all the childish beliefs in magical products. Let us roll up our sleeves and get down to serious business. There is no school like Old School. Whereas most fitness approaches are a mile wide and an inch deep, we are an inch wide and a mile deep. You can power your way out of the dank cocoon that physically envelopes you and emerge with a renovated body. You can undergo a physical metamorphosis and morph from what you are into what you want to be. The transformational trail has been blazed by the true Masters. Now it is time for you to turn words written on the pages of a book into your very own life-changing reality.

Rationalization, Visualization, Actualization

> ***People would like to see lions combed and scented like a marchioness's lapdogs.***
> **— Honoré de Balzac**

I recently had a client come visit me for one of my four hour Fitness Day Camps. It was the first trip up for this lady and in many ways she was typical of a certain type that continually seek me out. She was a 51 years old business executive who was quite successful. An empty nest mom with a husband and grown children, her bodyweight had ballooned upward over the past five years, and now, 50 pounds overweight, she was "desperate" to do something about it. On her visit she impressed me: she asked all the right questions, took notes and seemed engaged, sharp and determined.

I thought that by redirecting the drive that had made her successful in business towards fitness she would be able to reverse her physical disintegration. She had neglected herself while raising two kids and working fulltime. Now she had the time, money and desire to rectify her condition. With a minimum of determined effort and using the Purposefully Primitive methodology, I felt quite certain that she could realize a radical reduction in bodyweight within 60 days. She had discovered me when I wrote my weekly column for the *Washington Post.com.* Totally out of shape, completely ignorant of fitness-related systems or procedures, I had a blank slate, an empty canvas, to work with.

I knew from past experience that when a totally unfit individual suddenly institutes and executes our Purposefully Primitive methodology with the requisite consistency, the out-of-shape participant *invariably* experiences a quick burst of initial progress. This completely predictable initial burst is both physically exhilarating and psychologically empowering. I've supervised innumerable obese individuals as they underwent rapid and radical transformation using our ultra-basic methods. Sound methods need to be cubed with maximal physical effort. Transforming the body isn't magic: it is straightforward science, cause and effect, i.e., execute *this* procedure using these specific protocols for a specified period of time and *that* result *must* occur.

Changes occur quickly when the out-of-shape overweight person begins power walking. We insist they log cardio session frequency, time, distance, pace and heart rate. Simultaneously we have the obese individual institute our simplistic resistance program: we empower them with strength. Making an obese person stronger is a relatively easy task. The unnoticed upside is when the formerly weak obese person is made stronger they are able to power their bulk around with much greater ease. Climbing steps, getting up out of low chairs, arising from bed or in and out of bathtubs, tasks that were once difficult and demanding, suddenly are made much easier. The acquisition of newfound strength radically improves the overweight individual's quality of life. The obese weakling is empowered through an infusion of strength. The final piece of the transformation puzzle is nutrition. We insist the overweight clean up their food selections and adopt a dietary game plan.

Within a few weeks clothes start fitting loosely, within a month visible physical change is apparent; within three months total transformation becomes concrete reality. Again, this isn't magic, this is applied biology.

Anyway, my lady client requested a follow-up visit a few months later and indicated in her e-mail that she wasn't making any progress. I knew immediately she wasn't performing the program. I agreed to see her and when she showed up she looked identical. I had given her a three time-a-week weight training program consisting of three exercises: free weight squats, sumo deadlifts using a single kettlebell, and modified pushups. I had instructed her to walk at a local park in her neighborhood. I happened to know this park because I used to live in her neighborhood. It was a spectacular botanical garden with miles of lovely paths crisscrossing manicured grounds dotted with sculpted shrubs and ponds full of Koi carp. Serene and surreal, the park was an ideal spot for someone to fall in love with cardio walking. We'd agreed on her last visit that since she didn't report to work until 10 am, she would walk the park early every morning. Thrice weekly she would perform her three exercise/three set resistance training regimen. The training template, she agreed, was doable and user-friendly—assuming she actually pulled the trigger.

In fact she never completed a single day of full compliance. Her ingrained habits and slothful, self-indulgent lifestyle apparently had claws equal to those of a grizzly gripping a just-caught salmon. She felt it important to justify her laziness with abstract talk of self esteem and feeling good about herself. In reality she was a fitness poseur with zero pain tolerance and with no real desire to change any of her long-ingrained, exceedingly detrimental habits.

Let me count the ways I sought to accommodate this overconfident under-achiever: she had a sweet tooth so I had found her a sports nutrition bar that she absolutely loved. She agreed to use the substitution principle to wean herself away from sugar. Anytime the sweet tooth Jones hit, she was to eat a sport nutrition bar to satiate the sugar craving. She loved fish and shellfish and could afford all she wanted. I showed her how to make a variety of delicious fish and shrimp dishes, all of which could be prepared inside ten minutes. She had no problem eating salads and fibrous vegetables. When she left the first time she was enthused and fired up and I really thought she was going to succeed.

On her second visit I sat her down and before I could open my mouth she began talking a mile a minute, chockfull of rationalizations and excuses as to why she had fallen off the wagon. I pointed out that factually she had never gotten on the proverbial wagon to begin with. She seemed extremely practiced at excuse-giving. In my mind her problem started and ended with laziness. She told me with straight face that she was "unable" to wake up. She could not get it together to go to the park and walk. "I can't seem to get up in the morning. I like late night TV and consider it my quality time with my husband. I always feel tired in the morning." Some quality time. Her bitch list continued. "I can't seem to make time for the weight training program. It was so exciting when you were watching me and guiding me; at home it all seems so *boring*. I seem to have a lot of scheduling conflicts." There was more, much more. "I can't find time to get to the store and buy food...I don't like to grocery shop...I can't seem to get it together to prepare shellfish. They don't taste as good as when you made them...I made salmon one night and it stunk up my kitchen for days afterwards. I ate all my sport nutrition bars in three days and haven't gotten around to buying any more."

To my ears it was all "I can't, I won't, I refuse!" After she finished delivering her litany of excuses, I told her that there was nothing more I could do for her. She was baffled by this and explained that she needed *another* approach: this "primitive stuff" was "not for me." She wanted me to provide her something different. She suggested I teach her another form of exercise that was more "Pilates-like." As I unceremoniously escorted her to the door, I told her "I *can't* get results for those who can't implement the program." I told her that she should resign herself to physically spiraling downward for the rest of her life. She seemed mortally insulted and got a little testy. This bought out the testiness in me. I told her I was all out of "magical fairy dust" and thus, unable to sprinkle it on her, thereby allowing her to skip past all the disciplined effort. "Without magical fairy dust," I said, "I am unable to transform your *fat ass* into that svelte vision you envision." She left in a sanctimonious huff.

How much easier could I have made the process? She only needed to weight train three times a week for less than 20 minutes per session. She only needed to take a daily walk around a lovely public park in a surrealistic setting. She could eat once a day using the Warrior Diet, or she could graze, eating small mini-meals every three hours, using the Parrillo approach. She could eat out, often, if she obeyed our simple rules. To overcome her sweet addiction I introduced her to substitute nutritional supplements that she liked.

Factually, she didn't crave a new body more than she craved her self-indulgent habits and soft lifestyle. My simplistic approach was not nearly simple enough or easy enough for her.

I had another client who was in dire need of help: he needed a new attitude towards food and eating. He was in his late thirties and had added 35 pounds of pure body fat over the last 24 months. This was due to the metabolic slowdown that happens to men around this age. He had what I called the "cafeteria complex." He wanted to pick and choose amongst my strategies: he wanted to lose the body fat, but rejected every dietary approach I suggested for a variety of reasons. He didn't want to try the Warrior Diet because he HAD to eat during the day. He didn't want to use the Parrillo approach because eating 5 to 7 times a day was "too much hassle." He liked my weight training and couldn't get enough of that. He was consistent in his cardio and did it often. He generated excellent training intensity and I told him he had "NFL offensive lineman syndrome." He asked what I meant. I said, "Real strong, great cardio conditioning—yet still fat as a pregnant hippopotamus." He too became mortally offended.

What he really wanted was for me to suggest the slightest, mildest of modifications; tiny tweaks that would produce dramatic effects. In actuality the only changes that would net him the radical results he sought were radical changes that he was unwilling to embrace. He wanted to argue so I told him the same thing I had told the change-resistant lady. "Resign yourself to looking and staying the same—or getting fatter." Like an auctioneer he wanted me to rattle off a list of mild dietary strategies until I stumbled upon one to his liking. The diagnosis for his current condition was as plain as the nose on his chubby face: he was eating way too much of the wrong stuff at the wrong times. He wanted me to rearrange his dietary deck chairs ever so slightly, then pat him on the head, tell him how great he was doing and send him on his way. Then he would magically lose 35 pounds of fat in two weeks by cutting out the second piece of pie and switching to lite beer. He was another example of "I can't" or perhaps more accurately in his case, "I won't!" He was far more attached to his current habits and comforts than he was to the idea of building a new body.

In my experience unless the individual positively *burns* for transformation, unless they can mentally visualize themselves as a final finished physical product and use that vision to tantalize and induce self-motivation, nothing of any significant physical consequence is likely to occur. If a person approaches the transformational process with the approximate same level of motivation and commitment they muster for mowing the lawn or brushing their teeth, the whole effort is doomed to eventual failure. The internal vision must be so strong and so real that it motivates the person to actually drop bad habits. Vision enables a tired trainee to get out of bed when they don't really feel like it-then train with the savagery necessary to produce gains. Vision enables people to break the chains of bad habit and escape the ceaseless cycle of endless, mindless self-indulgence. Those individuals with strong inner vision are the ones likely to gain traction and eventually succeed in engineering a successful physical transformation.

"County Ron" had vision. When Ron first came to me I was unaware that he had been in a horrific industrial accident a few years prior: his leg and knee had been destroyed when a truck engine fell on him. One shoulder had to be reconstructed and in the accident aftermath the 5'9" 49 year old man had ballooned up to 240 pounds. Had I known he was damaged goods, I likely would have passed on working with him for fear of re-injuring his rebuilt body.

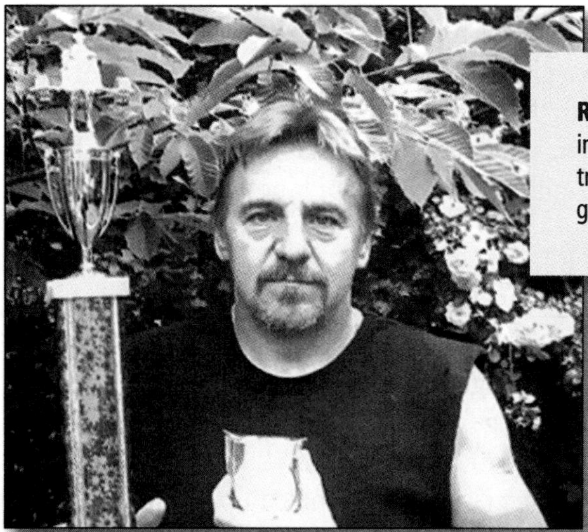

Ron Patterson: Had his body virtually destroyed in a factory accident. He underwent a complete transformation, losing 66 pounds of fat and gaining 10 pounds of muscle in 90 days.

Ron is classical country: stoic, dignified, resolute and steadfast. A man of few words, he was by nature a hard worker with a high pain tolerance. He never murmured a single complaint. His progress was breathtaking: for three straight months he improved in each lift in each session. His walking morphed into power walking, then trotting, then jogging and eventually running. His lovely wife Roxanne mixed up massive amounts of chicken, rice and vegetables that he would graze on throughout the day. He neither smoke nor drank, he never missed a workout despite working two jobs. For three straight months he performed the three powerlifts—and nothing else.

On day one he squatted 95 pounds for a few shaky reps; bench pressed 95 for five, and deadlifted 135 eight times. Fast forward to the AAU World Championships 89 days later: Ron squatted 253 (making 275, called on depth), bench pressed 226 and deadlifted 402. On day one working with me he weighed 241 pounds. Ninety days later at the competition he weighed an official 174 pounds, he had lost a staggering 66 pounds in 90 days. It was even better than that; he had added 10 pounds of muscle in those same 90 days. The 50 year old took third place in his age group and weight division, his first ever athletic competition, the Amateur Athletic Union world powerlifting championships.

Ron is a classical example of country can-do. You can replicate Ron's results; you too can undergo a radical transformation in a matter of months. Our methods work every single time. The only variable is the degree of application the user is able to generate. Visualize your body in final finished physical form. This vision will help power your ongoing efforts.

Those who burn for transformation now have a proven methodology of metamorphosis: the search is over...time for implementation!

Fitness from Big Pink

Taking Cues from Musical Purposeful Primitives, I Went to the Proverbial Woodshed

> *The Band came from nowhere specific and their evocations were indistinct...saloons with cracked windows and leaky ceilings, dancehall girls, hotel rooms with naked light bulbs, highways, deserts, great rivers, mountains, girls glimpsed once or left behind or revisited many times. Saturday afternoon outings, race track bets, traveling over country back roads in fourth-hand cars with a bottle passed hand to hand; truck stops, railroads, three cell jails, eternal dreams of wealth, bad debts, hangovers and movement—always movement—forever that sense of traveling back and forth across the land, trapped by its immensity and engulfed in never ending and infinite change.*
>
> —Nik Cohn

There was a time when I thought about calling this book, "Fitness from Big Pink." I didn't think many people would understand my abstract correlation so I shelved the idea. In 1967 a record was released called Music from Big Pink and it set off a counterrevolutionary shockwave. Eric Clapton quit his superstar group, The Cream, upon hearing the record. Michael Schumacher wrote in Clapton's biography,

> *The Band's unique song arrangements were deceptive; what appeared to be simple, back-to-the-basics music was in fact a complex, thoughtful layering of sound, devoid of flash.*

That's actually a pretty good description of the Purposefully Primitive philosophy. Clapton was playing in the biggest band in the world and upon hearing Music from Big Pink, he realized...

> *I felt we {The Cream} were dinosaurs and what we were doing was outdated and boring. Music from Big Pink bowled me over. Nothing was ever the same for me after that record.*

At the time, the popular music world resembled the current state of the fitness universe. Sonic overkill infected popular music as mindless pretension and needless nihilism was *de rigueur.* Music mired in muddled politics was passed off as social sophistication. Lyrical cynicism was melded with increasingly elaborate musical modes and the musical world was awash in Orwell's "smelly little orthodoxies." It seemed each new musical offering was louder, harsher, brasher, more derivative and pretentious than its competitive predecessor. Everyone sought the next "breakthrough."

Nowadays fitness "experts" and "industry leaders" enthrall and bedazzle the gullible public with the unquestioned contention that physical progress is all about what lies around the next corner. The unspoken assumption is that we live in an era of fitness miracles and "the march of progress" trumps into obsoleteness any and all things that came before. This fitness contention is as false and ridiculous as its musical corollary was back in 1967. The Band created music that pointed *backwards* while everyone else pointed forward. Primordial counterrevolutionaries, they honed their retro message in rural isolation, away from radio, pop culture trends and contemporary influences.

Musical Purposeful Primitives, they displayed deceptive degrees of sophistication and nuance. They strove for simplification while everyone else sought complication. The Band told stories while everyone else surface skimmed. They didn't confuse emotional immaturity with factual reality. They left space in their music and played with taste and restraint, speaking with clarity and conviction. They told tales that were at once interesting, humorous, profound, profane, emotional, wicked, angelic and always and forever rooted in personal experience.

Oddly, the public took their message to heart. People sensed the truth in their music and they achieved commercial success. When I first conceptualized this book I thought that I would construct a fitness equivalent of Music from Big Pink, "Fitness from Big Pink." This analogy was entirely appropriate. I too point backwards. While I pay homage to fitness Masters, Big Pink paid homage to ancient blues Masters.

I had the good fortune to have a farsighted publisher and editor, John Du Cane, who insisted my book be something more than the conventional "fitness cookbook." The cookbook fitness formula is all about making money. The fitness cookbook is a mercenary undertaking that coldly selects a large target demographic then assembles a series of softball exercises and easy-as-pie diet strategies that are then attached to happy-face sound bites used in purposefully deceptive ad campaigns. Bogus pabulum is boldly proclaimed as 'revolutionary' and 'breakthrough.' Dynamic, attention-grabbing adjectives lure naïve consumers to user-friendly, factually ineffective methods designed to sell units. Cookbooks are financially driven "projects" that play fast and loose with the truth.

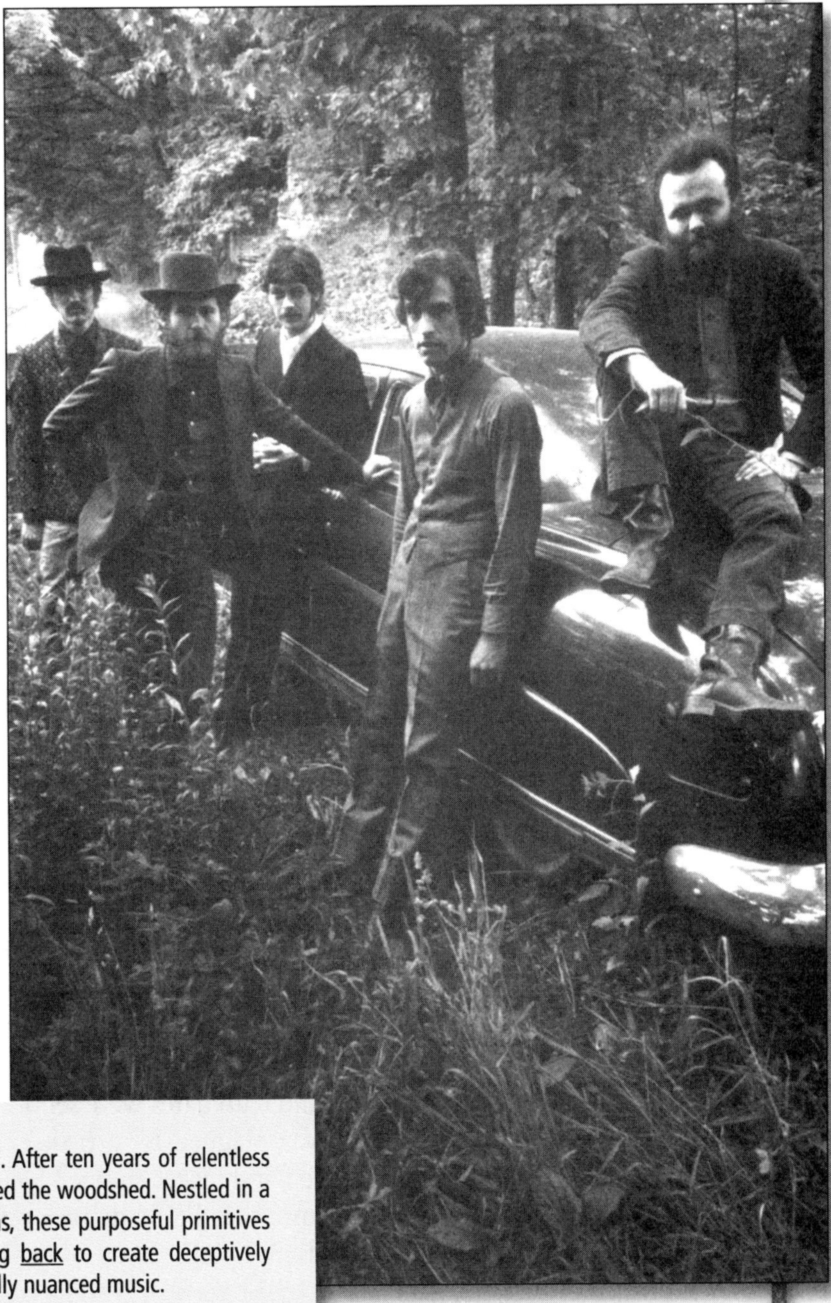

Retro Radicals: The Band circa 1967. After ten years of relentless touring the five grizzled veterans entered the woodshed. Nestled in a pink house in the Saugerties Mountains, these purposeful primitives sparked a retro revolution by reaching back to create deceptively simple, yet multi-layered and emotionally nuanced music.

John insisted we create something more, something with "eloquent gravitas." My idea was to champion an unpalatable message: I would reiterate to the public the fitness ultra-basics they likely never learned to begin with. Championing the harsh and unvarnished truth is always a tough sell.

People demand a method or product that will enable them to circumvent the harsh realities of the physical transformation process. Unscrupulous fitness hucksters are only too happy to provide the gullible public with pretend solutions, magical mystery products that provide product owners the fitness equivalent of a "get out of jail free card." When the sales curve plummets on the current magical mystery product, the product maker retires that particular product and introduces an even better magical mystery product, "Turbo X Cubed! Now with Supercharged Nitrous Mx3!!" The new magical mystery product is trotted out with a brand new ad campaign and the ceaseless cycle rolls ever onward....

I thought this book should be musically analogous to a plaintive Band song, or perhaps a John Coltrane solo or a Thelonious Monk composition. I would not pander to anyone. Like the iconic bebop jazz Masters, I might actually drive away potential audiences with the uncompromising nature of the harsh message. The message would remain true to what I knew to be true. Jazz at the highest level is the polar opposite of the modern Machiavellian corporate rock template where Svengalian puppet masters assemble Scandinavian songwriters to compose funk ditties played by mercenary studio musicians using genius studio wizards to gloss over vocal inadequacies of talent-less pop divas. Skilled choreographers are then assigned to teach rhythm-less spastics how to put on slickster shows for mind-numbed masses paying $150 for a ticket to watch a 50 foot video screen in a football stadium. I wanted to produce the fitness equivalent of a Keith Jarrett solo piano gig on a Friday night at the Village Vanguard circa 1975.

I think it not coincidental that in his previous life as a Cambridge undergraduate, John Du Cane had been a rabid jazz enthusiast and a film and literary critic The book took me the best part of a year to write, yet John never once pressured me. It was a testament to his intense artistic sensibilities. I isolated myself in rural seclusion and used a musician tactic known as "going to the woodshed" to write my data download. I took my artistic cues from a famous urban musical purposeful primitive...

In 1962 tenor saxophone colossus Sonny Rollins stood atop the Jazz universe. Acclaimed by critics and fans, his concerts and club dates were sellouts and his record sales were tops in the jazz industry. Yet Rollins was plagued by artistic self-doubt. He could not shake an intense dissatisfaction with himself and his technique. He felt a spiritual disconnect between himself and his playing. The music that he made was reflective of his life to that point in time, but that musical reflection bored him to tears. What he really wanted was a break from clubs, recording, touring and traveling the world so he could turn inward and recalibrate.

Introspection requires isolation, time and space to think and breathe and above all else, time to forget all that you've learned. To come upon something new an artist needs seclusion. So many wanted to see him play his music, so many depended on a working Sonny Rollins for the food for their families' table. An inactive Rollins would disappoint and deprive those who loved him most. The pressure was strangulating his creativity. Incongruously everyone in his orbit told him he was at the absolute peak of his awesome powers. He felt hemmed in and static, restrained by the constraints of the stylistic path he had blazed. The end came when Rollins repeatedly caught himself plagiarizing himself. He became painfully aware that he was continually and uncontrollably repeating certain ingrained phrase patterns. Tics and habits infected his improvisations and the very air he sucked in to power the horn on exhalation felt stale and lifeless; yet he was at the peak of his powers. He was plagiarizing himself. As Nick Tosches wrote "In the Hand of Dante,"

> ***"Above all I stole from myself. Words and phrases that enamored me, whether I had come upon them or they had come to me from within, were endlessly repeated and recycled: ridden like horses until they were dead. I became a fool, a thief who stole from himself."***

Suddenly and mysteriously Sonny Rollins dropped off the scene. For three years, five nights a week, he took his saxophone and trudged to the middle of the Williamsburg Bridge. He would stand mid-bridge on a catwalk, his back to a pillar, staring out over the river. He'd let his mind go blank and let his fingers mindlessly move over the keys of the horn. He would improvise from midnight until four. Then he would trudge back to his nearby apartment. The Bridge offered him seclusion and the ability to blow as loud and long as he wanted. By thrusting himself into a new and odd environment, he struck off in a new and odd musical direction. His odyssey, without purposeful direction, took his nightly practice sessions to strange new places. He strode boldly down an unmarked artistic trail; he had no idea where it might lead or where it would end or when it ended if it would end in an artistic dead-end, a dry hole.

As the months melted into years, Sonny underwent a musical detoxification. It was not all pleasant. It is difficult and counterintuitive to give up what you know and what made you famous and popular. Some nights deep into his improvisations Rollins would experience artistic vertigo, an odd sensation similar to stepping off the last step of a long staircase in the dark and missing the bottom step. His elaborate "no mind" improvisational flights often could find nowhere to "land" after extended and exhausting passages. Initially his practice sessions were unfocused and somewhat confused. Over the subsequent months and years, his practice sessions became increasingly and incrementally more focused and intense. Late into his third year of seclusion an internal 6th sense signaled to him that this phase had run its course. It was time for Sonny Rollins to renter the "real world."

Out of the despairing depths of artistic uncertainty a new musical vocabulary slowly revealed itself By purposefully isolating himself and allowing himself time to forget, new phrases and fresh musical ideas emerged, slowly and subtly. Rollins no longer plagiarized himself because he had purposefully forgotten how he used to play. Something strangely different was emerging and it was exhilarating—he was continually amazed at the oddness, the pure strangeness of what leapt from the bowels of his horn—the notes he played were now conceived within the deepest depths of his musical sub-consciousness. His transformation was complete. It became apparent during those explosive nightly practice sessions towards the end of his third and final year that it was time to end the woodshed phase.

It was time for Sonny Rollins to share with the public his musical discoveries: whether or not the public embraced or rejected his new language was irrelevant. His purposeful isolation and introspection had born strange fruit. Rollins had abandoned one musical style, invented another style and in doing so reinvented himself. After his self-imposed sabbatical he reemerged and went straight into the recording studio. He produced a groundbreaking album unlike anything he had done before. He titled his reentry record "The Bridge."

This book is my version of Music from Big Pink or The Bridge. Strange fruit honed in rural isolation, away from modern influences, the internet, magazines, TV and any and all contemporary fitness trends. I have consciously constructed this book using my own odd blend of personal experience, reflection and intense introspection. I have borrowed the musician's timeless woodshed template. My approach invokes The Band's retro message, the iconoclastic jazz musician's allegiance to artistic purity, and the scientist's cold recognition of factual reality. My approach stands in stark contrast to the modern fitness template where a rationale is reverse engineered to justify the existence of a (ineffectual) system or product.

Our stark, plaintive Purposefully Primitive method offers a limited menu of choices, but within the reduced selection exist a veritable universe of variations and variables; enough possibilities to keep a diligent man busy for the rest of his natural life. When balanced application of all the individual elements is achieved, synergistic critical mass is attained, causing transformational progress to accelerate dramatically.

Science and method need to be melded with physical and psychological fierceness: methodical consistency is the progress amplifier. Willpower jump starts the process. When enthusiasm takes over for willpower, intense training and disciplined eating become effortless and enjoyable. Tangible physical results continually stoke and refuel the fires of enthusiasm. The pace of progress accelerates in direct proportion to the degree of enthusiastic commitment the trainee is able to generate.

I would like to offer my heartfelt and sincere thanks to all the true Masters I have encountered on my long and circuitous life journey. These men were kind enough to share with me their profound discoveries. As a fitness Prometheus I now pass along to you the transformational fire of these true Masters. Make wise use of this incredible information. I wish you the best of luck in your own transformational efforts.

Marty Gallagher
February, 2008

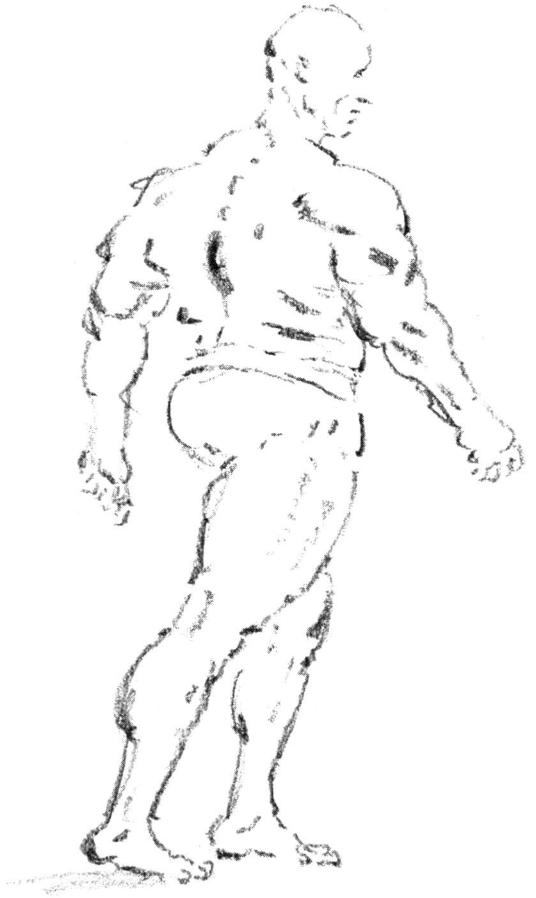

Reader Reference and Resource Guide

Want more information about the Masters spotlighted in this book? Here is a brief synopsis of how to learn more about these amazing individuals...not all are contactable.

Paul Anderson

Paul's legacy is found in books, tapes and old articles. He wrote articles for *Strength & Health* magazine in the sixties and was the author of a series of homemade books. The best of the lot was *Power by Paul.* I also liked his little 37 pager called *Secrets of My Strength.* You can find eleven books by or on Paul by heading to Rickey Dale Crain's website, www.crainsmuscleworld.com. Further information on Anderson books and tapes can be found by contacting Paul Anderson Youth Ministries. Google up Paul and take it from there. The best single book on Anderson is undoubtedly Randy Strossen's *The Mightiest Minister* a beautifully written biography/training treatise available through www.ironmind.com.

Bill Pearl

Bill Pearl Enterprises Inc. is the official locale for all things Pearl-related. Highly recommended is his retrospective book, *Beyond the Universe*, which at times is humorous and other times profound. Bill also created the King of weight training encyclopedias, the elephantine *Keys to the Inner Universe*. This 640+ page monster describes every weight training exercise known to man and is the last word on resistance possibilities. Bill has dozens of training and instructional DVDs, books, training charts, supplements and all things Old School. www.billpearl.com

Bob Bednarski

If you "Google up" Bob Bednarski you will be able to view a priceless, six minute YouTube black and white filmstrip footage showing Bob going through a Saturday workout in 1967. Shot at the old York gym, Bob Hoffman and other luminaries sit in folding chairs watching. The 9th Wonder is shown lifting at the absolute peak of his awesome capacity. No film commentary is provided as Barski works his way through limit presses, cleans, split snatches, squat snatches and clean & jerks. This footage provides a crystal clear picture of the man's youthful charisma and buoyant personality. He really was a lifting rock star. www.youtube.com/watch?v=0pqWIRoANus

Hugh Cassidy

Hugh is retired and living in Maryland.

Mark Chaillet

Mark lives in York, Pennsylvania. He is the founder and president of the International Powerlifting Association and runs a state-of-the-art personal training facility in suburban York. He remains active as a powerlifting promoter. Anyone seeking phone consultations, personal training, or IPA information can reach him at 717-767-6481.

Doug Furnas

Doug currently lives in Tucson, Arizona.

Ed Coan

Ed Coan recently retired from powerlifting. He still resides in Chicago and his series of tapes on the squat, bench press and deadlift remain the best powerlifting videos ever made. In each tape you are treated to Ed discussing in detail the technical aspects of each lift. His technical demonstrations are pure iron poetry. Ed talks at length about his approach towards assistance exercises and lays out his exact training template and shows you how to customize your own program using Ed Principles. Priceless information presented professionally. In addition, Ed makes staggering lifts in the gym and in competition. My book on *Ed, Coan: The Man, The Myth, The Method*, along with Ed's tapes, is available through Quads Gym: www.quadsgym.com

Ken Fantano

Ken lives in Connecticut and has retired from powerlifting.

Dorian Yates

The Mighty Diesel is still active, though no longer competing. I unhesitatingly recommend *Blood & Guts*, the best training video ever made, and his seminal book, *A Warrior's Story*, written with muscle super scribe (and *Muscle & Fitness* editor in chief) Peter McGough. Both documents are as relevant and important as the day they were released. Dorian has a line of supplements, Dorian Yates' Ultimate Formula, that are no doubt as potent as any supplements available anywhere. For further information contact www.dorianyates.net or www.dorianyates.eu

Kirk Karwoski

Kirk is active in his family business in suburban Washington DC. Karwoski spliced together a training and competitive retrospective entitled *From Cadet to Captain* that is positively awe inspiring. See him squat 900x5, 940x3, 960x2 and 1,000x2 in four successive weeks; watch him dead-stop double 775 in the deadlift; see as he bench presses 560x2. Footage stretches back to his teen lifting years. Dramatic stuff, his world record lifts make for fabulous viewing. www.smpgkirk@hotmail.com

Krishnamurti

His books are available everywhere. The Krishnamurti Foundation of America website is a treasure trove of books, tapes and DVDs. Go to the local used bookstore and pick up copies of his books. Go online and purchase tapes and videos of The Great One guiding you into mindless alertness. www.kfa.org

Aladar Kogler

Is a fencing coach at Columbia University in New York. See if you can find (on eBay?) either of his two seminal books, *Clearing the Path to Victory* or *Yoga for Every Athlete*. Powerful stuff, scientific plain-speak; perfectly worded and textbook-like.

Len Schwartz

Go to Heavyhands website and contact the good doctor directly. He will answer questions and queries about how best to use his amazing system. Still vibrant and engaged at age 82, he remains an anti-aging role model and the best possible example of the terrific benefits of his amazing exercise system. www.heavyhandsfitness.com

John Parrillo

John runs an expansive empire and is located in suburban Cincinnati, Ohio. Parrillo Performance Products has a huge corporate headquarters and manufactures potent nutritional supplements onsite. Parrillo conducts nutrition workshops and certifies personal trainers. John custom constructs training equipment and puts out a monthly magazine: *The Parrillo Performance Press*. At age 60 Parrillo remains as innovative and physically fit as he was twenty years ago. www.parrillo.com

Ori Hofmekler

Ori's website is the meeting place for followers of his iconic approach towards nutrition and training. Highly recommended are his two revolutionary books, *The Warrior Diet* and *The Anti-estrogenic Diet*. Ori produces a complete line of all natural supplements; these are designed to augment and amplify his unique approach towards health and fitness. Ori has a militaristic approach and the goal is to develop "survival skills." www.warriordiet.com

Steve Justa

Make sure to purchase a copy of Justa's amazing book, *Rock, Iron, Steel…The Book of Strength*. This is the most iconic strength book I have read in ten years. The prose, approach and subject matter is deceptively profound. Justa predicted, personified and pre-dated the "sustained strength" revolution by a decade: I give this 105 page booklet my highest recommendation. www.ironmind.com

MILO

Journal for Serious Strength Athletes: This is the classiest publication in all of muscle-dom, MILO is published quarterly and features any and all things strength related. Devoid of hyperbole and flash, MILO is a must. Randy Strossen is the hands-down finest Olympic lift/weightlifting photographer to ever strap on a Nikon. Strossen's uncompromisingly non-commercial stance serves as a foundation of saneness in an insane world. www.ironmind

Powerlifting USA

Mike Lambert is powerlifting's stoic, stolid, steadfast backbone. Ours is a sport intent on eternal suicide and Lambert's immutability and responsibility have served as the safe haven for all things powerlifting-related for three decades. Mike is the finest powerlift photographer of all time. Mike *is* powerlifting. It is impossible to imagine the sport without Powerlifting USA...not that he's planning on going anywhere…www.usapowerlifting.com

Planet Muscle

Jeff Everson, PhD, is the personification of all things Iron…a nationally ranked collegiate track & field athlete, a collegiate national weightlifting champion with a 340 pound snatch, national master bodybuilding champion, runner up at the Masters Mr. Universe, (Damn you Roy Duval!) ex-husband and mentor to the greatest Ms. Olympia in history, Corey Everson, inventor of the innovative Planet Muscle, Jeff was, is and shall remain the sharpest tool in the muscle magazine toolbox. www.planetmuscle.com

The Weightlifting Encyclopedia

If stranded on a desert island and allowed one weightlifting reference guide, I would pick Art Drechsler's *Weight Lifting Encyclopedia*, 550 pages of meat and potatoes without a hint of fluff or filler. Purchase a copy at www.atomicathletic.com

Special thanks to...

Chuck Miller: A lawyer with a degree in journalism, AAU national powerlifting champion, master of rest and recovery, Chuck graciously posed for the exercise photos.

Dean Turner: The Dean of Magic took the superb outdoor photos and converted my incoherent babblings into photogenic reality.

John Goodie: Friend and bench presser extraordinary, John was instrumental in preserving my sanity during this grueling, extended project.

Pavel Tsatsouline: True friend, trusted advisor, his heart is huge, his aim is true.

John Du Cane: The man who made it all possible and put up with my periodic temperamental tantrums straight out of Spinal Tap, ("I'm an artist – I'll rise above it!") He successfully kept the Mad Irish from flying completely off the rails at several critical junctures.

About the Cover Illustration

The Prototypical Purposefully Primitive Man is a pencil sketch by internationally famous satirical artist **Ori Hofmekler***. Ori is also one of our fifteen featured Masters. His scathing political portraits of major world political leaders have been published in The New York Times, Newsweek, US News & World Report, Rolling Stone, The Washington Post, der Spiegel, The London Times and Time Magazine to name just a few. Ori was so moved upon reading this book that he created our Prototypical Purposefully Primitive Man expressly for this book. He and author Marty Gallagher have been fast friends for many years.*

Index

A

ab wheel (as basic equipment), 154. *See also* equipment
abdominal exercises, 425–426, 428
aerobic exercise. *See* cardiovascular training
Ali, Muhammad, 25–26
anabolism, 145, 399–402, 422. *See also* nutrition
Anderson, Paul, 11–16
  career of, 12, 13, 14, 459
  training methods of, 12, 13, 14–16, 101
Anti-Estrogenic Diet, The (Hofmekler), 376–377
autovisualization (AV), 236–237, 239–240
AV. *See* autovisualization

B

back exercises, 123–124, 179–185
back muscles, 180
Bagalino, Bobby, 199–200
barbell row/rowing, 124, 183
basal metabolic rate (BMR), 401
base strength, 186–187
Bass, Clarence, 12
Bednarski, Bob, 25–30
  career of, 25, 26–27, 30, 459
  training methods of, 27–29, 101
bench (as basic equipment), 153. *See also* equipment
bench pressing, 110–111
bicep curls, 115
biological imperatives, 6, 99, 166, 170
Blood & Guts (film), 78, 79
BMR. *See* basal metabolic rate
body fat
  burning of, 6, 105, 288, 370–371, 392–393, 401, 416–420, 429
  desire to lose, 4, 98, 99
  measurement of, 368
  spot reduction and, 425–429
  storage of, 426–427
body fat percentages, 136, 166, 378, 400, 417–419, 427
bodybuilding, 17, 18, 20. *See also* resistance training
BodyStat kit, 368
brain (functions of), 223
Brain Train, 235, 236, 240, 242–244, 266–268
Bridges, Mike, 56
burst cardio, 302. *See also* interval cardio

C

calf raises, 118
calories
  burning of, 6, 105–106, 166, 310, 314–315, 328–329, 333, 337–339, 386, 387, 391, 401–402, 428–429
  intake of, 105, 150, 181, 310, 320, 360, 363–365, 366, 367, 368, 374, 379–380, 385, 391–392, 399–402, 419–420, 422–423, 427–428
  muscle and, 106, 150, 394, 400, 416, 427
cardiovascular training, 285–296, 299–315
  benchmarks of, 288, 311, 312, 313
  benefits of, 285–286, 287–288, 418
  calorie burning during, 337–339
  equipment for, 288, 302–303, 310–311, 312, 314–315, 326
  fight training and, 349–352. *See also* martial arts/artists
  gender and, 319
  goals of, 288, 289, 299, 335
  indoor options for, 326–327
  intensity of, 289, 305, 310, 311, 313, 331
  jogging as, 291–292, 314
  logging results of, 288
  modes of, 286, 299–307, 309
  nutrition and, 286, 288, 311, 320, 330, 387
  outdoor options for, 257, 268, 314–315, 321, 330, 341. *See also* jogging; walking
  oxygen consumption and, 292–293, 294–295, 299, 302

periodization and, 310–311, 312, 313
physical transformation and, 6–7, 220, 319
resistance training and, 20, 166, 288, 295–296, 305, 306
training schedule for, 286–287, 310–311, 312, 313
variety in, 257, 287, 300, 302, 326
weight loss and, 166
Casey, Pat, 18
Cassidy, Hugh, 31–36
career of, 31–32, 460
as mentor, 149
training methods of, 33–36, 37, 51, 101, 125
CFT. *See* Controlled Fatigue Training
Chaillet, Mark, 37–45
career of, 37–38, 88, 460
"House of Pain" of, 41–444
training methods of, 38–42, 43, 44, 52, 102, 125, 209
chest exercises, 121–122
Chicago YMCA, 26
Clay, Cassius. *See* Ali, Muhammad
Clearing the Path to Victory (Kogler), 229
Coan, Ed, 55–64
career of, 55–60, 86, 89, 460
training methods of, 51, 52, 53, 60–64, 81, 90, 91, 92, 102, 129, 130
Coleman, Mark, 347–348, 352
Coleman, Ron, 18
Columbo, Franco, 18
Controlled Fatigue Training (CFT), 375, 377, 378. *See also* Warrior Diet
conventional deadlifts, 183. *See also* deadlifts
creeping incrementalism, 134, 233, 255–256, 288, 310, 313, 390
curls, 115, 120

D

deadlifts, 112–113, 183, 184
decline sit-ups, 119
deep muscle fatigue (DMF), 176
Deluxe, Chuck, 341–343, 345–346
detoxification (and diet), 360, 374, 376, 377, 380–381, 409. *See also* Warrior Diet
Dimiduk, Mark, 33
dips (variations of), 122
direct muscle soreness (DMS), 176
DMF. *See* deep muscle fatigue
DMS. *See* direct muscle soreness
Du Cane, John, 453-454
dumbbell flyes, 122
dumbbells (as basic equipment), 153. *See also* equipment

E

Eder, Marvin, 18
endorphins, 221, 257
equipment
for cardiovascular training, 288, 302–303, 310–311, 312, 314–315, 326. *See also* heart rate monitors
machines as, 151–152, 188–191, 320, 331
for resistance training, 151–155
fraudulent claims about, 287

F

fad diets, 360, 391, 392, 400. *See also* nutrition
Fantano, Ken, 65–74
career of, 65–67, 200, 460
training methods of, 68–74, 87, 102
fasting, 409–410. *See also* nutrition; Warrior Diet
fight training, 349–352. *See also* martial arts/artists
fish (cooking of), 433–435
flee phenomenon, 85–86
Flex (magazine), 77, 79
Food Network, 437
food preparation techniques, 431–436. *See also* nutrition
Fortenbaugh, Bob, 210
free weight exercises, 106–132. *See also* resistance training
auxiliary exercises, 119–124
effectiveness of, 188–191
equipment needed for, 107
machine-type exercises and, 151–152, 188–191
overview of, 106–107
partners for, 162–163
primary exercises, 108–113
secondary exercises, 114–116

tertiary exercises, 117–118
training schedules for, 125–132
front squats, 119. *See also* squats
Furnas, Doug, 45–54
career of, 45–48, 50–53, 55–56, 57, 88, 89, 460
training methods of, 46, 48–51, 52, 53–54, 61, 91, 92, 102
Furnas, Mike, 47, 48–49, 50, 51

G

Gajda, Bob, 26
Grimek, John, 18
Gurdjieff, G. I., 3, 7
gyms (clientele of), 192–196. *See also* specific gyms

H

habits
breaking of, 219–220
nutritional types of, 222, 256–257. *See also* nutrition
Hackleman, John, 348, 350–351
Haney, Lee, 76, 77
health clubs (resistance training at), 100, 151. *See also* machine-type exercises
heart rate monitors
aerobic mode and, 302–303, 314–315
calorie counting by, 337–339
cardiovascular training and, 288, 310–311, 312
walking and, 321, 325
Heavyhands, 291–293, 294, 295, 306, 322
Heavyhands, The Ultimate Exercise (Schwartz), 293
high pulls, 182, 184
Hilligen, Roy, 8
Hoffman, Bob, 26
Hofmekler, Ori, 305, 306, 351, 352, 360, 361, 373–375, 405–406, 461. *See also* Warrior Diet
holidays (and eating), 421–424
hunger (and nutrition), 407–410
hybrid cardio, 286, 305–307, 309, 326. *See also* cardiovascular training
hypertrophy, 79, 100, 104, 106, 157–160, 176, 180, 257, 265, 360, 367, 400, 403, 405, 445

I

incline press, 121
interval cardio, 286, 302–304, 309, 323. *See also* cardiovascular training
isotonometrics, 324, 325

J

Jacboy, Dave, 211–212
jazz musicians (mental state of), 252, 253
jogging, 291–292, 314
jump rope (as basic equipment), 153. *See also* equipment
Justa, Steve, 353–355, 462

K

Karwoski, Kirk, 85–94
career of, 85–87, 92–94, 210, 212–213, 280–281, 460–461
training methods of, 87–91, 103, 128, 130, 209
Kazmaier, Bill, 61
Ketogenic Diet, The (McDonald), 106
Kogler, Aladar, 219, 223, 229–231, 242–244, 461
Kono, Tommy, 16
Krishnamurti, Jiddu, 219, 223, 225–227, 252, 253, 461
Kuc, John, 277–279

Lancaster, Robert, 146
layoffs (from training), 273–276
leg exercises, 119–120
Liddell, Chuck, 351
logging
of cardiovascular training results, 288
of periodization entries, 136–139. *See also* periodization
of resistance training results, 221, 269
lying leg curls, 120
machine-type exercises, 151–152, 188–191, 320, 331. *See also* equipment

M

March, Bill, 27
Maryland Athletic Club, 85, 161
martial arts/artists, 347–348, 349–352
McDonald, Lyle, 106
meat (cooking of), 431–433
meditation, 250. *See also* mental amalgamation
Meetings with Remarkable Men (Gurdjieff), 3, 7
mental amalgamation, 235–241. *See also* psychology
  approaches to, 236–241
  foundations of, 235
metabolism, 320, 366, 367–368, 379–380, 400, 418
Middleton, Glenn, 32
Mills, Joe, 26, 27
mind/muscle connection, 258–262. *See also* psychology
Mr. America, 23
Mr. Olympia, 23, 76–77, 81–82, 335, 365, 408
Mr. Universe, 23
MMA. *See* martial arts/artists
momentum (in training), 269
Moran, Lee, 91
motivation
  nutrition and, 219, 222, 390, 408–409
  for training, 219–221, 277–279. *See also* psychology
Muscle & Fitness (magazine), 14, 80, 211, 277, 335
Muscle Factory, 66, 68, 71, 72, 200–204
muscle fibers, 307–308
muscles
  building of, 4, 98, 99, 100, 105–106, 370–371, 392–393, 418–419
  calorie burning and, 106, 150, 394, 400, 416, 427
  fibers of, 307–308
  soreness/fatigue of, 176–179, 185
music
  Purposefully Primitive philosophy and, 451–453, 454–456
  working out and, 257, 266, 267, 268, 324
musicians (mental state of), 252, 253, 254

N

National Championships, 30, 32, 39, 51–52, 56, 57, 85, 86, 89, 280
NEB. *See* negative energy balance
negative energy balance (NEB), 6, 385, 429
nutrition, 359–362, 385–393
  approaches to, 359–362, 385–386. *See also* Parrillo nutritional system; Warrior Diet
  bad habits in, 222, 256–257, 411–415
  caloric intake and. *See* calories, intake of
  cardiovascular training and, 286, 288, 311, 320, 330, 387
  commitment to, 388–389, 390–393, 444
  detoxification and, 360, 374, 376, 377, 380–381, 409. *See also* Warrior Diet
  discipline and, 255–256
  fad diets and, 360, 391, 392, 400
  fasting and, 409–410
  food preparation techniques and, 431–436
  goals for, 386–388, 392–393
  guidelines for improvement of, 256
  health/lifestyle and, 386, 388
  holidays and, 421–424
  hunger and, 407–410
  metabolism and, 320, 366, 367–368, 379–380, 400, 418
  motivation and, 219, 222, 390, 408–409
  periodization and, 361
  physical transformation and, 6–7
  post-workout environment and, 403–404, 405–406
  psychology and, 389–390
  resistance training and, 387
  supplements and, 368–369
  taste and, 407–410, 430–436
  variety in, 171
  weight loss and, 166
nutritional supplements, 368–369. *See also* nutrition

O

obese individuals
  dieting by, 400, 402
  exercise programs for, 164–167, 320, 386, 388, 447
  health issues of, 374

metabolism of, 320, 333, 427
walking/jogging by, 289, 314, 333
Oliva, Sergio, 18, 23
Olympic barbells (as basic equipment), 153. *See also* equipment
Olympic weight-lifting, 17, 18
overcompensation (in training), 175
overhead press, 114
oxygen consumption, 292–293, 294–295, 299, 302

P

Pacifico, Larry, 38, 57, 58
Park, Reg, 18–19, 23
Parrillo, John, 305, 306, 351, 352, 361, 363, 461. *See also* Parrillo nutritional system
Parrillo nutritional system, 363–371. *See also* nutrition
application of, 385–386, 387, 391, 393
foundations of, 364–371, 394
metabolism and, 367–368
origins of, 363–364
supplements and, 368–369
Warrior Diet versus, 359, 360. *See also* Warrior Diet
partners (for resistance training), 161–163
Patmalnee, Roy, 145, 146, 147
Pearl, Bill, 17–24
as anti-aging role model, 22, 23–24
career of, 18–19, 23–24, 459
training methods of, 19–22, 101, 130, 219
Peck, Marshall "Doc," 33, 35, 37
performance (and psyche), 277–279, 280–282. *See also* psychology
periodization, 133–139
ability and, 127, 133, 135–136
cardiovascular training and, 310–311, 312, 313
definition of, 133
logging of entries for, 136–139
nutrition and, 361
training schedule and, 98, 99, 133–134, 135–136, 138–139, 310–311
Phase I training, 69
Phase II training, 70–71, 73
physical transformation
cardiovascular training and, 6–7, 220, 319
case studies of, 446–451
nutrition and, 6–7
overview of, 4–7
psychology of, 6–7, 149–150, 219. *See also* psychology
tools for, 220, 445–446
post-workout nutrition, 403–404, 405–406. *See also* nutrition
power clean, 123, 182
power rack (as basic equipment), 153. *See also* equipment
power walking. *See* walking
powerlifting, 17, 18
Presley, Elvis, 11, 413
progressive pulls, 179–185
effectiveness of, 179
lifts for, 182–185
poundage for, 180, 181
psyche, 266–268. *See also* psychology
psychology
of champion athletes, 269–272
layoffs from training and, 273–276
maintaining progress and, 269–272
mental amalgamation and, 235–242
mind/muscle connection and, 258–262
motivation and, 219–221, 277–279
nutrition and, 389–390
performance and, 277–279, 280–282
personal weak points and, 263–266
of physical transformation, 6–7, 149–150, 219. *See also* physical transformation
psyche and, 266–268
purposeful mindlessness and, 249–254
willpower, 220, 255–257
purposeful mindlessness, 249–254. *See also* psychology
Purposefully Primitive training amalgamation
adaptation of, 164–167
cardiovascular training and. *See* cardiovascular training
foundations of, 97–99, 106, 443–446
free weight exercises for, 106–107. *See also* free weight exercises
guidelines for, 104–105
modes/methods of, 100–103, 443
motivation and, 220

muscle building with, 105–106
nutrition. *See* nutrition
periodization and, 133–139. *See also* periodization
psychology and. *See* psychology
resistance training and. *See* resistance training
templates for, 98
trainee level and, 125–132
training schedules for, 125–132, 166. *See also* periodization
weight loss and, 164–167. *See also* obese individuals
push-pull strategy, 324, 325

R

reality TV, 205–208
repetitive motion injuries, 331
resistance training
breaks from, 273–276
cardiovascular training and, 20, 166, 288, 295–296, 305, 306
evolution of, 18
forms of, 17–18
goal of, 98, 99
health clubs/YMCAs and, 100
intensity of, 157, 158, 159–160, 162, 172
maintaining progress in, 168–175, 269–272
nutrition and, 387
partners for, 161–163
periodization cycle of. *See* periodization
physical transformation and, 6–7
poundage for, 98, 130
regularity of, 172
time available for, 97–98, 99, 156
training schedule for, 156–160
variety in, 171, 173, 174
warming up for, 157
weight loss and, 166
rice (cooking of), 435
Rock, Iron, Steel: The Book of Strength (Justa), 353
Rollins, Sonny, 454–456
Romanian deadlifts, 117
running. *See* jogging; walking
Russian literature, 148

S

Samadhi state, 251, 253
Schmidt, Julian, 79, 82
Schwartz, Leonard (Len), 291–296, 305, 306, 324, 338, 351, 352, 461
Schwarzenegger, Arnold, 18, 23, 130
Scully, Sean, 210, 212
sense gates, 223
Shikantaza, 237–239, 240
sit-ups, 118
Smart Bomb, 403–404
smoked foods, 437–440
spot reduction, 425–429
spotters (for lifting), 162–163. *See also* partners
squats, 108–109, 119
steady-state cardio, 286, 299–301, 309, 323, 326. *See also* cardiovascular training
stiff-legged deadlifts, 183, 184. *See also* deadlifts
Strength & Health (magazine), 26, 126, 144, 176, 179, 469
Strossen, Randy, 14, 16
supplements (nutritional), 368–369. *See also* nutrition

T

taste (and nutrition), 407–410, 430–436. *See also* food preparation techniques; nutrition
Temple Street Gym, 78
tricep extensions, 116

V

vacation (and exercise), 273, 275–276
vegetables (cooking of), 435–436
Vilmi, Kyosti, 93
visualization, 267
Vlasov, Yuri, 12

W

walking
efficiency of, 328–332, 333
intensity of, 322–325
in outdoors, 330–331, 341
results from, 447
variety in, 323

warm-up for, 321
Warrior Diet, 359–360, 373–381. *See also* nutrition
application of, 385–386, 388, 391, 393, 410
detoxification and, 360, 374, 376, 377, 380–381, 410
foundations of, 359–360, 373, 375–380, 395
Parrillo nutritional system versus, 359, 360. *See also* Parrillo nutritional system
weight training. *See* resistance training
willpower, 220, 255–257
World Championships, 30, 32, 51–52, 57, 85, 86–87, 89, 280, 281
World Team Championships, 209–214
Wright, Dennis, 46, 48–49, 50–51, 61

Y

Yates, Dorian, 75–84
career of, 18, 75–80, 334, 460
training methods of, 20, 21, 79, 80–84, 103, 128, 130, 131, 335, 419–420
YMCAs (resistance training at), 100
York Barbell Lifting Club, 26, 30

Z

Zen principles. *See* mental amalgamation
Zone, The, 226, 227, 235, 270

ABOUT THE AUTHOR

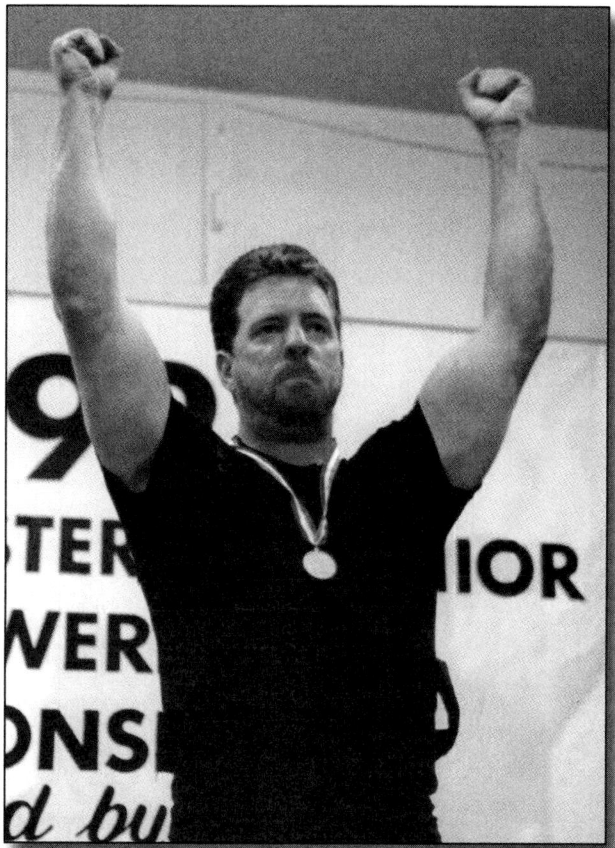

Three-time World Master Powerlifting Champion, Teenage National Olympic Lift Champion, Marty Gallagher coached Black's Gym to four National team titles and in 1991 coached the United States squad to victory at the World Powerlifting Championships.

Marty's highly-acclaimed 230+ weekly Live Online columns for ***Washington Post.com*** created a legion of followers for his Purposefully Primitive Fitness philosophy. Over the last thirty years he has had over 1,000 articles appear in two dozen fitness publications.

Marty Gallagher can be reached at **www.martygallagher.com**

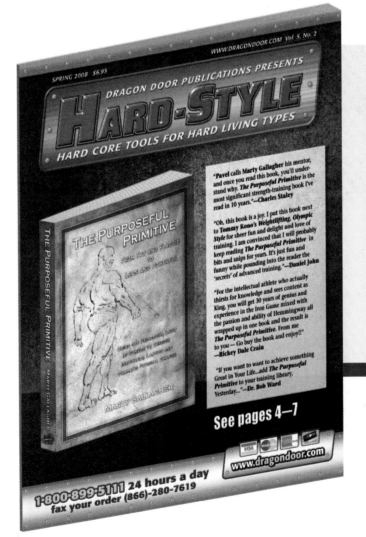